# Spine Disorders

# Spine Disorders

Editor: Rickon Hamill

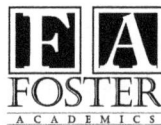

FA FOSTER
ACADEMICS

www.fosteracademics.com

www.fosteracademics.com

**FA** **FOSTER** ACADEMICS

Cataloging-in-Publication Data

Spine disorders / edited by Rickon Hamill.
   p. cm.
Includes bibliographical references and index.
ISBN 978-1-63242-758-8
1. Spine--Diseases. 2. Spine--Instability. 3. Spine--Puncture--Complications.
I. Hamill, Rickon.
RD768 .S65 2019
616.73--dc23

Foster Academics,
118-35 Queens Blvd., Suite 400,
Forest Hills, NY 11375, USA

ISBN 978-1-63242-758-8 (Hardback)

# Contents

# Preface

The spinal cord is a tubular structure consisting of nervous tissue. It extends from the medulla oblongata to the lumbar region. Its primary function is to transit nerve signals from the motor cortex to the sensory cortex. There are 8 cervical segments, 12 thoracic segments, 51 lumbar segments, 5 sacral segments and 1 coccygeal segment in the human spinal cord. The conditions, which impair the functioning of the backbone, are known as spinal diseases. Some common examples include ankylosing spondylitis, spina bifida, spinal muscular atrophy, osteoporosis, lumbar spinal stenosis, spinal tumors, etc. This book includes some of the vital pieces of work being conducted across the world, on various topics related to spinal disorders. It elucidates new diagnostic and treatment techniques and their applications. For all readers who are interested in spinal disorders, the case studies included in this book will serve as an excellent guide to develop a comprehensive understanding.

After months of intensive research and writing, this book is the end result of all who devoted their time and efforts in the initiation and progress of this book. It will surely be a source of reference in enhancing the required knowledge of the new developments in the area. During the course of developing this book, certain measures such as accuracy, authenticity and research focused analytical studies were given preference in order to produce a comprehensive book in the area of study.

This book would not have been possible without the efforts of the authors and the publisher. I extend my sincere thanks to them. Secondly, I express my gratitude to my family and well-wishers. And most importantly, I thank my students for constantly expressing their willingness and curiosity in enhancing their knowledge in the field, which encourages me to take up further research projects for the advancement of the area.

**Editor**

# Change of sagittal spinal alignment and its association with pain and function after lumbar surgery augmented with an interspinous implant

Rebecca J. Crawford[1,2]*, Quentin J. Malone[3] and Roger I. Price[4,5]

## Abstract

**Background:** Interspinous spacer/implants like the Device for Intervertebral Assisted Motion (DIAM™) are controversially yet commonly used in the surgical treatment of lumbar degenerative pathologies. Criticism is based on ill-defined indications, lack of superiority over decompression, and a poorly understood mechanical effect. Yet, continued use by surgeons implies their perceived clinical merit. We examined radiographic spinal alignment for 12 months, and pain and function for 24 months, after DIAM-augmented surgery to improve the understanding of the mechanical effect relating to clinical outcomes in patients.

**Methods:** We undertook a single-surgeon prospective, longitudinal study of 40 patients (20 F, 20 M) who received DIAM-augmented surgery in treatment of their symptomatic lumbar degenerative condition. Outcomes measured included sagittal spinal alignment (lumbar lordosis, sacral inclination, primary (PDA), supradjacent (SDA) disc angles, and regional sagittal balance (RSB; standing lateral radiographs), and back and leg pain (visual analogue scale; VAS) and function (Oswestry Disability Index; ODI). Responders were identified as those with clinically meaningful improvement to pain (>20%) and function (>15%) at 24 months postoperatively; features of sagittal spinal alignment between responders and non-responders were examined.

**Results:** Sagittal alignment was unchanged at 12 months. At 6 weeks postoperatively, PDA (mean (SD)) reduced by 2.2° (4.0°; $p < 0.01$) and more-so in back pain non-responders (3.8° (3.2°)) than responders (0.7° (4.4°); $p < 0.05$). Positive preoperative RSB in responders (26.7Rmm (42.3Rmm); Rmm is a system-relative measure) decreased at 6 weeks (by 3.1Rmm (9.1Rmm)). Non-responders had a negative RSB preoperatively (−1.0Rmm (32.0Rmm)) and increased at 6 weeks (11.2Rmm (15.5Rmm); $p < 0.05$). Clinically meaningful improvement for the whole cohort for back pain and function were observed to 24 months (back pain: 25.0% (28.0); function: 15.4% (17.6); both $p < 0.0001$).

**Conclusions:** Unaltered sagittal alignment at 12 months was not related to symptoms after DIAM-augmented lumbar surgery. Subtle early flattening at the index disc angle was not maintained. Preoperative and early post-operative sagittal alignment may indicate response after DIAM-augmented surgery for mixed lumbar pathologies. Further investigation toward defining indications and patient suitability is warranted.

**Keywords:** Interspinous implant, DIAM, Spinal alignment, Low back pain, Clinical outcomes, Radiological outcomes

* Correspondence: Rebecca.crawford@zhaw.ch
[1]Institute for Health Sciences, School of Health Professions, Zürich University of Applied Sciences, Technikumstrasse 81, Winterthur CH-8401, Switzerland
[2]Faculty of Health and Exercise Sciences, Curtin University, Perth, Australia
Full list of author information is available at the end of the article

## Background

Interspinous implants are controversially used in the surgical treatment of lumbar degenerative pathologies [1]. An inadequate etiological understanding, ill-defined indications, and lack of superiority compared to more cost-effective decompression, have drawn their utility into question [2–6]. Second generation and perhaps the most commonly used and investigated interspinous implants include the X-Stop™ [7], Wallis™ [8], DIAM™ [9], and Coflex™ [10] devices, which provide a non-fusion surgical option in the treatment of lumbar segment disease [11]. These spacer devices vary in design and employ compressible (DIAM and Wallis) or rigid (X-Stop and Coflex) composite materials; they are surgically introduced into the interspinous space using differential access and insertion techniques that aim toward closest approximation to the deep spinous process and laminae in order to induce distraction of the posterior elements [11]. An increasing number of interspinous devices are available and appear to have wide international adoption, with promising new evidence emerging for their benefit in discreet diagnoses and indications [12, 13]. Interspinous implants may have relevance in safely ameliorating back and associated leg pain in an ageing society where co-morbidities necessitate minimised invasive interventions. Identifying features of patients with superior clinical outcomes is fundamental to optimising the successful application of these devices.

For the purposes of this paper examining a single device, and in light of the vast literature dedicated to the many individual interspinous implants, we subsequently refer to studies reporting the Device for Intervertebral Motion (DIAM; Medtronic Sofamor Danek, Memphis, USA). The DIAM is an X-shaped elastomeric interspinous spacer with developer-purported indications including lumbar spinal stenosis, herniated and degenerated disc, facet joint pain syndrome and minor degenerative spondylolisthesis [9]. Low lumbar implantation predominates in augmenting decompression [5, 6, 14–17]. Evidence reports meaningful reduction in pain and function [9, 15–17], yet effect can be variable. Few studies examine the relationship between pain and function, and sagittal spinal alignment as related determinants of postoperative outcome after surgeries involving DIAM implantation [16, 18, 19].

Developer guidelines for the application of the DIAM [9] direct that the largest possible device be implanted to optimise therapeutic effect by maximally-tensioning the supraspinous ligament without imposing actual segmental kyphosis. Subtle relative kyphosis at the index segment has been shown with DIAM in cadaveric spines [20, 21], and in the early postoperative period in patients [16, 18]. However, no studies that we are aware of have attempted to identify pre- or post-operative skeletal features of sagittal alignment that may be prognostic for successful patient-reported outcomes. We therefore evaluated the effect in-vivo on sagittal spinal alignment of DIAM-augmented surgery at regional, operated, and supradjacent levels, and in relation to clinically meaningful improvement in self-reported pain and function.

## Methods

### Study overview

This study assessed 40 patients (mean age: 54 years; SD: 13 years) including 20 women (mean age: 56 years; SD: 9 years), and 20 men (mean age: 51 years; SD: 14 years) from a larger prospective, longitudinal, effectiveness investigation examining clinical outcomes for 2 years after DIAM-augmented lumbar surgery from a single-surgeon practice [17]. Outcome measures included patient-reported pain and function, in addition to measures of skeletal spinal curvature using standing lateral radiography, respectively. The study received institutional ethics and review board approvals from the University of Western Australia and complied with the Declaration of Helsinki. Patients were consecutively recruited with informed consent after the surgical author (QM) made the clinical decision for DIAM-augmented surgery. Patients with previous lumbar spinal surgery and an inability to communicate in English (for completion of questionnaires) were excluded. The 40 patients examined for the radiographic analysis described in the present paper were all of the subjects from the larger study that had complete and usable radiographs. Preoperative questionnaires and radiographs were completed within 1 week of surgery; postoperative radiographs were undertaken at 6 weeks and 12 months, and questionnaires at 6 weeks, 12 months and 24 months.

The surgeon's (QM) preoperative diagnoses of lumbar spinal stenosis ($n = 27$), facet joint pain syndrome ($n = 3$), and minor degenerative spondylolisthesis ($n = 10$) were based on patient case-notes, clinical examinations, static and functional imaging, facet joint injections, diagnostic blocks, and/or discography (as relevant). Intended vertebral levels, number of implants, and the primary (in case of multiple) index segment were recorded preoperatively by the surgical author (QM), and verified postoperatively via case-note audit (by author RJC). All DIAMs were implanted at or caudal to L3/4. Twenty-two patients received a single DIAM, 15 had two implants, and three received three devices. The primary (index) level for the implant was L4/5 ($n = 26$), L5/S1 ($n = 12$) and L3/4 ($n = 2$).

### Surgical procedure

Subjects underwent DIAM-augmented lumbar surgery according to routine supraspinous ligament-sparing procedure for the device without ligatures [9]. Briefly regarding device implantation, a mid-sagittal incision is made and muscle tissue retracted from the spinous process bilaterally, the interspinous space is prepared approximating the laminae as close as possible, with subsequent excision of interspinous ligamentous tissue and applied distraction to optimise the size of implanted device, and then employing device-specific instruments, the DIAM is inserted from one side.

## Pain and function

Evaluations of patient-reported back and leg pain, and function, were made using visual analogue scales (VAS) [22] and Oswestry Disability Index (ODI) [23], respectively.

## Responder analysis

Within-subject absolute changes for back pain, leg pain, and function between 12 months and preoperative timepoints were used to establish outcome at 1 year after surgery. Subjects were categorised into three groups [moderate-, minimal-, non-responders] based on definitions for minimal clinically important differences [24]. Improvement was deemed moderate with >30% reduction in ODI or VAS, minimal 15–29% ODI and 20–29% VAS, and non-response ODI <15% and pain <20%.

## Radiographic evaluation

The standardised procedure for lateral views involved: 100 cm film-tube distance, centred at L3, and barefoot standing in the clavicle position (elbows flexed with lightly clenched fists resting over their ipsilateral clavicles) to optimise visualisation of lumbar vertebral landmarks [25]. Lumbar skeletal alignment was measured from digital [JPEG, 1200dpi] images using a bespoke programme. Vertebral bodies (L1-S1) were defined with

a standardised four-point quadrilateral system based on an established method [26]. Computed radiographic variables included: lumbar lordosis (referencing superior end-plates of L1 and S1) [27]; sacral inclination (referencing superior end-plate of S1 and the horizontal); disc angles (referencing the inferior end-plate of the upper vertebra and superior end-plate of the lower vertebra) PDA and SDA; and RSB defined as the horizontal distance between plumb-line from the centroid of L1,and the posterior corner of the S1 superior end-plate [28]. Radiographic methods are schematically illustrated in Fig. 1.

Correction for magnification between serial radiographs was necessary for the non-angular variable RSB. Projected areas of the L2, L3 and L4 vertebral bodies enabled correction-factor calculation. Ratios between postoperative and preoperative images were scaled according to the square root of the combined L2-4 vertebral body areas of the baseline image. The magnification metric was unknown so RSB is denoted by system-relative millimetres (Rmm).

## Statistical analysis

Data were analysed using Microsoft Excel and StatView (Abacus Concepts, Berkley, 1992). Descriptive statistics trichotimised by responder category (moderate, minimal or non) reported mean (±SD) lumbar lordosis, sacral inclination, PDA, SDA, and RSB at baseline, and change scores between baseline and 6 weeks. Change was assessed according to response and categorisation using unpaired t-tests. Repeated measures ANOVA with Scheffe's post-hoc tested serial change. Box-plots present data indicating 10th, 25th, 50th, 75th and 90th

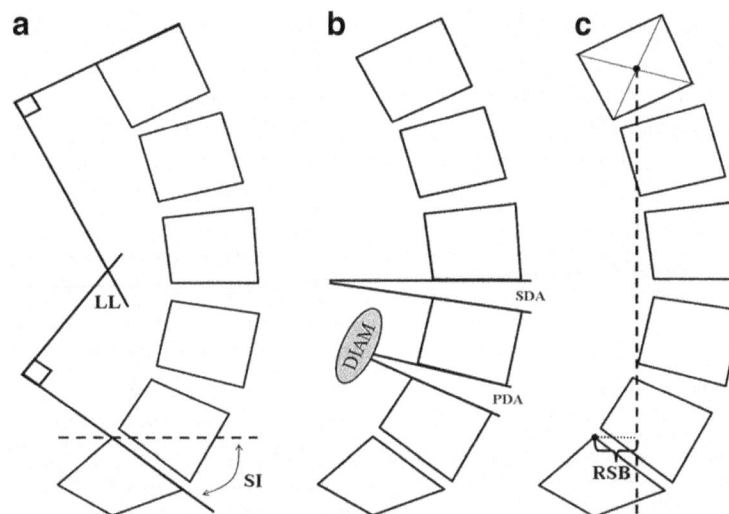

**Fig. 1** Schematic representation of the methods employed to measure lumbar sagittal alignment from standing lateral radiographs showing: (**a**) Lumbar lordosis and sacral inclination; (**b**) Primary and supradjacent disc angle; and (**c**) Regional sagittal balance. Footnote: *LL* lumbar lordosis, *SI* sacral inclination, *PDA* primary disc angle, *SDA* supradjacent disc angle, and *RSB* regional sagittal balance

percentiles. Association between radiographic variables, pain and function were tested using Pearson's correlation coefficient [r]. Statistical significance was $p < 0.05$.

### Repeatability of the measurement technique

Intrarater repeatability of radiographic data was assessed with repeated measurements (1 week apart) of ten baseline images (Table 1). No significant difference for any variable was noted but was lowest for PDA compared to the other variables.

### Results

No change in lumbar lordosis, sacral inclination, SDA, or RSB was shown at either 6 weeks or 12 months. PDA flattened by 2.2° (4.0°; $p < 0.01$) at 6 weeks, and remained 1.5° (4.7°) flatter at 12 months (not significant) (see Table 2 and Fig. 2). Back pain, leg pain and function meaningfully improved at all post-operative time-points ($p < 0.0001$; Table 2 and Fig. 3). Best back pain (mean (SD)) improvement was observed at 6 weeks (32.1% (32.0)), and then 29.0% (27.8) at 12 months and 25.0% (28.0) at 24 months (decline not significant; Fig. 3 left). Best leg pain improvement was observed at 6 weeks (27.4% (32.0)), and then 23.8% (34.0) at 12 months and 19.1% (32.8) at 24 months (decline not significant; Fig. 3 middle). Best improvement to function was observed at 12 months (17.1% (15.8)), and 15.0% (17.0) at 6 weeks and 15.4% (17.6) at 24 months (decline not significant; Fig. 3 right). The proportion of responders versus non-responders for each subjective outcome was equivalent at yearly time-points (Fig. 3 bottom).

### Outcomes according to responder groups

*Baseline*: Only RSB significantly differed preoperatively between responder groups; subjects with moderate response for function had positive RSB preoperatively (26.7Rmm (42.3Rmm)), while non-responders were negative (–1.0Rmm (32.0Rmm); $p < 0.05$) (Table 3).

*Six weeks postoperative change*: PDA flattened by 0.7° (4.4°) in back pain responders while non-responders flattened more (by 3.8° (3.2°); $p < 0.05$). RSB (–3.1Rmm (9.1Rmm)) reduced in leg pain responders, while non-responders increased (11.2Rmm (15.5Rmm); $p < 0.05$). PDA minimally flattened (by 1.8° (3.8°)) in function

**Table 1** Repeat measurements (mean (SD)) of the same baseline lateral radiographs for ten surgical cases

| | Test 1 | Test 2 | Difference | 2-tail $t$-test |
|---|---|---|---|---|
| Lumbar Lordosis (°) | 57.1 (11.4) | 57.0 (12.2) | –0.15 (2.32) | $p = 0.86$ |
| Sacral Inclination (°) | 37.4 (5.2) | 37.3 (6.2) | 0.07 (1.56) | $p = 0.90$ |
| Primary Disc Angle (°) | 15.6 (6.8) | 16.1 (7.5) | 0.50 (1.09) | $p = 0.20$ |
| Regional Sagittal Balance (Rmm) | 2.3 (27.9) | 2.0 (27.5) | 0.31 (1.92) | $p = 0.62$ |

**Table 2** Mean (standard deviation) values for lumbosacral sagittal alignment, and back pain, leg pain and function

| | B | 6w | 12 m | 24 m |
|---|---|---|---|---|
| LL (°) | 53.3 (12.3) | 53.3 (10.6) | 55.3 (9.2) | |
| SI (°) | 36.4 (7.3) | 35.9 (7.0) | 36.7 (6.6) | |
| PDA (°) | 9.2 (5.7) | 7.0 (4.5) | 7.7 (4.8) | |
| SDA (°) | 9.9 (4.9) | 9.8 (4.1) | 10.5 (4.4) | |
| RSB (Rmm) | 5.6 (38.0) | 11.1 (33.7) | 9.5 (38.7) | |
| Back Pain (VAS%) | 49.2 (27.4) | 17.1 (18.5) | 20.3 (21.3) | 23.9 (28.0) |
| Leg Pain (VAS%) | 40.1 (33.5) | 12.7 (19.4) | 16.4 (23.4) | 21.0 (30.1) |
| Function (ODI%) | 36.9 (14.7) | 21.9 (18.0) | 19.8 (16.4) | 21.5 (19.6) |

*B* preoperative baseline, *6w* 6 weeks, *12 m/24 m* 12/24 months postoperative, *LL* lumbar lordosis, *SI* sacral inclination, *PDA* primary disc angle, *SDA* supradjacent disc angle, *RSB* regional sagittal balance, *VAS* visual analogue scale, *ODI* Oswestry Disability Index

responders while non-responders flattened more (by 3.6° (3.1°)), while RSB decreased in responders (by 6.2Rmm (31.7Rmm)) and increased in non-responders (by 10.6Rmm (15.0Rmm); $p < 0.05$) (Table 3).

*Serial change in primary disc angle*: When serial change in PDA was split according to sex, diagnosis, number of implanted DIAMs, and responder groups, differences between sub-groups were noted (Fig. 4). Females ($n = 20$), lumbar spinal stenosis cases ($n = 27$), single DIAM surgeries ($n = 22$), and non-responders in back pain ($n = 17$), leg pain ($n = 21$) and function ($n = 25$) all showed significant early flattening at PDA compared to their sub-group counterparts who were unchanged. Subjects receiving a single DIAM had significantly flatter PDA at 12 months.

### Associations between variables

*Pre-operative*: Lumbar lordosis associated with sacral inclination (–0.62, $p < 0.0001$), PDA (–0.48, $p < 0.01$), SDA (–0.54, $p < 0.001$) and RSB (–0.33, $p < 0.05$). PDA was additionally associated with SDA (0.40, $p < 0.01$) and RSB (–0.56, $p < 0.001$). SDA and RSB were weakly associated with function (–0.31, $p < 0.05$) and leg pain (0.42, $p < 0.01$), respectively. Back pain showed a moderate correlation with leg pain (0.54, $p < 0.001$) and function (0.52, $p < 0.001$); leg pain and function associated weakly (0.36, $p < 0.05$).

*Post-operative*: Early changes (6 weeks; Table 4) in RSB and SDA were weakly related to change in symptoms (RSB: back pain (0.33; $p < 0.05$), leg pain (0.40; $p < 0.05$), function (0.43; $p < 0.01$); SDA: leg pain (–0.38; $p < 0.05$), function (–0.35; $p < 0.05$)). Change in lumbar lordosis at 12 months (Table 5) related to change in all other variables, ranging from strong associations with sacral inclination (–0.70; $p < 0.0001$) and SDA (0.64; $p < 0.0001$) to weak associations with PDA (0.40; $p < 0.05$), back pain (–0.40; $p < 0.05$), leg pain (–0.35; $p < 0.05$) and function

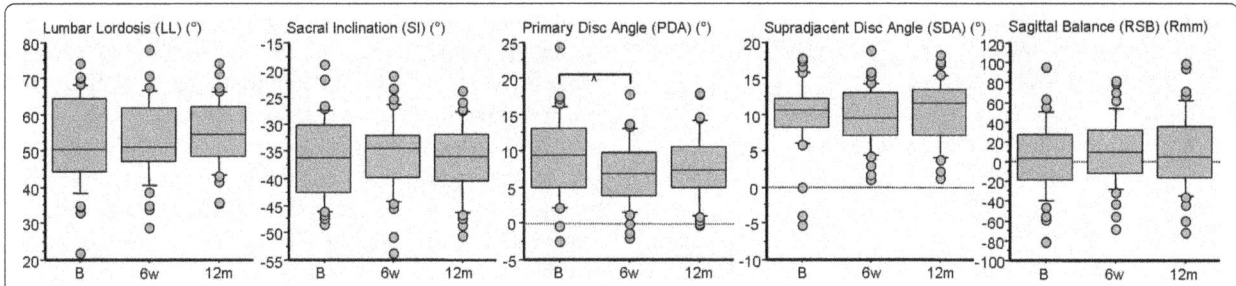

**Fig. 2** Box-plots with outliers revealing serial change in lumbar lordosis, sacral inclination, primary disc angle, supradjacent disc angle and regional sagittal balance. Footnote: *B* preoperative baseline, *6w* 6 week time-point, *12 m* 12 month time-point, *LL* lumbar lordosis, *SI* sacral inclination, *PDA* primary disc angle, *SDA* supradjacent disc angle, and *RSB* regional sagittal balance; * = $p < 0.01$

($-0.32$; $p < 0.05$). Relationships between change in back and leg pain and function were equivalent in the early postoperative period (0.67 (back and leg pain), 0.71 (back pain and function), 0.73 (leg pain and function)) than at 1 year (0.49 (back and leg pain); $p = 0.23$, NS); 0.57 (leg pain and function; $p = 0.47$, NS), 0.64 (back pain and function; $p = 0.30$, NS).

## Discussion

Our study examined sagittal alignment, pain, and function in 40 adults after lumbar surgery augmented with the DIAM, and showed an early postoperative reduction in the index disc angle (by 2.2°) that was not sustained out to 1 year. This subtle and transient change to spinal alignment observed in the postoperative period was apparently unrelated to the improvement in pain and function that was demonstrated at each serial time-point out to 2 years postoperatively. However, preoperative sagittal balance and the early postoperative changes observed for angulation of the index segment were

different between patients with and without meaningful improvement. This may point to characteristics of skeletal spinal curvature with prognostic and/or indication-defining potential.

The subtle angulation change to the index segmental angle was expected based on previous biomechanical studies reporting DIAM and other interspinous implants with ex-vivo evidence for an induced posterior element distraction [21, 29] due to reduced posterior disc annular pressure [10], facet joint unloading [30], and limited lumbar extension [20, 21, 29]. In agreement with Sobottke et al. [18], the initial flattening at the index segment (by 3.8° (4.6°) in their DIAM cases) was not sustained and appeared to revert toward preoperative values by 6 to 12 months. This reversion may signify diminished biomechanical effect over time, irrespective of symptoms, which may be secondary to device-settling after resuming habitual upright postures. Our results showing no change to lumbar lordosis and the supradjacent disc angle throughout the postoperative year

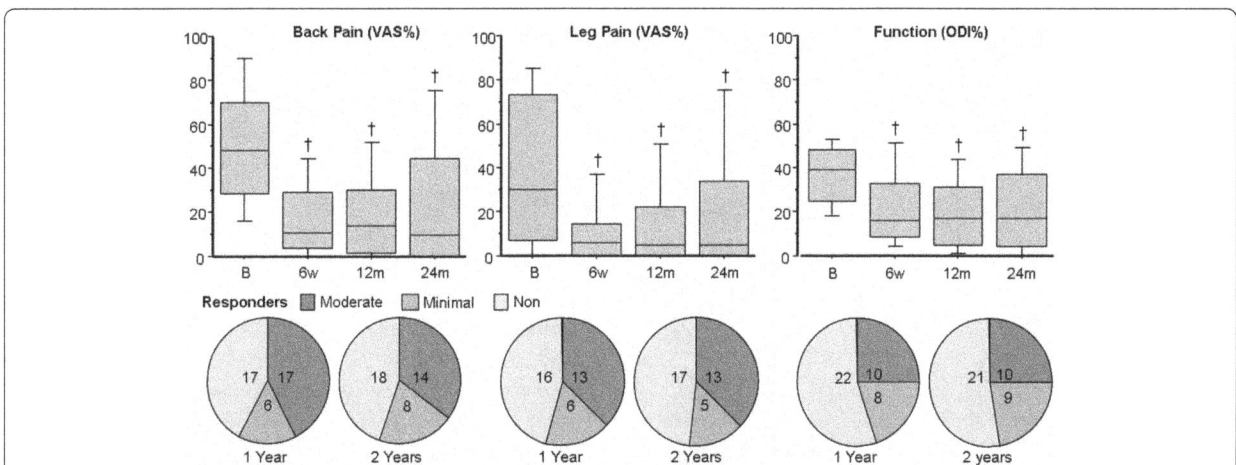

**Fig. 3** Box-plots (*top*) and pie-charts (*bottom*) revealing patient-reported change in back pain, leg pain and function for 40 cases out to 2 years after DIAM-augmented surgery. Box-plots reveal serial change with significant differences compared to baseline values noted at each time-point. Pie-charts indicate the number of cases in responder groups for each measure at 1 and 2 years postoperatively. Footnote: *B* preoperative baseline, *6w* 6 week time-point, *12 m* 12 month time-point, *LL* lumbar lordosis, *SI* sacral inclination, *PDA* primary disc angle, *SDA* supradjacent disc angle, and *RSB* regional sagittal balance; * = $p < 0.0001$

**Table 3** Mean (standard deviation) values at baseline (top) and change at 6 weeks (bottom) for sagittal alignment according to responder group

| Case Numbers | | Total | Moderate | Minimal | Non |
|---|---|---|---|---|---|
| Back Pain | | 40 | 17 | 6 | 17 |
| Leg Pain | | 35 | 13 | 6 | 16 |
| Function | | 40 | 10 | 8 | 22 |
| **Baseline** | | | | | |
| LL (°) | Back | 50.9 (13.6) | 54.6 (14.8) | 55.2 (10.3) | |
| | Leg | 54.2 (14.3) | 46.7 (11.5) | 54.5 (11.1) | |
| | Function | 47.9 (14.6) | 56.2 (7.4) | 54.8 (11.9) | |
| SI (°) | Back | 36.1 (8.4) | 36.2 (6.9) | 36.7 (6.7) | |
| | Leg | 37.1 (8.1) | 33.8 (4.4) | 36.6 (7.6) | |
| | Function | 35.4 (8.5) | 33.9 (9.1) | 37.3 (6.6) | |
| PDA (°) | Back | 8.0 (5.1) | 10.8 (4.4) | 9.9 (6.6) | |
| | Leg | 7.4 (5.8) | 9.8 (5.1) | 10.2 (5.8) | |
| | Function | 7.7 (5.3) | 7.0 (5.8) | 10.3 (5.8) | |
| SDA (°) | Back | 9.3 (5.5) | 13.4 (2.4) | 9.3 (4.6) | |
| | Leg | 10.8 (4.6) | 7.0 (6.6) | 10.3 (4.5) | |
| | Function | 9.6 (4.7) | 10.2 (3.5) | 10.0 (5.4) | |
| RSB (Rmm) | Back | 17.2 (43.3) | 2.3 (45.7) | −4.8 (27.1) | |
| | Leg | 10.6 (38.3) | 17.3 (43.2) | −0.8 (37.0) | |
| | Function | **26.7 (42.3)** | −3.4 (48.1) | **−1.0 (32.3)** | |
| **6 weeks – Baseline** | | | | | |
| LL (°) | Back | 2.6 (11.9) | −1.9 (5.9) | −1.8 (6.5) | |
| | Leg | 3.3 (13.2) | −0.7 (3.9) | −1.7 (6.6) | |
| | Function | **5.4 (15.2)** | −0.2 (3.3) | **−2.0 (5.6)** | |
| SI (°) | Back | −0.9 (5.4) | 1.6 (3.1) | 1.5 (4.2) | |
| | Leg | −1.6 (4.4) | 1.1 (3.4) | 1.6 (4.9) | |
| | Function | −0.9 (5.1) | −0.8 (4.3) | 1.3 (4.5) | |
| PDA (°) | Back | **−0.7 (4.4)** | −1.9 (3.5) | **−3.8 (3.2)** | |
| | Leg | −1.2 (4.4) | −1.7 (2.2) | −3.0 (4.1) | |
| | Function | −0.9 (4.7) | **1.8 (3.8)** | **−3.6 (3.1)** | |
| SDA (°) | Back | 0.1 (4.7) | −2.3 (2.2) | 0.3 (4.4) | |
| | Leg | 1.1 (4.5) | 1.0 (4.2) | −0.7 (4.4) | |
| | Function | 1.2 (4.7) | −1.3 (4.3) | −0.5 (4.2) | |
| RSB (Rmm) | Back | 1.6 (26.2) | −0.3 (13.3) | 11.5 (15.2) | |
| | Leg | 0.2 (28.7) | **−3.1 (9.1)** | **11.2 (15.5)** | |
| | Function | **−6.2 (31.7)** | 3.7 (5.9) | **10.6 (15.0)** | |

Moderate = responders improving more than 30% in one or more variable; Minimal = responders improving 20–29% for pain and 15–29% for function; Non non-responders with less than minimal improvement (or actual deterioration), LL lumbar lordosis, SI sacral inclination, PDA primary disc angle, SDA supradjacent disc angle, and RSB regional sagittal balance, Rmm system relative metric for RSB. Significant differences are indicated in bold ($p < 0.05$)

implantation with the Wallis interspinous implant, and radiographically showed a subtle reduction to sagittal range of motion of the full lumbar region at their first (up to 10 days; by 3.9°), second (3 months; by 2.8°), and fourth (12 months; by 3.5°) post-operative time-points, yet no statistical difference at 6 or 24 months (approximately 2.5°). It would seem that the skeletal mechanical effects of interspinous implants are short-lived, directing any biomechanical rationale for symptom improvement toward other tissues or physiological processes.

Repeat radiographic evaluation at 24 months was not justified or undertaken in our study for ethical reasons; however, PDA reversion toward baseline at 12 months may indicate a need for longer follow-up wherein non-ionising imaging (like MRI) might be preferable. We showed that non-responders flattened more at the index level than cases who improved, while lumbar lordosis subtly flattened in non-responders yet increased in responders (refer to Table 3 and Fig. 4). This finding suggests that relative kyphosis at either the index segment or lumbar region is not beneficial, which does not support maximising interspinous distraction by inserting the largest device possible as is recommended [9].

As an alternative rationale to altered angulation, the mechanical effect of DIAM in-vivo may instead relate to subtle change to tensile load in local connective and muscle tissues. Further, responders had more positive regional sagittal balance preoperatively that reduced with surgery, while non-responders started negative and became positive. Therefore clinically, preoperative forward trunk inclination might indicate potential for positive response to this surgery, and point to patients that describe relief in flexed postures (a common symptom in lumbar spinal stenosis). The potential influence of a stress-shielding phenomenon wherein soft, or osseous, tissues adapt to tensile loads via Davis' or Wolff's Laws, respectively, may provide explanation. Further investigation using appropriate imaging to concurrently examine paravertebral muscles and skeletal recovery under physiological conditions appears warranted to better understand DIAM's etiology.

Meaningful improvements were observed at 12 and 24 months for back pain and function, while response in terms of leg pain was variable. Therefore, patients describing predominant back pain might be expected to respond better to DIAM-augmented surgery than those with predominant leg pain. However, in assessing absolute change in pain and function we emphasise those with highest preoperative pain scores and limit generalisability to patients with lower levels of pain. Variable pain and function demonstrated by broad standard deviations in our cohort indicate diverse responses that challenge investigators and clinicians to identify patient characteristics leading to best effect. Moreover, it could

provide support for a localised mechanical effect at the index segment alone that does not relate to symptoms. Interestingly, and in tacit agreement with our results, Daentzer et al. [13] followed ten patients after

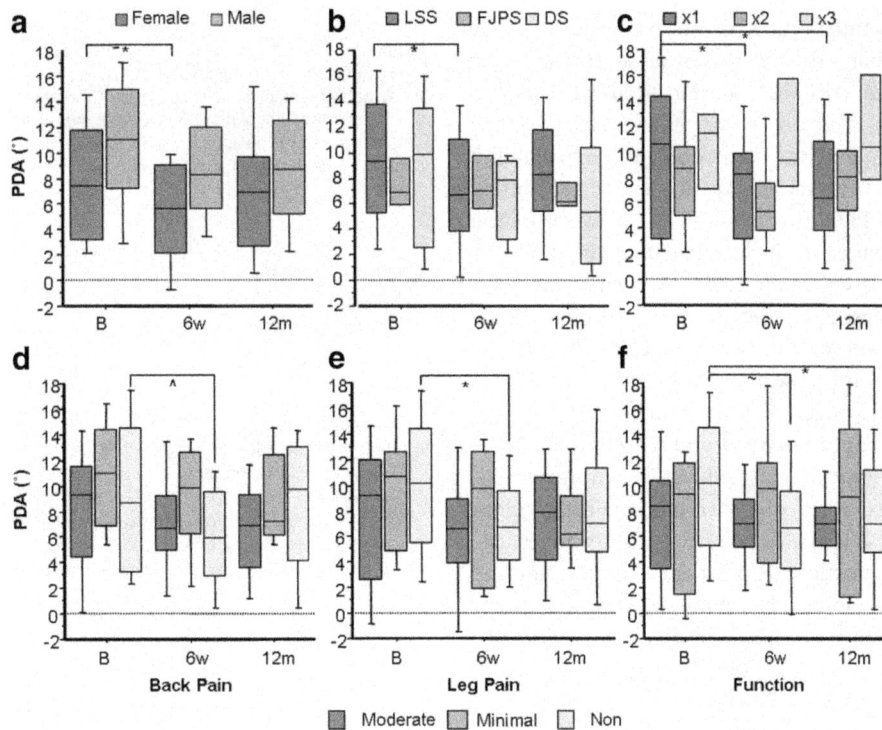

**Fig. 4** Box-plots revealing serial change in primary disc angle for 40 cases according to sex (**a**), diagnosis (**b**), number of implanted DIAMs (**c**); and responder groups according to back pain (**d**), leg pain (**e**) and function (**f**) (sub-group sample sizes indicated in Table 3). Footnote: *B* preoperative baseline, *6w* 6 week time-point, *12 m* 12 month time-point, *LL* lumbar lordosis, *SI* sacral inclination, *PDA* primary disc angle, *SDA* supradjacent disc angle, and *RSB* regional sagittal balance, *LSS* spinal stenosis, *FJPS* facet joint pain syndrome, *DS* degenerative spondylolisthesis

be argued that lumbar spinal stenosis represents an inclusive diagnosis that requires sub-classification to be meaningful in determining specific response. While our results point to differential diagnosis responses, unfortunately the insufficient power of our sample size did not accommodate multiple sub-group comparisons.

Our results should be interpreted in light of the study limitations. We examined outcomes after DIAM-augmented surgery in a heterogeneous patient group from a single centre. While this may reflect the broad

clinical (and global) reality of interspinous implant surgeries, examining discreet patient-groups with fewer covariates would offer improvement. Further, providing suitable distinction between the influences of DIAM in contrast to the surgery it augmented was not addressed and is relevant when equitable outcomes for interspinous implant-augmented decompression versus decompression-alone are shown [3, 16, 18, 31, 32]. As a single-surgeon effectiveness study our sample size was understandably small. However, our findings offer new insights and hint at

**Table 4** Matrix representing relationships [*r*-values] between sagittal alignment, pain and function according to change at 6 weeks

|  | LL | SI | PDA | SDA | RSB | BP | LP |
|---|---|---|---|---|---|---|---|
| SI | **−0.65** | | | | | | |
| PDA | **0.49** | **−0.32** | | | | | |
| SDA | **0.57** | −0.15 | −0.03 | | | | |
| RSB | **−0.69** | 0.20 | **−0.52** | −0.38 | | | |
| BP | **−0.37** | 0.23 | −0.27 | −0.24 | **0.33** | | |
| LP | −0.26 | 0.05 | −0.19 | **−0.38** | **0.40** | **0.67** | |
| Function | **−0.45** | 0.24 | −0.24 | **−0.35** | **0.43** | **0.71** | **0.73** |

*LL* lumbar lordosis, *SI* sacral inclination, *PDA* primary disc angle, *SDA* supradjacent disc angle, and *RSB* regional sagittal balance, *BP* back pain, *LP* leg pain. Statistically significant relationships are indicated in bold (*p* < 0.05)

**Table 5** Matrix representing relationships [*r*-values] between sagittal alignment, pain and function according to change at 12 months

|  | LL | SI | PDA | SDA | RSB | BP | LP |
|---|---|---|---|---|---|---|---|
| SI | **−0.70** | | | | | | |
| PDA | **0.40** | −0.20 | | | | | |
| SDA | **0.64** | −0.23 | 0.27 | | | | |
| RSB | **−0.44** | 0.06 | **−0.52** | **−0.42** | | | |
| BP | **−0.40** | 0.27 | −0.07 | −0.08 | −0.01 | | |
| LP | **−0.35** | 0.28 | −0.12 | −0.14 | 0.17 | **0.49** | |
| Function | **−0.32** | 0.21 | −0.22 | −0.13 | 0.14 | **0.64** | **0.57** |

*LL* lumbar lordosis, *SI* sacral inclination, *PDA* primary disc angle, *SDA* supradjacent disc angle, and *RSB* regional (lumbar) sagittal balance, *BP* back pain, *LP* leg pain. Statistically significant relationships are indicated in bold (*p* < 0.05)

potential identifiers for patients who may best respond to DIAM (and other) interspinous or lumbar surgeries. Our radiographic imaging was undertaken at several sites for patient convenience. Although routine protocol, it is not ideal in serial analysis of subtle changes to vertebral alignment that is dependent on methodological repeatability and where potential for variable quality exists. Our intrarater reliability for PDA was low and is indicative of the subtlety of small change to single-segment angulation.

Results of the present study reveal women, cases with lumbar spinal stenosis, or those who receive single DIAM-augmented surgery, show a significant alteration to disc angle at the index segment, albeit brief. Despite change in segmental angulation, its influence on patient's pain and function appears limited and therefore probably does not explain meaningful subjective improvement. While this study examines objective and subjective measures out to 1 and 2 years, respectively, further investigation of discreet diagnostic categories aimed at isolating the influence of DIAM appear necessary. Sagittal alignment and additional imaging features of functional significance like muscle quality warrant further investigation for interspinous implant or other minimally-invasive surgeries.

## Conclusions

Improvements in back, leg pain and function at 6 weeks and 12 months after DIAM-augmented surgery in patients with varied indications were not reflected in change to skeletal alignment. Subtle radiographic changes at 6 weeks differed according to response, which should be investigated further to identify modifiable risks. Preoperative sagittal balance and posture may have a bearing on outcome.

## Abbreviations

ANOVA: Analysis of variance; DIAM™: Device for intervertebral assisted motion; F: Female; M: Male; NS: Not significant; ODI: Oswestry disability index; PDA: Primary disc angle; Rmm: System-relative measurement for RSB (regional sagittal balance); SD: Standard deviation; SDA: Supradjacent disc angle

## Acknowledgements

The authors would like to thank Dr. Kevin P. Singer, PhD for his significant contribution to study delivery; Mr. Livio Mina for developing the digitising programme employed in radiographic assessments; the 14 radiology practices that adopted the standardised procedure for the cohort; the University of Western Australia and the National Health and Medical Research Council (NHMRC; Australia) for supporting the first author; and importantly to the patients for their cooperation. Study was undertaken at the University of Western Australia, Perth, Australia.

## Funding

RJC received personal funding (Australian Postgraduate Award and NHMRC Biomedical scholarship) in support of her PhD candidature.

## Authors' contributions

All three authors have: made substantial contributions to conception and design, acquisition of data, and analysis and interpretation of data; been involved in drafting the manuscript or revising it critically for important intellectual content; given final approval of the version to be published; and agreed to be accountable for all aspects of the work in ensuring that questions related to the accuracy or integrity of any part of the work are appropriately investigated and resolved.

## Competing interests

QM is a part patent holder of a competitor interspinous implant. RJC and RIP have no competing interests.

## Author details

[1]Institute for Health Sciences, School of Health Professions, Zürich University of Applied Sciences, Technikumstrasse 81, Winterthur CH-8401, Switzerland. [2]Faculty of Health and Exercise Sciences, Curtin University, Perth, Australia. [3]Centre for Neurological Surgery, Perth, Australia. [4]Department of Medical Technology and Physics, Sir Charles Gairdner Hospital, Perth, Australia. [5]School of Physics, University of Western Australia, Perth, Australia.

## References

1. Gazzeri R, Galarza M, Alfieri A. Controversies about interspinous process devices in the treatment of degenerative lumbar spine diseases: past, present, and future. 2014. p. 975052.
2. Wu AM, Zhou Y, Li QL, Wu XL, Jin YL, Luo P, Chi YL, Wang XY. Interspinous spacer versus traditional decompressive surgery for lumbar spinal stenosis: a systematic review and meta-analysis. PLoS One. 2014;9:e97142.
3. van den Akker-van Marle ME, Moojen WA, Arts MP, Vleggeert-Lankamp CL, Peul WC. Interspinous process devices versus standard conventional surgical decompression for lumbar spinal stenosis: cost utility analysis. Spine J. 2014; 16:702–10.
4. Lee SH, Seol A, Cho TY, Kim SY, Kim DJ, Lim HM. A systematic review of interspinous dynamic stabilization. Clin Orthop Surg. 2015;7:323–9.
5. Gazzeri R, Galarza M, Neroni M, Fiore C, Faiola A, Puzzilli F, Callovini G, Alfieri A. Failure rates and complications of interspinous process decompression devices: a European multicenter study. Neurosurg Focus. 2015;39:E14.
6. Siewe J, Selbeck M, Koy T, Rollinghoff M, Eysel P, Zarghooni K, Oppermann J, Herren C, Sobottke R. Indications and contraindications: interspinous process decompression devices in lumbar spine surgery. J Neurol Surg A Cent Eur Neurosurg. 2015;76:1–7.
7. Siddiqui M, Smith FW, Wardlaw D. One-year results of X Stop interspinous implant for the treatment of lumbar spinal stenosis. Spine. 2007;32:1345–8.
8. Senegas J. Mechanical supplementation by non-rigid fixation in degenerative intervertebral lumbar segments: the Wallis system. Eur Spine J. 2002;11 Suppl 2:S164–9.
9. Taylor J, Pupin P, Delajoux S, Palmer S. Device of intervertebral assisted motion: technique and initial results. Neurosurg Focus. 2007;22:E6 1-6.
10. Wilke HJ, Drumm J, Haussler K, Mack C, Steudel WI, Kettler A. Biomechanical effect of different lumbar interspinous implants on flexibility and intradiscal pressure. Eur Spine J. 2008;17:1049–56.
11. Crawford RJ, Price RI, Singer KP. Surgical treatment of lumbar segment disease with interspinous implant: review. J Musculoskelet Res. 2009;12:153–67.
12. Roder C, Baumgartner B, Berlemann U, Aghayev E. Superior outcomes of decompression with an interlaminar dynamic device versus decompression alone in patients with lumbar spinal stenosis and back pain: a cross registry study. Eur Spine J. 2015;24:2228–35.
13. Daentzer D, Hurschler C, Seehaus F, Noll C, Schwarze M. Posterior dynamic stabilization in the lumbar spine - 24 months results of a prospective clinical and radiological study with an interspinous distraction device. BMC Musculoskelet Disord. 2016;17:90.
14. Sur YJ, Kong CG, Park JB. Survivorship analysis of 150 consecutive patients with DIAM implantation for surgery of lumbar spinal stenosis and disc herniation. Eur Spine J. 2011;20:280–8.

15.  Mariottini A, Pieri S, Giachi S, Carangelo B, Zalaffi A, Muzii F, Palma L. Preliminary results of a soft novel lumbar intervertebral prosthesis (DIAM) in the degenerative spinal pathology. Acta Neurochirurgica [Suppl]. 2005;92:129–31.

16.  Kim KA, McDonald M, Pik JH, Khoueir P, Wang MY. Dynamic intraspinous spacer technology for posterior stabilization:case-control study on the safety, sagittal angulation, and pain outcome at 1-year follow-up evaluation. Neurosurg Focus. 2007;22:E7 1-9.

17.  Crawford RJ, Malone Q, Price RI. A prospective study for two years after lumbar surgery augmented with DIAM interspinous implant. J Musculoskelet Res. 2012;15:1250018.

18.  Sobottke R, Schluter-Brust K, Kaulhausen T, Rollinghoff M, Joswig B, Stutzer H, Eysel P, Simons P, Kuchta J. Interspinous implants (X Stop, Wallis, Diam) for the treatment of LSS: is there a correlation between radiological parameters and clinical outcome? Eur Spine J. 2009;18:1494–503.

19.  Crawford RJ, Price RI, Singer KP. The effect of interspinous implant surgery on back surface shape and radiographic lumbar curvature. Clin Biomech. 2009;24:467–72.

20.  Phillips F, Voronov L, Gaitanis I, Carandang G, Havey R, Patwardhan A. Biomechanics of posterior dynamic stabilizing device (DIAM) after facetectomy and discectomy. Spine J. 2006;6:714–22.

21.  Schilling C, Pfeiffer M, Grupp TM, Blomer W, Rohlmann A. The effect of design parameters of interspinous implants on kinematics and load bearing: an in vitro study. Eur Spine J. 2014;23:762–71.

22.  Mannion AF, Balague F, Pellise F, Cedraschi C. Pain measurement in patients with low back pain. Nat Clin Pract Rheumatol. 2007;3:610–8.

23.  Fairbank JCT, Pynsent PB. The Oswestry Disability Index. Spine. 2000;25:2940–53.

24.  Ostelo RWJG, Deyo RA, Stratford P, Waddell G, Croft P, Von Korff M, Bouter LM, de Vet HC. Interpreting change scores for pain and functional status in low back pain: towards international consensus regarding minimal important change. Spine. 2008;33:90–4.

25.  Horton WC, Brown CW, Bridwell KH, Glassman SD, Suk S-I, Cha CW. Is there an optimal patient stance for obtaining a lateral 36" radiograph? A critical comparison of three techniques. Spine. 2005;30:427–33.

26.  Spencer P, Steiger S, Cummings H, Genant H. Placement of points for digitising spine films. J Bone Miner Res. 1990;5 Suppl 2:S247.

27.  Singer KP, Edmonston SJ, Day RE, Breidahl WH. Computer-assisted curvature assessment and Cobb angle determination of the thoracic kyphosis. Spine. 1994;19:1381–4.

28.  Kawakami M, Tamaki T, Ando M, Yamada H, Hashizume H, Yoshida M. Lumbar sagittal balance influences the clinical outcome after decompression and posterolateral spinal fusion for degenerative lumbar spondylolisthesis. Spine. 2002;27:59–64.

29.  Richards JC, Majumdar S, Lindsey DP, Beaupre GS, Yerby SA. The treatment mechanism of an interspinous process implant for lumbar neurogenic intermittent claudication. Spine. 2005;30(4):744–9.

30.  Wiseman CM, Lindsey DP, Fredrick AD, Yerby SA. The effect of an interspinous process implant on facet loading during extension. Spine. 2005;30:903–7.

31.  Marsh GD, Mahir S, Leyte A. A prospective randomised controlled trial to assess the efficacy of dynamic stabilisation of the lumbar spine with the Wallis ligament. Eur Spine J. 2014;23:2156–60.

32.  Crawford RJ, Lynn JM, Malone Q, Price RI. Pain and function one year after decompressive disc surgery: cases augmented with the DIAM interspinous implant versus those receiving microdiscectomy. J Musculoskelet Res. 2012; 15:1250013.

# 2

# Revisiting the psychometric properties of the Scoliosis Research Society-22 (SRS-22) French version

Jean Théroux[1,2]* 🔾, Norman Stomski[2], Stanley Innes[2], Ariane Ballard[1,3], Christelle Khadra[1,3], Hubert Labelle[1,4] and Sylvie Le May[1,3]

## Abstract

**Background:** Adolescent idiopathic scoliosis (AIS) is among the most common spinal deformities affecting adolescents. The Scoliosis Research Society-22 questionnaire is commonly used to assess health-related quality of life in AIS patients, including pain.
The objective of this study is to verify the psychometric properties of the Scoliosis Research Society-22 French version (SRS-22fv) questionnaire.

**Methods:** A prospective methodological design was used to verify the psychometric properties of the French version of the SRS-22fv. Participants were initially recruited from the orthopaedic scoliosis department at Sainte-Justine Hospital (Montreal, Canada) and completed the SRS-22fv and the SF-12 questionnaire. The SRS-22fv's structure was evaluated through principal component analysis (PCA). Linear regression was used to assess convergent validity between the SRS-22fv and the SF-12.

**Results:** Data was available from 352 participants with AIS. Most participants were female (87%, $n = 307$), and the average age was 14.3 (SD = 1.8) years. The mean thoracic and lumbar Cobb angles were 27.9° (SD = 3.3) and 23.6° (SD = 9.4), respectively. Overall, 71.4% ($n = 252$) of the participants presented with spinal pain. About one-third (29%) reported thoracic pain, and almost half (44%) experienced lumbar pain. The PCA identified four redundant items, which resulted in a modified 18-item questionnaire. In comparison to the original questionnaire, the modified version showed higher levels of internal consistency for four of the five factors, explained a greater proportion of the total variance (63.3%), and generated higher inter-item total correlations.

**Conclusion:** We propose a shorter version of the SRS-22fv, thus the Canadian SRS-18fv, which showed an improved internal consistency and scale structure compared to the original SRS-22fv. We believe that this modified version would be better suited to assess the quality of life of adolescents with idiopathic scoliosis.

**Keywords:** SRS-22, Adolescent idiopathic scoliosis, Reliability, Validity, Psychometrics

* Correspondence: j.theroux@murdoch.edu.au
[1]Research Center, Sainte-Justine University Hospital Center, Montreal, QC, Canada
[2]School of Health Profession, Murdoch University, 90, South Street, Murdoch, WA 6150, Australia
Full list of author information is available at the end of the article

## Background

Adolescent idiopathic scoliosis (AIS) is among the most common spinal deformities affecting children and adolescents [1]. This deformity is defined as a three-dimensional structural lateral deviation of the spine greater than 10° with an associated prevalence of 2–3% in adolescents [2].

Initially developed by Haher et al. [3] and the Scoliosis Research Society (SRS), the initial SRS-24 questionnaire was designed to evaluate disease-specific health-related quality of life (HRQoL) in AIS patients who were scheduled to undergo spinal fusion surgery. The original version of this questionnaire contained 24 items with an underlying structure of six different factors (pain, general self-image, postoperative self-image, postoperative function, function from back condition, general level of activity, and satisfaction). The SRS-24 underwent further refinement [4] and was modified to a 23-item questionnaire with five factors instead of six.

To obtain a more reliable disease-specific instrument, the SRS questionnaire was further modified to a 22-item version [5, 6]. The final version of this questionnaire (SRS-22r) was revised in 2006. [7] The SRS-22r includes 22 items distributed among five different factors (pain, self-image/appearance, function/activity, mental health, and satisfaction with management). Each component includes five items, except for the "satisfaction with management", which only contains two items.

The SRS-22 has become one of the most widely used instruments in assessing the quality of care for individuals with scoliosis and has been validated in adolescent and adult populations [8, 9]. It has been translated and adapted in multiple languages over the last decade [10–26], among which a French-Canadian version (SRS-22fv) was developed and validated by Beauséjour et al. [18] in 2009. Several issues arise from that French validation study, particularly cross-loading of numerous items and items loading in factors that differed from the original English version. Hence, we consider that it would be important to reassess the psychometric properties of the SRS-22fv. The aim of this study was to verify the structure, reliability, and construct validity of the SRS-22fv.

## Methods

The present study is part of a larger prospective study examining back pain [27]. Overall, 500 consecutive participants were enrolled in the study, but the completed SRS-22fv questionnaire data were only obtained from 352 participants, which met the requirement for factor analysis. The study took place at Sainte-Justine University Hospital Centre (Montreal, Canada) which is the largest mother and child centre in Canada and received approval by the Institutional Research Ethics Board of Sainte-Justine's Research Centre. Questionnaires were completed by patients on their first or subsequent visit at the scoliosis orthopaedic clinic from October 2014 until May 2015. Patients were included if they were aged between 10 and 17 years and had received a diagnosis of adolescent idiopathic scoliosis with a spinal curve (Cobb angle) of at least 10°. Patients were excluded if they had (1) a spinal deformity other than AIS, (2) a congenital or acquired spinal abnormality, (3) previous spinal surgery, (4) a diagnose of mental disability, or (5) sustained a significant spinal trauma within the last 12 months.

## Analyses

All analyses were performed with SPSS v22 (IBM, Armonk, NY, USA). According to instrument validation guidelines [28], 10 participants per item are needed to undertake a robust factor analysis. Considering that the SRS-22fv has 22 items, a minimum sample size of 220 participants was required.

The adapted French-Canadian SRS-22fv was summed and scored in agreement with the original English version on a five-point Likert scale (5 = best; 1 = worst). As such, the minimum and maximum score range is from 5 to 25, except for the "satisfaction with management" domain which contains only two items. Mean scores, internal consistency, and ceiling and floor effects were calculated for each factor. Construct validity was assessed with multiple regression comparing corresponding factors of the SRS-22fv and SF-12 [29, 30].

Principal component analysis [31] with a promax rotation was used to explore the structure of SRS-22fv. Items with loadings below 0.45, cross-loadings above 0.32, or inter-item correlations below 0.30 were individually deleted, and the component solution was then re-extracted [32]. Internal consistency was examined by calculating Cronbach's alpha for each factor and the total questionnaire score.

## Results

### Characteristics of participants

More than 70% (352/500) of the participants returned a completed questionnaire and thus were eligible for analysis. Participants' characteristics are described in Table 1. Most participants were female (87%) ($n = 307$), with a mean age of 14.3 (SD = 1.8) years, and had a mean thoracic and lumbar Cobb angles of 26.6° (SD = 12.8) and 23.6° (SD = 9.4), respectively. About one-third (31%, $n = 109$) of the participants attended the orthopaedic clinic for the first time, and almost half (40%, $n = 142$) were using braces.

### Mean score of SRS-22fv factors

Mean scores for each of the factors of the SRS-22fv are presented in Table 2. The total mean SRS-22fv score (4.14 [SD = 0.45]) indicated that the participants, in general, had a high level of well-being. No floor effects

**Table 1** Characteristics of participants

|  | All (n = 352) | Girls (n = 307) | Boys (n = 45) |
|---|---|---|---|
| Age (mean) (SD) | 14.26 (1.76) | 14.25 (1.73) | 14.33 (1.93) |
| Brace (yes) n (%) | 142 (40) | 125 (41) | 17 (38) |
| First visit (yes) (%) | 109 (31) | 92 (30) | 17 (38) |
| Mean Cobb angle (SD) in degrees |  |  |  |
| Thoracic principal | 27.87° (13.30) | 27.93° (13.37) | 26.64° (12.81) |
| Thoraco-lumbar | 23.93° (11.14) | 24.38° (11.19) | 21° (10.90) |
| Lumbar | 23.61° (9.40) | 23.72° (9.15) | 22.88° (11.20) |
| Angle of trunk rotation in degrees |  |  |  |
| Dorsal | 8.52° (4.16) | 8.40° (4.15) | 9.60° (4.18) |
| Lumbar | 7.2° (4) | 7° (3.81) | 8.60° (5.4) |

There were no statistical differences on all the variables between genders

were observed but moderate ceiling effects were noted for two factors (satisfaction with management and self-image).

**Psychometric properties of the SRS-22fv**

The psychometric properties of the SRS-22fv were considered through examining the loading of each item on discrete factors, item cross-loading between factors, inter-item correlations, item floor and ceiling effect, and communality values. The initial principal component analysis (PCA) (Table 3) revealed that item 15 had an inter-item correlation below 0.30. That item was deleted, and the factors were re-extracted, which showed that item 12 cross-loaded and that item 18 did not load on any component. Item 18 was deleted, and PCA was performed once again, which demonstrated that item 12 cross-loaded. After removing item 12 and re-extracting the factor solution, it was found that item 19 was redundant since its inter-item correlation fell below 0.30. The next iteration of the PCA revealed that all remaining items strongly loaded on discrete factors and all inter-item correlations exceeded 0.30. This resulted in a revised 18-item questionnaire (Table 4) that explained more of the variance than the original SRS-22fv item questionnaire (63.3% compared to 55.7%). In addition, four of the scales, derived from the final factor solution, demonstrated higher levels of internal consistency than the corresponding scales in the SRS-22fv (Table 5).

Finally, for the revised 18-item questionnaire, the Kaiser-Meyer-Olkin value (0.87) was well above the minimum criterion of 0.5, and the Bartlett test of sphericity was statistically significant ($p = 0.000$).

Table 6 displays the results of linear regression analysis undertaken to examine the convergent validity of the revised 18-item SRS. Results showed that the scales in the revised questionnaire were significantly associated with conceptually similar scales in the SF-12. These findings provide additional support to the factor structure of the revised questionnaire.

**Discussion**

This study reexamined the psychometric properties of the adapted French-Canadian version of the SRS-22. Our results identified four redundant items in the SRS-22fv, which after deletion improved the total variance explained by the five factors, while also enhancing the internal consistency of four of the five factors. Hence, our proposed SRS-18fv is more parsimonious and psychometrically robust than the SRS-22fv.

Adolescent idiopathic scoliosis evaluation is no longer viewed solely based on treatment procedures (observation, bracing, or surgery), but also requires assessment of health-related quality of life [7, 33]. The original SRS-22 questionnaire is currently widely utilised to assess HRQoL in adolescents with scoliosis, [10–26, 30, 34–41] but the findings of the present study indicate that our revised SRS-18fv may be more appropriate for the French-Canadian adolescent population.

Our findings were consistent with the previous study by Beauséjour et al. [18] that validated the SRS-22 in a French-Canadian population. Both our results and Beauséjour's [18] identified several cross-loading items and several items that loaded on factors that differed from the English version of the SRS-22. But Beauséjour et al. [18] did not delete poorly fitted items and re-extract the factors, which is inconsistent with psychometric guidelines [32]. The authors also noted that the SRS-22 was suitable to use without any revisions. In our view, however, the identification of poorly performing items in the present study and the previous study underlines the need to use a revised questionnaire that defines health-related quality of life constructs of

**Table 2** Mean scores among all the factors of the SRS-22fv (n = 352)

|  | Pain | Self-image | Function | Mental health | Satisfaction with management | Total (1–22) |
|---|---|---|---|---|---|---|
| Mean score (SD) | 4.32 (0.65) | 3.93 (0.62) | 4.32 (0.41) | 4.14 (0.66) | 3.75 (0.89) | 4.14 (0.45) |
| SEM | 0.034 | 0.033 | 0.021 | 0.035 | 0.048 | 0.02 |
| % floor | 0 | 0 | 0 | 0 | 1.7 |  |
| % ceiling | 22.8 | 5.4 | 0.9 | 11.1 | 17.1 |  |

SEM standard error of the mean

**Table 3** Factor structure of the SRS-22fv

| | 1 | 2 | 3 | 4 | 5 |
|---|---|---|---|---|---|
| Q3: During the past 6 months, have you been a very nervous person?[a] | *.757* | .168 | −.063 | −.082 | −.076 |
| Q7: In the past 6 months, have you felt so down in the dumps that nothing could cheer you up? | *.682* | .007 | .034 | .055 | −.046 |
| Q13: Have you felt calm and peaceful during the last six months? | *.753* | .087 | −.114 | −.034 | .095 |
| Q16: In the past six months, have you felt down hearted and blue? | *.845* | −.026 | .070 | .008 | .052 |
| Q20: Have you been a happy person during the past six months? | *.699* | −.030 | .174 | −.100 | .026 |
| Q1: Which of the following best describes the amount of pain you have experienced during the past 6 months? | .204 | *.766* | −.147 | .102 | −.038 |
| Q2: Which one of the following best describes the amount of pain you have experienced over the last month? | .179 | *.807* | −.165 | .126 | −.001 |
| Q8: Do you experience back pain when at rest? | .050 | *.717* | .016 | −.103 | −.127 |
| Q11: Which one of the following best describes your medication usage for your back? | −.174 | *.479* | .076 | .196 | .096 |
| Q17: In the past three months, have you taken any sick days from work/school due to back pain and, if so, how many? | −.166 | *.333* | .001 | .267 | (.458) |
| Q4: If you had to spend the rest of your life with your back as it is right now, how would you feel about it? | −.002 | (.486) | *.367* | .029 | .008 |
| Q6: How do you look in clothes? | .152 | −.110 | *.673* | .183 | −.029 |
| Q10: Which of the following best describes the appearance of your trunk, defined as the human body except for the head and extremities? | .021 | .088 | *.730* | .055 | .000 |
| Q14: Do you feel that your condition affects your personal relationships? | .275 | −.093 | *.383* | .196 | .176 |
| Q19: Do you feel attractive with your current back condition? | −.047 | −.172 | *.441* | .095 | .181 |
| Q5: What is your current level of activity? | −.031 | −.052 | .060 | *.766* | −.105 |
| Q9: What is your current level of work/school activity? | −.076 | .130 | .051 | *.759* | .009 |
| Q12: Does your back limit your ability to do things around the house? | .036 | (.358) | −.003 | *.539* | .038 |
| Q15: Are you and/or your family experiencing financial difficulties because of your back? | .112 | −.230 | .117 | −.023 | (.777) |
| Q18: Does your back condition limit your going out with friends/family? | .029 | −.165 | .078 | *.544* | (−.585) |

**Table 3** Factor structure of the SRS-22fv *(Continued)*

| | 1 | 2 | 3 | 4 | 5 |
|---|---|---|---|---|---|
| Q21: Are you satisfied with the results of your back management? | −.117 | (.422) | (.583) | −.198 | *−.102* |
| Q22: Would you have the same management again if you had the same condition? | −.066 | (.480) | (.484) | −.181 | *−.018* |

Italicized data indicates items of the original questionnaire
Items in parenthesis () represent items loading on the inappropriate factor as compared to the original English version
[a]Questions from the original English version

importance to adolescents with scoliosis in a clearly delineated manner.

Regarding the internal consistency, only one factor, "function", in the SRS-18fv had a Cronbach alpha value below 0.70, the minimally acceptable level [42]. Other studies of the original SRS-22 and SRS-22fv also reported Cronbach alpha values for the function factor that fell below the accepted value. [12, 26, 30, 35, 39] This suboptimal level of internal consistency suggests that items within this component may not all be clearly tapping the same construct. The lack of clear conceptual delineation might arise from the inclusion of terms like "labor" and "work" in the phrasing of the items. This wording may not be readily comprehended or deemed

**Table 4** Factor structure of the SRS-18fv

| | 1 | 2 | 3 | 4 | 5 |
|---|---|---|---|---|---|
| | MH | Pain | SI | Func | Satis |
| Q3 | .726 | | | | |
| Q7 | .749 | | | | |
| Q13 | .764 | | | | |
| Q16 | .837 | | | | |
| Q20 | .584 | | | | |
| Q1 | | .877 | | | |
| Q2 | | .863 | | | |
| Q4 | | .439 | | | |
| Q8 | | .795 | | | |
| Q11 | | .476 | | | |
| Q6 | | | .849 | | |
| Q10 | | | .779 | | |
| Q14 | | | .719 | | |
| Q5 | | | | .749 | |
| Q9 | | | | .795 | |
| Q17 | | | | .599 | |
| Q21 | | | | | .846 |
| Q22 | | | | | .850 |

% explained variance 63.30%
Residual ≥0.05, 31%; determinant = 0.0001
*MH* mental health, *SI* self-image, *Func* function, *Satis* satisfaction with management

**Table 5** Internal consistency comparison

| Factor | Beauséjour [18] | Current study | |
|---|---|---|---|
| | | SRS-22fv | SRS-18fv |
| Pain | 0.79 | 0.76 | 0.80 |
| Self-image | 0.67 | 0.66 | 0.74 |
| Function | 0.68 | 0.60 | 0.61 |
| Mental health | 0.79 | 0.83 | 0.83 |
| Satisfaction with management | 0.69 | 0.71 | 0.71 |

relevant by children and adolescents, particularly considering that one-third of our sample was aged 13 years or below.

Notably, items 4 and 17 of the SRS-18fv loaded on different factors than in the English version of the SRS-22, which may be influenced by differences in interpretation of the items following translation from English to French. Item 4: "If you had to spend the rest of your life with your back shape as it is right now, how would you feel about it?" originally associated with "self-image" loaded on the "pain" component. This inconsistency could be related to the meaning attributed to the term "back shape" in French. In the translated French version, the adolescents' interpretation of this item might be more closely associated with "pain" than the actual "shape" of their back. Hence, item 4 in the French translation could be revised to be more congruent with the initial English meaning. Item 17: "In the last 3 months have you taken any days off of work, including household work, or school because of back pain" originally associated with "pain" loaded on the "function" component. This divergence in loading may result from the interpretation that pain and function are conceptually similar since they are related to physical limitations. These interpretation issues suggest that it might be worthwhile to reexamine the content validity of the initial French version of the SRS-22.

In the previous validation study of the SRS-22fv [18], construct validity was examined by performing Pearson correlations between the related SRS-22 and the SF-12 domains. However, the use of such correlations does not control for covariance and also increase the risk of type II errors [43]. In the present study, we established construct validity using linear regression, which controls for covariance and adjusts for multiple comparisons which result in a more robust assessment.

### Study limitations

Several caveats should be considered in interpreting this study's findings. First, this study enrolled participants from a single institution, which may impact on the generalisability of the results. However, the institution from which participants were recruited is the most important mother and child centre in Canada and therefore receives a diversified adolescent population from many different regions of this province. Second, participants were all pre-surgical cases with a Cobb angle inferior to 45°. Consequently, results should be interpreted with caution in a population with more severe Cobb angles. Third, the test-retest reliability of our revised questionnaire warrants examination in further studies. Finally, the construct validity of our revised questionnaire was assessed with the SF-12 questionnaire which has yet to be validated in a French adolescent population.

### Conclusion

Our revised questionnaire is briefer and more psychometrically robust than the original version of the SRS-22fv. It provides clinicians and researchers with a better tool to understand the impact of scoliosis on adolescents' health-related quality of life.

**Table 6** Construct validity of the SRS-18fv with corresponding SF-12 factors

| SF-12 | SRS-18fv (β; 95% CI) | | | | |
|---|---|---|---|---|---|
| | Pain | Self-image | Function | Mental health | Satisfaction with management |
| Physical functioning | 0.67; 0.19–1.15 | 0.59; 0.30–0.88 | | | |
| Role functioning | 0.70; 0.31–1.08 | 0.54; 0.31–0.77 | | | |
| Bodily pain | 1.00; 0.56–1.43 | 0.36; 0.10–0.62 | | | 0.45; 0.17–0.73 |
| General health perception | | 0.39; 0.17–0.62 | −0.30; −0.49 to −0.11 | | |
| Vitality | | 0.64; 0.31–0.96 | | | |
| Social functioning | | 0.62; 0.33–0.92 | | 0.59; 0.14–1.04 | |
| Role emotional | | 0.52; 0.29–0.75 | | | |
| Mental health | | 0.47; 0.25–0.69 | −0.28; −0.46 to −0.09 | 0.68; 0.34–1.02 | |

Results not reported were not significant

## Abbreviations
AIS: Adolescent idiopathic scoliosis; HRQoL: Health-related quality of life; PCA: Principal component analysis; SD: Standard deviation; SRS: Scoliosis Research Society

## Acknowledgements
Not applicable.

## Funding
Not applicable.

## Authors' contributions
JT and SL design the study. JT collected the data. JT and NS analysed the data and interpreted the results. JT and NS drafted the manuscript. SL, SI, AR, CK, and HL revised the article and table for content and accuracy. All authors approved the final manuscript.

## Competing interests
The authors declare that they have no competing interests.

## Author details
[1]Research Center, Sainte-Justine University Hospital Center, Montreal, QC, Canada. [2]School of Health Profession, Murdoch University, 90, South Street, Murdoch, WA 6150, Australia. [3]Faculty of Nursing, University of Montreal, Montreal, QC, Canada. [4]Faculty of Medicine, University of Montreal, Montreal, Canada.

## References
1. Goldberg MS, Mayo NE, Poitras B, Scott S, Hanley J. The Ste-Justine Adolescent Idiopathic Scoliosis Cohort Study. Part I: description of the study. Spine (Phila Pa 1976). 1994;19(14):1551–61.
2. Weinstein S, Dolan L, Cheng J, Danielsson A, Morcuende J. Adolescent idiopathic scoliosis. Lancet. 2008;371:1527–37.
3. Haher TR, Gorup JM, Shin TM, Homel P, Merola AA, Grogan DP, Pugh L, Lowe TG, Murray M. Results of the Scoliosis Research Society instrument for evaluation of surgical outcome in adolescent idiopathic scoliosis. A multicenter study of 244 patients. Spine (Phila Pa 1976). 1999;24(14):1435–40.
4. Asher MA, Min Lai S, Burton DC. Further development and validation of the Scoliosis Research Society (SRS) outcomes instrument. Spine (Phila Pa 1976). 2000;25(18):2381–6.
5. Asher M, Min Lai S, Burton D, Manna B. The reliability and concurrent validity of the scoliosis research society-22 patient questionnaire for idiopathic scoliosis. Spine (Philadelphia, Pa 1976). 2003;28(1):63–9.
6. Asher M, Min Lai S, Burton D, Manna B. Discrimination validity of the scoliosis research society-22 patient questionnaire: relationship to idiopathic scoliosis curve pattern and curve size. Spine (Philadelphia, Pa 1976). 2003;28(1):74–8.
7. Asher MA, Lai SM, Glattes RC, Burton DC, Alanay A, Bago J. Refinement of the SRS-22 health-related quality of life questionnaire function domain. Spine (Phila Pa 1976). 2006;31(5):593–7.
8. Glattes RC, Burton D, Lai S, Frasier E, Asher M. The reliability and concurrent validity of the Scoliosis Research Society-22r patient questionnaire compared with the Child Health Questionnaire-CF87 patient questionnaire for adolescent spinal deformity. Spine (Philadelphia, Pa 1976). 2007;32(16):1778–84.
9. Bridwell KH, Cats-Baril W, Harrast J, Berven S, Glassman S, Farcy JP, Horton WC, Lenke LG, Baldus C, Radake T. The validity of the SRS-22 instrument in an adult spinal deformity population compared with the Oswestry and SF-12: a study of response distribution, concurrent validity, internal consistency, and reliability. Spine (Phila Pa 1976). 2005;30(4):455–61.
10. Bago J, Climent JM, Ey A, Perez-Grueso FJ, Izquierdo E. The Spanish version of the SRS-22 patient questionnaire for idiopathic scoliosis: transcultural adaptation and reliability analysis. Spine (Phila Pa 1976). 2004;29(15):1676–80.
11. Monticone M, Carabalona R, Negrini S. Reliability of the Scoliosis Research Society-22 Patient Questionnaire (Italian version) in mild adolescent vertebral deformities. Europa medicophysica. 2004;40(3):191–7.
12. Alanay A, Cil A, Berk H, Acaroglu RE, Yazici M, Akcali O, Kosay C, Genc Y, Surat A. Reliability and validity of adapted Turkish version of Scoliosis Research Society-22 (SRS-22) questionnaire. Spine (Phila Pa 1976). 2005; 30(21):2464–8.
13. Zhao L, Zhang Y, Sun X, Du Q, Shang L. The Scoliosis Research Society-22 questionnaire adapted for adolescent idiopathic scoliosis patients in China: reliability and validity analysis. J Child Orthop. 2007;1(6):351–5.
14. Cheung KM, Senkoylu A, Alanay A, Genc Y, Lau S, Luk KD. Reliability and concurrent validity of the adapted Chinese version of Scoliosis Research Society-22 (SRS-22) questionnaire. Spine (Phila Pa 1976). 2007;32(10):1141–5.
15. Hashimoto H, Sase T, Arai Y, Maruyama T, Isobe K, Shouno Y. Validation of a Japanese version of the Scoliosis Research Society-22 Patient Questionnaire among idiopathic scoliosis patients in Japan. Spine (Phila Pa 1976). 2007; 32(4):E141–6.
16. Glowacki M, Misterska E, Laurentowska M, Mankowski P. Polish adaptation of Scoliosis Research Society-22 questionnaire. Spine (Phila Pa 1976). 2009; 34(10):1060–5.
17. Antonarakos PD, Katranitsa L, Angelis L, Paganas A, Koen EM, Christodoulou EA, Christodoulou AG. Reliability and validity of the adapted Greek version of Scoliosis Research Society-22 (SRS-22) questionnaire. Scoliosis. 2009;4:14.
18. Beausejour M, Joncas J, Goulet L, Roy-Beaudry M, Parent S, Grimard G, Forcier M, Lauriault S, Labelle H. Reliability and validity of adapted French Canadian version of Scoliosis Research Society Outcomes Questionnaire (SRS-22) in Quebec. Spine (Phila Pa 1976). 2009;34(6):623–8.
19. Niemeyer T, Schubert C, Halm HF, Herberts T, Leichtle C, Gesicki M. Validity and reliability of an adapted German version of Scoliosis Research Society-22 questionnaire. Spine (Phila Pa 1976). 2009;34(8):818–21.
20. Rosanova GC, Gabriel BS, Camarini PM, Gianini PE, Coelho DM, Oliveira AS. Concurrent validity of the Brazilian version of SRS-22r with Br-SF-36. Rev Bras Fisioter. 2010;14(2):121–6.
21. Mousavi SJ, Mobini B, Mehdian H, Akbarnia B, Bouzari B, Askary-Ashtiani A, Montazeri A, Parnianpour M. Reliability and validity of the Persian version of the Scoliosis Research Society-22r questionnaire. Spine (Phila Pa 1976). 2010; 35(7):784–9.
22. Lee JS, Lee DH, Suh KT, Kim JI, Lim JM, Goh TS. Validation of the Korean version of the Scoliosis Research Society-22 questionnaire. Eur Spine J. 2011; 20(10):1751–6.
23. Leelapattana P, Keorochana G, Johnson J, Wajanavisit W, Laohacharoensombat W. Reliability and validity of an adapted Thai version of the Scoliosis Research Society-22 questionnaire. J Child Orthop. 2011;5(1):35–40.
24. Danielsson AJ, Romberg K. Reliability and validity of the Swedish version of the Scoliosis Research Society-22 (SRS-22r) patient questionnaire for idiopathic scoliosis. Spine (Phila Pa 1976). 2013;38(21):1875–84.
25. Schlosser TP, Stadhouder A, Schimmel JJ, Lehr AM, van der Heijden GJ, Castelein RM. Reliability and validity of the adapted Dutch version of the revised Scoliosis Research Society 22-item questionnaire. Spine J. 2014;14(8):1663–72.
26. Haidar RK, Kassak K, Masrouha K, Ibrahim K, Mhaidli H. Reliability and validity of an adapted Arabic version of the Scoliosis Research Society-22r Questionnaire. Spine (Phila Pa 1976). 2015;40(17):E971–7.
27. Theroux J, Le May S, Hebert JJ, Labelle H. Back pain prevalence is associated with curve-type and severity in adolescents with idiopathic scoliosis: a cross-sectional study. Spine (Phila Pa 1976). 2016.
28. Worthington RL, Whittaker TA. Scale development research: a content analysis and recommendations for best practices. Couns Psychol. 2006;34(6):806–38.
29. Beausejour M, Roy-Beaudry M, Goulet L, Labelle H. Patient characteristics at the initial visit to a scoliosis clinic: a cross-sectional study in a community without school screening. Spine (Phila Pa 1976). 2007;32(12):1349–54.
30. Lonjon G, Ilharreborde B, Odent T, Moreau S, Glorion C, Mazda K. Reliability and validity of the French-Canadian version of the scoliosis research society 22 questionnaire in France. Spine (Phila Pa 1976). 2014;39(1):E26–34.

31. Beavers AS, Lounsbury JW, Richards JK, Huck SW, Slolits GJ, Esquivel SL. Practical considerations for using exploratory factor analysis in educational research. Practical Assessment, Res Eval. 2013;18(6):1-13.

32. Hair JF, Black WC, Barry BJ, Anderson RE. Multivariate data analysis. 7th ed. Upper Saddle River: Prentice Hall; 2010.

33. Graham B, Green A, James M, Katz J, Swiontkowski M. Measuring patient satisfaction in orthopaedic surgery. J Bone Joint Surg. 2015;97(1):80–4.

34. Climent JM, Bago J, Ey A, Perez-Grueso FJ, Izquierdo E. Validity of the Spanish version of the Scoliosis Research Society-22 (SRS-22) Patient Questionnaire. Spine (Phila Pa 1976). 2005;30(6):705–9.

35. Monticone M, Baiardi P, Calabro D, Calabro F, Foti C. Development of the Italian version of the revised Scoliosis Research Society-22 Patient Questionnaire, SRS-22r-I: cross-cultural adaptation, factor analysis, reliability, and validity. Spine (Phila Pa 1976). 2010;35(24):E1412–7.

36. Li M, Wang CF, Gu SX, He SS, Zhu XD, Zhao YC, Zhang JT. Adapted simplified Chinese (mainland) version of Scoliosis Research Society-22 questionnaire. Spine (Phila Pa 1976). 2009;34(12):1321–4.

37. Camarini PM, Rosanova GC, Gabriel BS, Gianini PE, Oliveira AS. The Brazilian version of the SRS-22r questionnaire for idiopathic scoliosis. Braz J Phys Ther. 2013;17(5):494–505.

38. Adobor RD, Rimeslatten S, Keller A, Brox JI. Repeatability, reliability, and concurrent validity of the scoliosis research society-22 questionnaire and EuroQol in patients with adolescent idiopathic scoliosis. Spine (Phila Pa 1976). 2010;35(2):206–9.

39. Qiu G, Qiu Y, Zhu Z, Liu Z, Song Y, Hai Y, Luo Z, Liu Z, Zhang H, Lv G, et al. Re-evaluation of reliability and validity of simplified Chinese version of SRS-22 patient questionnaire: a multicenter study of 333 cases. Spine (Phila Pa 1976). 2011;36(8):E545–50.

40. Sathira-Angkura V, Pithankuakul K, Sakulpipatana S, Piyaskulkaew C, Kunakornsawat S. Validity and reliability of an adapted Thai version of Scoliosis Research Society-22 questionnaire for adolescent idiopathic scoliosis. Spine (Phila Pa 1976). 2012;37(9):783–7.

41. Potoupnis M, Papavasiliou K, Kenanidis E, Pellios S, Kapetanou A, Sayegh F, Kapetanos G. Reliability and concurrent validity of the adapted Greek version of the Scoliosis Research Society-22r Questionnaire. A crosssectional study performed on conservatively treated patients. Hippokratia. 2012;16(3): 225–9.

42. DeVellis RF. Scale development : theory and applications. 3rd ed. Los Angeles: SAGE; 2012.

43. Cohen J, Cohen P, West SG, Aiken LS. Applied multiple regression/ correlation analysis for the behavioral sciences. Mahwah, N.J., L. Erlbaum Associates; 2003.

# 3

# Asymmetrical pedicle subtraction osteotomy for progressive kyphoscoliosis caused by a pediatric Chance fracture

Satoshi Suzuki, Nobuyuki Fujita, Tomohiro Hikata, Akio Iwanami, Ken Ishii, Masaya Nakamura, Morio Matsumoto and Kota Watanabe[*] (ID)

**Abstract**

**Background:** Although most pediatric Chance fractures (PCFs) can be treated successfully with casting and bracing, some PCFs cause progressive spinal deformities requiring surgical treatment. There are only few reports of asymmetrical osteotomy for PCF-associated spinal deformities.

**Case presentation:** We here report a case of a 10-year-old girl who suffered an L2 Chance fracture from an asymmetrical flexion-distraction force, accompanied by abdominal injuries. She was treated conservatively with a soft brace. However, a progressive spinal deformity became evident, and 10 months after the injury, examination showed segmental kyphoscoliosis with a Cobb angle of 36°, a kyphosis angle of 31°, and a coronal imbalance of 30 mm. Both the coronal and sagittal deformities were successfully corrected by asymmetrical pedicle subtraction osteotomy.

**Conclusions:** Initial kyphosis and posterior ligament complex should be evaluated at some point when treating PCFs. Asymmetrical pedicle subtraction osteotomy can be a useful surgical option when treating rigid kyphoscoliosis associated with a PCF.

**Keywords:** Chance fracture, Flexion-distraction injury, Kyphoscoliosis, Asymmetrical pedicle subtraction osteotomy, Case report

## Background

Chance fractures, which are flexion-distraction injuries of the spine, were defined by George Quentin Chance in 1948 as a fracture line passing transversely through the spinous process, laminae, and pedicle and then into the vertebral body [1]. Chance fractures account for 5–11% of the acute thoracolumbar spinal injuries in adults [2, 3]. Although pediatric spinal injuries are more unusual, affecting only 0.3–4% of the pediatric population, they have become more common due to mandatory seat-belt laws [4–6]. Of these injuries, about 43–50% consist of pediatric Chance fractures (PCFs) [5]. The treatment of these fractures depends on the fracture pattern as well as neurologic status [5]. Purely osseous injuries with minimal deformity, and even those involving ligamentous injuries, have been treated conservatively, and these injuries have a good prognosis in pediatric patients [7]. However, in some cases, surgery is required to correct a kyphotic deformity or to halt neurological deterioration or a progressive deformity [5, 7]. Surgeries to treat chronic, rigid deformities caused by PCF are rare [8–10]. We here report a case of a 10-year-old girl with rigid, chronic-phase kyphoscoliosis caused by a PCF. The kyphoscoliosis was successfully treated by asymmetrical pedicle subtraction osteotomy (PSO) at the affected vertebra.

## Case presentation

A 10-year-old girl was traveling in the back seat of a car, wearing a 3-point restraint, when the car was involved in a collision at an intersection. The girl was transported to a nearby hospital, where she complained of abdominal

* Correspondence: kw197251@keio.jp
Department of Orthopaedic Surgery, Keio University School of Medicine, 35 Shinanomachi, Shinjyuku, Tokyo 160-8582, Japan

and back pain. After clinical and radiographic examination, the diagnoses were perforations in the duodenal and transverse colon, a fracture of the right wrist, and an L2 Chance fracture without neurologic deficit. Radiographs of the lumbar spine revealed local lumbar scoliosis at L1–L3 with a Cobb angle of 18° in a supine position (Fig. 1). CT images

showed a horizontal split in the right L2 pedicle (Fig. 2b), a collapse of the right anterior vertebral column (Fig. 2a, b), and splitting of the L2 left transverse processes, the left L2 pedicle, and the middle of the L2 vertebral column (Fig. 2c), resulting in asymmetrical kyphoscoliosis. The girl underwent emergency surgery for the abdominal injury and wrist fracture. The Chance fracture was treated conservatively with 4 weeks of bed rest, after which the patient was allowed to walk with a soft brace. However, the deformity gradually deteriorated, and the girl was referred to our hospital. Physical examination showed that her trunk was leaning to the left side, and standing whole spine radiographs revealed kyphoscoliosis at the thoracolumbar area with a Cobb angle of 36° at L1–L3 (Fig. 3a), a kyphosis angle of 31° at L1–L3 (Fig. 3b), and a coronal imbalance of 30 mm (the distance between the C7 plumb line and the center of the sacrum) to the left (Fig. 3c). The kyphotic angle decreased to 2.4° over a bolster (Fig. 3d). MR images did not show any soft tissue injury or spinal cord damage when she was transferred to our hospital (data not shown). CT images revealed that the fractures had fused (Fig. 4a).

Ten months after the injury, we performed correction and fusion surgery using asymmetrical PSO at L2. After exposing the posterior elements through a posterior midline approach, we placed pedicle screws bilaterally at T12, L1, and L3 and at the right L2 pedicle. We next removed the upper one third of the elongated left L2 pedicle, the left upper and posterior portion of the vertebra, and the L1/L2 intervertebral disc (Fig. 5a). After local bone graft into L1/L2 disc space, we applied compression force between the L1 and L3 pedicle screws on the left side while

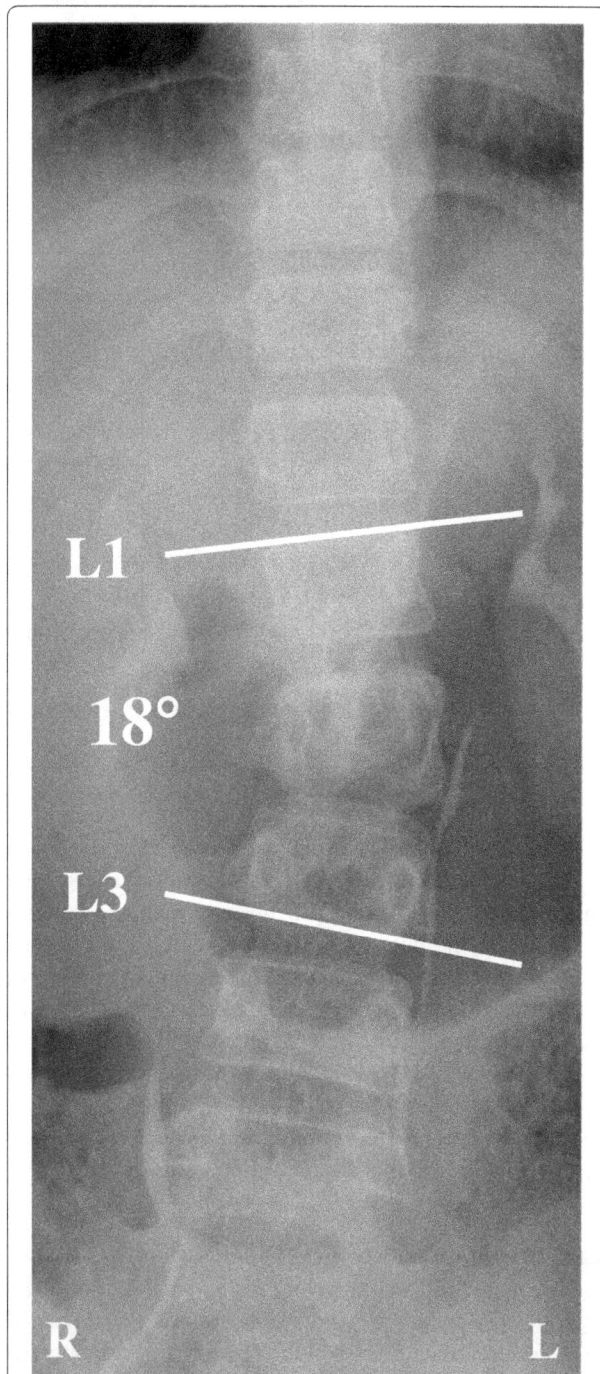

**Fig. 1** Radiographs at the time of injury. Radiographs obtained immediately after the injury revealed an L2 fracture with local lumbar scoliosis at L1–L3 of 18° (AP view)

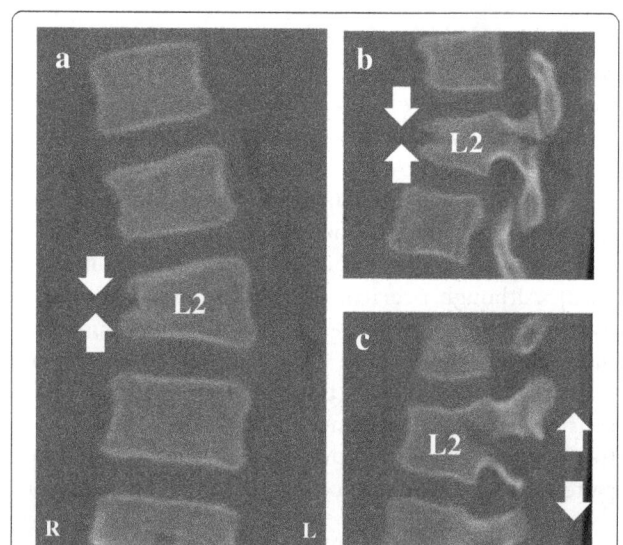

**Fig. 2** CT images at the time of injury. CT images revealed a Chance-type injury with an associated L2 compression fracture of the right vertebral body (**a**), a horizontal split of the right L2 pedicle (**b**), and the splitting and distraction of the left L2 transverse processes, left L2 pedicle, and the L2 middle column (**c**), resulting in asymmetrical kyphoscoliosis

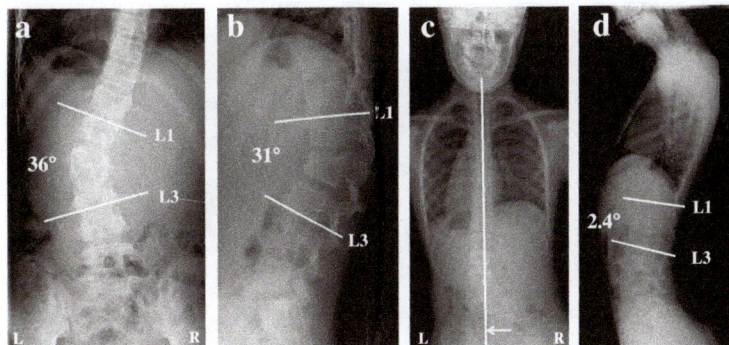

**Fig. 3** Radiographs at the time of surgery. Lumbar radiographs revealed segmental kyphoscoliosis with a Cobb angle of 36° (**a**) and a kyphosis angle of 31° (**b**). A standing AP view of the entire spine showed a 30-mm leftward shift of the C7-central sacral vertical line (**c**). The kyphotic angle decreased to 2.4° on a lateral radiograph over a bolster (**d**)

monitoring motor-evoked potentials (Fig. 5a). The facet joints of T12/L1 and L2/L3 and transverse processes of T12, L1, L2, and L3 were decorticated. The remaining local bone graft was placed along the decorticated bones. The intraoperative time was 91 min; the estimated blood loss was 220 ml (Fig. 5b).

The scoliosis was corrected from 36° to 1° and the kyphosis from 31° to 1° (Fig. 6a, b). At the 2-year follow-up, radiographs showed excellent coronal balance, no instrument failure or loss of correction, and osseous continuity between the vertebrae (Fig. 6c).

## Discussion

In 1948, George Quentin Chance characterized a type of fracture with "horizontal splitting of the spine and neural arch [1]." Nicoll proposed the term "Chance fracture" in 1949 [11]. Most cases are associated with a flexion-distraction injury obtained in a motor vehicle accident [12]. In children, however, 2-point restraints and improperly used restraints have increased the incidence of PCFs at the lumbar spine, often at L2 or L3 [7]. As a result of anatomical characteristics, Chance injuries are more likely to cause neurological issues in children than in adults: 15–43% of PCFs involve neurological deficits [7, 13, 14].

### PCF post-traumatic deformities

Delayed displacement and progressive deformities have been reported after conservative therapy for PCF [7, 8, 13, 15, 16]. To summarize the reports, in Chance fractures, the threshold of kyphosis angle for surgical indication was ranged from 15° to 22°. However, taking standing radiographs for assessing initial kyphosis will be difficult in the situation of an acute spinal injury. Additionally, more attention will be paid for the possible concomitant injuries

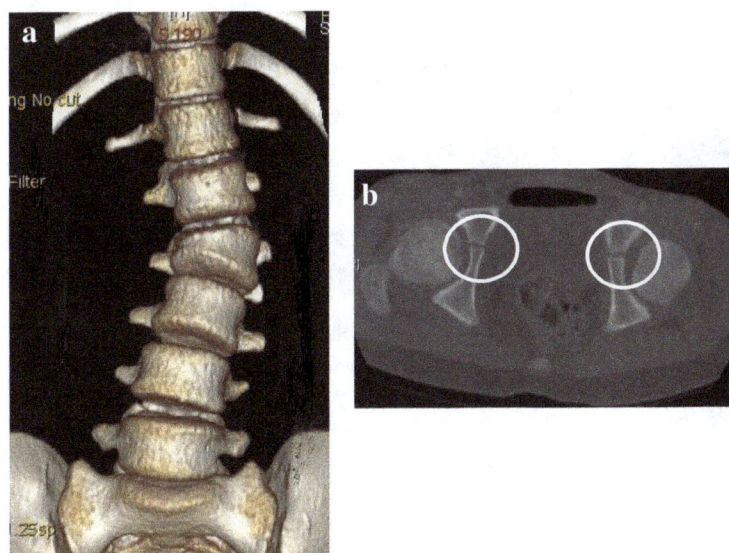

**Fig. 4** CT images at the time of surgery. A reconstructed three-dimensional CT image showing kyphoscoliosis due to the affected L2 vertebra (**a**). CT images revealed an opening of bilateral Y-shaped cartilage (**b**)

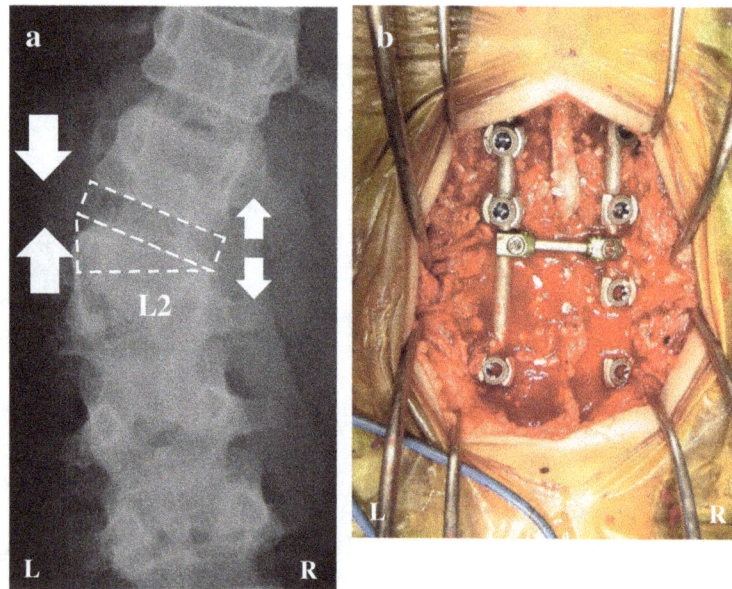

**Fig. 5** Intraoperative findings. The deformity was corrected by L1/L2 intervertebral disc resection and osteotomy of the upper one third of the elongated L2 pedicle and vertebral body, followed by compression to the left side and distraction to the right side (**a**). An intraoperative photograph just after the correction is shown in (**b**)

including abdominal viscera and vascular injuries at the time of injury. In our patient's case, the initial lumbar scoliosis at L1–L3 was 18° in a supine position. Based only on the scoliosis, conservative treatment was a reasonable choice. Additionally, since treatments for abdominal injuries had the priority in this case, the delay in the evaluations for kyphosis angle and damages of posterior ligament complex were inevitable. The case report is therefore an important lesson of what can happen if an unstable asymmetrical

Chance fracture is not well managed in the acute phase after trauma.

### Treatment of PCFs

Outcomes of conservative therapy for PCFs are relatively good; however, some PCFs should be treated surgically to correct an initial kyphotic deformity or to prevent further neurological deterioration or a progressive deformity [17]. Since the injury of PCFs is mainly the

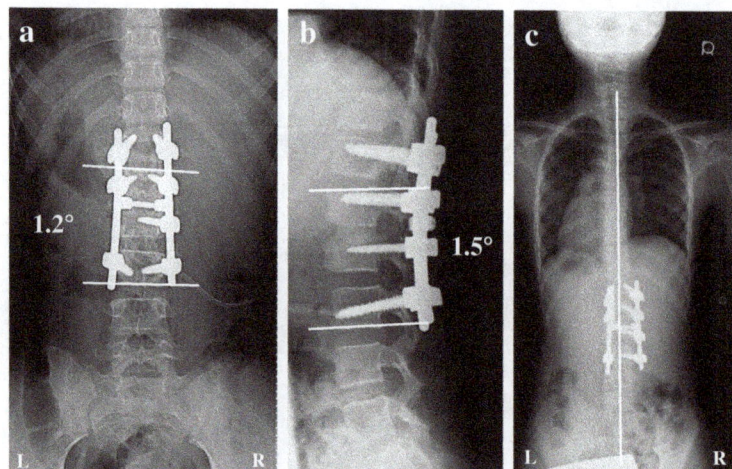

**Fig. 6** Postoperative radiographs and CT images. Postoperative radiographs revealed that the L1–L3 scoliosis was corrected to 1.2° (**a**) and the kyphosis to 1.5° (**b**). A radiograph and CT image obtained at the 2-year follow-up showed good global coronal balance with no instrument failure or loss of correction (**c**)

posterior osteoligamentous complex, reduction and stabilization with posterior instrumentation should be considered [18]. When treating acute PCFs surgically, pedicle screw instrumentation, which extended one or two levels above and below the affected vertebra, seems to be a popular treatment [19]. With a recent progress of spinal instrumentations, percutaneous pedicle screw fixation may have evolved as an alternative approach for PCFs [5, 20]. On the other hand, there are only a few reports of surgical treatment for chronic deformities due to PCFs, including combined anterior and posterior fusion surgery, transforaminal thoracic interbody fusion, and transpedicle wedge osteotomy and posterior fusion [8, 21, 22]. Asymmetrical PSO, which was first reported in 2012 by Sathya et al. [23], is not a novel technique; however, it seems to be rare rerated to a report of asymmetrical PSO for a chronic pediatric Chance fracture. Our patient's spinal deformity was caused by a deformity of the fractured L2 vertebra, so we judged that short fusion with asymmetrical PSO was sufficient to correct the affected vertebra. Our osteotomy procedure included partial resection of the pedicle, vertebral body, and adjacent disc in an applied grade 4 osteotomy, according to the classification system of anatomically based spinal osteotomies proposed by Schwab et al. [24]. In this case, we intended to fuse from T12 to L3 for the maintenance of spinal alignment after correction of scoliosis and kyphosis. The application of without fusion technique at L2/L3 fact joints and future removal of the spinal implants might be another option to preserve motion segment at L2/L3. However, we have removed posterior ligamentous complex at L2/L3 during the surgery and were afraid of the occurrence of distal junctional problem after removal of the implants.

## Conclusions

Initial kyphosis and posterior ligament complex should be evaluated at some point when treating PCFs. Asymmetrical PSO is not a novel technique; however, there are only few reports of asymmetrical osteotomy for PCF-associated spinal deformities. Asymmetrical pedicle subtraction osteotomy can be a useful surgical option when treating rigid kyphoscoliosis associated with a PCF.

**Abbreviations**
CT: Computed tomography; MR: Magnetic resonance; PCF: Pediatric Chance fracture; PSO: Pedicle subtraction osteotomy

**Acknowledgements**
Not applicable

**Funding**
Not applicable

**Authors' contributions**
All authors read and approved the final manuscript. KW conceived the study, participated in the design of the study, helped to write the manuscript, and revised it critically. SS participated in its design and drafted the manuscript. NF, TH, AI, KI, and NM participated in the study design and helped to draft the manuscript. MM conceived, designed, and coordinated the study and drafted the final manuscript.

**Competing interests**
The authors declare that they have no competing interests.

**References**
1. Chance GQ. Note on a type of flexion fracture of the spine. Br J Radiol. 1948;21:452–3.
2. Denis F. The three column spine and its significance in the classification of acute thoracolumbar spinal injuries. Spine. 1983;8:817–31.
3. Gumley G, Taylor TK, Ryan MD. Distraction fractures of the lumbar spine. J Bone Joint Surg (Br). 1982;64:520–25.
4. Campbell DJ, Sprouse 2nd LR, Smith LA, Kelley JE, Carr MG. Injuries in pediatric patients with seatbelt contusions. Am Surg. 2003;69:1095–99.
5. Le TV, Baaj AA, Deukmedjian A, Uribe JS, Vale FL. Chance fractures in the pediatric population. J Neurosurg Pediatr. 2011;8:189–97.
6. Lutz N, Nance ML, Kallan MJ, Arbogast KB, Durbin DR, Winston FK. Incidence and clinical significance of abdominal wall bruising in restrained children involved in motor vehicle crashes. J Pediatr Surg. 2004;39:972–75.
7. Glassman SD, Johnson JR, Holt RT. Seatbelt injuries in children. J Trauma. 1992;33:882–6.
8. Campbell A, Yen D. Late neurologic deterioration after nonoperative treatment of a Chance fracture in an adolescent. Can J Surg. 2003;46:383–5.
9. Keene JS, Lash EG, Kling Jr TF. Undetected posttraumatic instability of "stable" thoracolumbar fractures. J Orthop Trauma. 1988;2:202–11.
10. Reid AB, Letts RM, Black GB. Paediatric Chance fractures: association with intraabdominal injuries and seat belt use. J Trauma. 1990;30:384–91.
11. Nicoll EA. Fractures of the dorso-lumbar spine. J Bone Joint Surg (Br). 1949;31:376–94.
12. Louman-Gardiner K, Mulpuri K, Perdios A, Tredwell S, Cripton PA. Pediatric lumbar Chance fractures in British Columbia: chart review and analysis of the use of shoulder restraints in MVAs. Accid Anal Prev. 2008;40:1424–9.
13. Arkader A, Warner Jr WC, Tolo VT, Sponseller PD, Skaggs DL. Pediatric Chance fractures: a multicenter perspective. J Pediatr Orthop. 2011;31:741–4.
14. Rumball K, Jarvis J. Seat-belt injuries of the spine in young children. J Bone Joint Surg (Br). 1992;74:571–4.
15. Bouliane MJ, Moreau MJ, Mahood J. Instability resulting from a missed Chance fracture. Can J Surg. 2001;44:61–2.
16. Reilly CW. Pediatric spine trauma. J Bone Joint Surg Am. 2007;89 Suppl 1:98–107.
17. Vaccaro AR, Silber JS. Post-traumatic spinal deformity. Spine. 2001;26:S111–8.
18. Wood KB, Li W, Lebl DR, Ploumis A. Management of thoracolumbar spine fractures. Spine J. 2014;14:145–64.
19. Daniels AH, Sobel AD, Eberson CP. Pediatric thoracolumbar spine trauma. J Am Acad Orthop Surg. 2013;21:707–16.
20. Phan K, Rao PJ, Mobbs RJ. Percutaneous versus open pedicle screw fixation for treatment of thoracolumbar fractures: systematic review and meta-analysis of comparative studies. Clin Neurol Neurosurg. 2015;135:85–92.
21. Huang RC, Meredith DS, Taunk R. Transforaminal thoracic interbody fusion (TTIF) for treatment of a chronic Chance injury. HSS J. 2010;6:26–9.
22. Okuyama K, Sasaki H, Kido T, Chiba M. A chronic flexion-distraction injury with a "fistulous wither" on the split spinous process of the L1 vertebra—a case report of a modified transpedicle wedge osteotomy. Eur Orthop Traumatol. 2013;4:253–7.
23. Thambiraj S, Boszczyk BM. Asymmetric osteotomy of the spine for coronal imbalance: a technical report. Eur Spine J. 2012;21:S225–9.
24. Schwab F, Blondel B, Chay E, Demakakos J, Lenke L, Tropiano P, et al. The comprehensive anatomical spinal osteotomy classification. Neurosurgery. 2014;74:112–20.

# 4

# Adolescents with idiopathic scoliosis and their parents have a positive attitude towards the Thermobrace monitor

Sabrina Donzelli[1*], Fabio Zaina[1], Gregorio Martinez[2], Francesca Di Felice[1], Alberto Negrini[1] and Stefano Negrini[3]

## Abstract

**Background:** A temperature monitor is used to objectively measure brace wear time in adolescent idiopathic scoliosis. The reliability of this device have been demonstrated, and some specialists introduced the use of a compliance monitor as a standard of care in everyday clinical practice, as we did since 2010 with the Thermobrace (TB). The attitude towards these objective monitors has never been investigated.

The present study aims to investigate the attitude of parents and patients towards the use of temperature sensors for measuring brace wear compliance.

**Methods:** Three hundred one consecutive girls and 63 boys and their parents have been interviewed. The inclusion criteria were as follows: brace wear full-time prescription at first visit and at least one visit with download and discussion of TB data.

Usefulness, acceptability, reliability, and feeling related to data download were the investigated domains. Patients were invited by the administrative staff to complete anonymously the questionnaire. The European Commission was informed about the present survey and approved it (ICT-37-2015-1). Descriptive statistic was used to present the results.

**Results:** Among the 364 invited patients and parents, 336 adhered by completing it (rate of responders was 93.2%). The mean age was 14.65 (SD 2.36), the mean Cobb angle was 34.18 (SD 13.57), and the average brace wear prescription was 21.76 h per day (SD 2.53). We did not ask parents about their age, profession, nor other personal data.

Globally, the interviewed patients and parents showed a very positive attitude towards the TB monitor: the mean rate of parents stating a completely or at least partially positive attitude towards this electronic device was 94.0% while among patients, it was 85.6%.

**Conclusions:** This is the first study investigating the attitude of parents and patients towards a brace wear compliance monitor. People who experienced this objective monitoring are aware of the advantages related to it and support its usefulness not only for clinicians but also for patients and parents to respect the hours prescribed without any affection on the children and parents or the patient-physician relationship. The present results should encourage the spread of these tools in daily clinical practice.

**Keywords:** Compliance monitor, Brace, Scoliosis

* Correspondence: sabrina.donzelli@isico.it
[1]ISICO, Via R Bellarmino 13/1, 20141, Milan, Italy
Full list of author information is available at the end of the article

## Background

Adherence is defined as the degree to which a patient acts in accordance to the prescription of a health care provider. It has unquestionable implications on the effect of a therapy and as a consequence on the results of clinical research [1]. The harder the treatment, the higher the risks for non-adherent patients. Brace wear for scoliosis is a very hard and complex therapy; indeed, in this field, adherence can be very challenging due to the difficulties associated with wearing plastic for a long time and during one of the most critical phases of life: adolescence [2, 3]. Many brace studies in the past disregarded adherence to the prescribed regimen or considered referred adherence obtained from surveys and clinical assessments [4] notwithstanding their already recognized low reliability [5].

In recent years, the use of electronic devices was introduced in various research studies; after demonstrating the reliability of temperature sensors, the main topic of the investigation turned to the effects of adherence on results [5–10]. Brace efficacy was recently confirmed by a multicenter RCT [11, 12]; in the same study, adherence was assessed by using objective monitors and a relation between dosage and results was found, thus confirming previous researches: the more the brace wear, the better the results [4, 9–11, 13, 14]. The Thermobrace (TB) is a temperature compliance monitor introduced in everyday clinical activity as a standard of care since 2010, and today, 2579 patients are currently monitored during brace treatment. According to our experience, this device is very helpful in everyday clinical activity, because it offers a valuable help in therapeutic choices, without undermining the relationship with patients and their families [15]. The standardized use of TB contributes by improving the quality of the treatment through an optimization of the dosage, and recently, Karol and colleagues showed that providing patients with feedback about their real dosage increases adherence [16]. Our experience at ISICO is that open discussions based on objective data strengthen the mutual trust needed for the patient-physician relationship and increases compliance. The TB use showed to contribute also to the cognitive behavioral approach needed to enhance compliance [17]. Figure 1 shows the Thermobrace inside a brace.

Even if the usefulness of these electronic monitoring devices in research is widely recognized, in everyday clinical activity, it is still debated with many of the clinicians showing reluctance to its use, despite the clear indication of the SOSORT-SRS consensus [18]. The main reasons they advocate are the fear to harm the patient-physician relationship or to affect the relationship between parents and children being already very fragile at adolescents' age, but while the trust issue can be sometimes present also among parents who decide not to adopt the Thermobrace, the main reason is probably economic.

The aim of the present study is to investigate, in a population of TB-experienced subjects, the attitude of parents and patients towards the use of temperature sensors for measuring brace wear compliance and to verify the differences between parents and their children in the following domains: understanding of the device, usefulness, acceptance, reliability, and the feeling related to the moment of data reading and discussion.

## Methods

### Participants and procedure

The survey was conducted in a tertiary referral center specialized in scoliosis conservative treatment; the data collection lasted from May 2015 to July 2015. We applied a convenience sampling, inviting all the patients who used a brace and a Thermobrace for at least 4 months. The recruitment was done at the end of each visit; the doctor provided explanations and aims of the

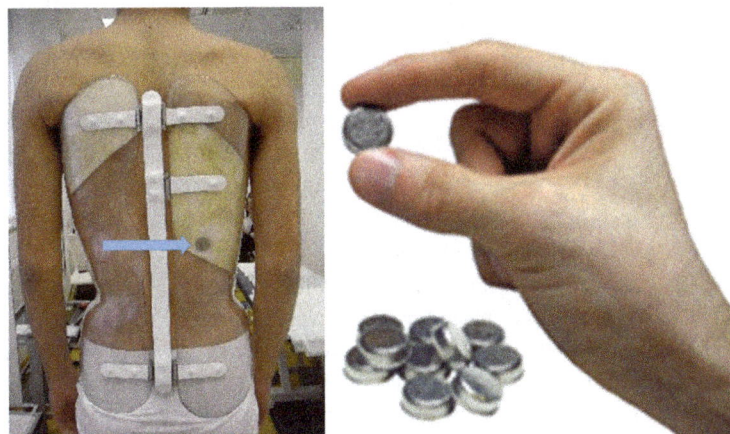

**Fig. 1** A Thermobrace sensor inside a Sforzesco brace is shown

survey study and then invited all the participants to fulfill the questionnaire in the waiting room. To allow the maximum rate of responders and considering the sensitive topics treated in the questionnaire, the completion was anonymous. The completed questionnaires were collected by the administrative staff before the patient and the family left our center.

Inclusion criteria were a brace prescription at first visit and at least one visit with download and discussion of TB data, which means at least 4 months of experience with the temperature monitor device and one shared analysis.

All the involved patients were aware of the monitoring device, which was embedded into the brace at the first brace check. Actually, since 2010, the Thermobrace sensor is prescribed to all patients who need a brace to treat their scoliosis. The standardized procedure includes that at the end of the visit, the doctor discusses with the patient and his family the main aim of the treatment and presents the TB as a useful tool able to guide clinical choices and finally to improve the results of the therapy. After these explanations, the parents who accept to buy the Thermobrace automatically agree to accept the monitoring device. At each physiotherapy session (every 3 months) and at each visit (usually every 6 months), the Thermobrace data are analyzed and discussed together to improve brace wear and to understand the main difficulties faced by each patient.

### Thermobrace temperature sensor

To measure the actual brace wear, we used a commercially available device called the "iButton™ DS1922LF5#" (http://www.maxim-ic.com/datasheet/index.mvp/id/4088/t/al) (Maxim Integrated Products, Inc.; 120 San Gabriel Drive, Sunnyvale, CA 94086), which we called for this specific use "Thermobrace." It is a small temperature data logger to be installed within each orthosis, and it includes a temperature sensor, a battery, and a memory. The sensor is meant to measure the brace temperature, and it is not placed in direct contact with the patient's skin but within a pressure pad, inside the brace. A reliability study has validated this specific instrument [19].

### Reading software

A specific software program to elaborate the data has been developed and is now freely available online, after a free registration on the website (http://www.scoliosismanager.org/thermobrace). The algorithm used to determine whether a sample corresponds to the brace being worn/not worn, and details concerning the reliability of collected and processed data, has already been described in a previous published paper [15]. This specific software has been integrated with our clinical system;

for further details, check also the freely accessible website (www.scoliosismanager.org).

### Survey construction

The conception of the questionnaire was entrusted to SN and SD who have 5 years of experience in using the Thermobrace sensor as a standard of care in braced patients. They decided to use a self-administered questionnaire, mainly composed of multiple-choice questions, to make the completion easier and quicker. Only one question was open, to let the responders share their thoughts freely in respect to what they had understood about the TB sensor. The choice to submit the questionnaire directly at the end of the visit is justified by the optimization of the number of responders; for the same reason, it was agreed that the doctor was responsible for the invitation, as this approach guaranteed a better compliance to questionnaire completion.

The 5 years' experience with an objective compliance monitor led to the definition of the following main items of the questionnaire:

*Usefulness and function* of the Thermobrace sensor: the aim was to investigate what the patients and their families understood about these devices.
*Perceived effect* of the Thermobrace on patients' behavior (in particular adherence to the treatment), with their brace from both the patients' and parents' point of view.
*Trust affection*: in this item, we aimed to investigate if the awareness of being monitored has any impact on the trust and the patient-parent relationship.
*Perceived reliability* of the device, which is related to the effective brace wear measured by the device and the declared and perceived mean time of brace wear of patients and parents.
*Discomfort feelings* related to the moment of data download, reading, and discussion. In these items, all the following feelings are included: awkwardness, anxiety, and being bothered.
*Satisfaction with the electronic device*: in this item, we aimed to investigate if the participants were happy with the choice of the objective monitoring of brace wear, if they would recommend this use to others, and if they would repeat again their choice.

After a pilot study involving 10 patients, a final version of the questionnaire was defined. Two external investigators, not directly involved in the clinical activity, reviewed the questionnaires and analyzed the data (AN and GM). The decision to make the questionnaire anonymous is justified by the fact that the questionnaire deals with personal and sensitive issues and to avoid the risk that respondents may refuse to answer some questions. It was not possible for parents to see the answers of their children nor vice versa.

## Statistics

For the present study, descriptive statistic was used; in fact, due to the choice of the anonymous completion of the questionnaire, it was not possible to make any kind of correlations with the clinical and demographic data of the included subjects (Additional file 1).

## Results

Among 364 invited patients to complete anonymously the questionnaire, 336 adhered by completing it; therefore, globally, the rate of responders was very high (93.2%), and most of them completed all the required sections of the questionnaire. The mean age of the recruited patients was 14.65 (SD 2.36), the mean Cobb angle was 34.18 (SD 13.57), and average brace wear prescription was 21.76 h per day (SD 2.53). We did not ask parents about their age, profession, nor other personal data.

Globally, the interviewed patients and parents showed a very positive attitude towards the TB monitor; in fact, the mean percentage of parents stating a completely or at least partially positive attitude towards this electronic device was 94.0% while among patients it was 85.6%. The rates of fully positive replies together with the partially positive ones, for each question's number, for parents and patients are shown in Fig. 2.

The first section of the parents' questionnaire comprises an open-ended question aimed to investigate the comprehension of the usefulness of the TB sensor. Among the 336 invited parents, seven did not answer to the first question (2.4%). All the answers have been evaluated and classified into three categories: the group of parents who wrote a very detailed description of the TB and its advantages, thus illustrating a very good understanding of the usefulness of the device (8.1%), the group who understood at least partially the usefulness of the TB sensor (88.0%), and those who completely misunderstood the significance and use of the TB sensor (1.5%).

A second question aimed to deepen the usefulness of the TB sensor; in fact, responders had to decide to whom the TB is most useful; multiple choices were allowed. This question showed a rate of responders of 100%. 35.3% of the responders consider the TB useful for parents, 56.9% consider it useful for patients, and

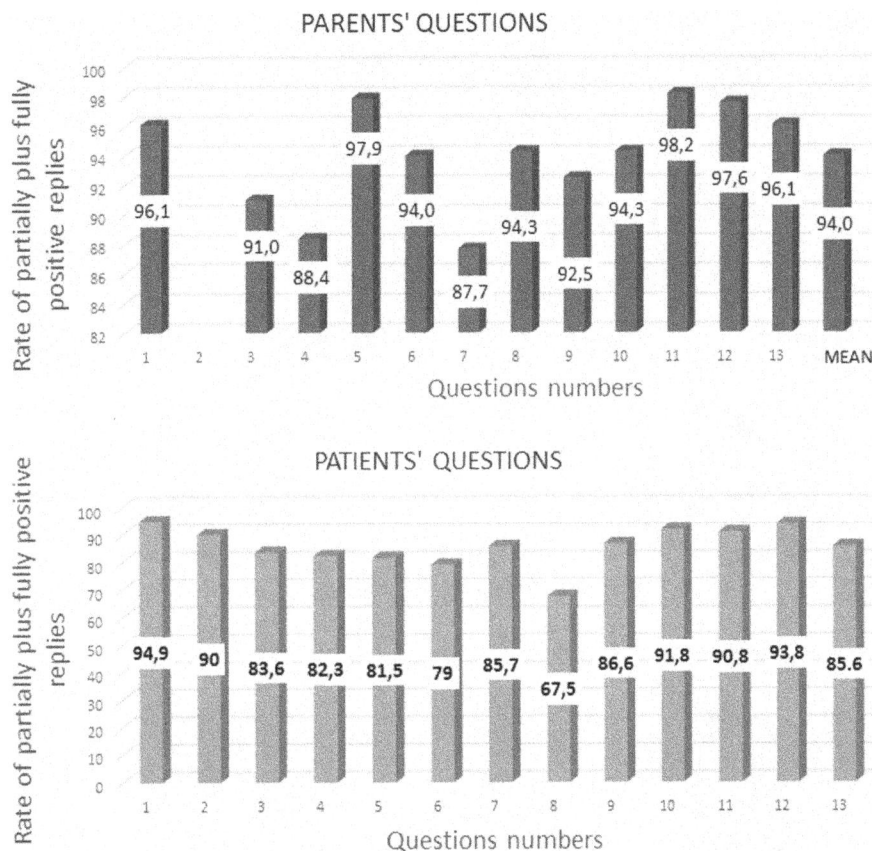

**Fig. 2** Rates of partially plus fully positive replies obtained from parents' and patients' questionnaires (*upper* and *lower parts*, respectively), according to question number and to survey's items

86.5% state that the TB sensor is useful for physicians. Only 0.6% answered "for none" and 1.2% answered "others." When considering the combined answers, we obtained the following rates: the TB is considered useful for both parents and patients by 22.5% of responders, for physicians and patients by 46.5% of responders, and for physicians and parents by 31.1% of responders. Among those declaring that they do not consider the TB helpful, most of them declare that it is useful for patients and physicians (the percentages are respectively 3.6 and 9.3%). The non-responder rate is 0.8%.

Also, patients were asked about the perceived usefulness; Fig. 3 shows the main results obtained by parents and patients for the usefulness item.

The results concerning the items on trust of parents and patients are shown in Fig. 4.

Table 1 summarizes the rate of answers related to the reliability of the TB sensor and the discomfort feelings related to the moment of data download.

In questions 12 and 13, the parents were asked respectively if they would accept again to use the TB sensor and if they would recommend its use to other people. 91.2% answered that they surely would accept again the TB, 6.0% would have some doubts, and 1.5% answered "no" (non-responder rate 0.9%). 91.3% of parents would recommend TB use to other patients, 2.7% declare that they would not recommend the TB use, and 4.8% would recommend the use of TB only in particular situations, for example, if the patient is not accepting the therapy, in very anxious subjects, and in non-compliant patients and if it was possible to check TB data at home by parents (non-responder rate 1.2%).

## Discussion

This is the first study investigating the attitude of scoliosis patients and their family towards a monitoring device able to measure objectively the number of hours of brace wear. The use of compliance monitors in everyday clinical practice is still highly debated among expert clinicians, with very few promoting their use [16, 20, 21], and most of them ignoring their functioning or advantages or simply refusing their use by advocating reasons related to the trust affection and damages to the mutual relationship between patient and physician.

As physicians, we strongly agree that it is fundamental that the new system does not affect negatively the mutual trust needed for the patient-doctor and patient-parent relationship, but after experiencing its use, it is possible to state that the new device provides objective data for open discussions, thus allowing to increase adherence to treatment but without disturbing or making the patient feel worry. This is confirmed by the answers given by the patients and parents involved in the present survey related to the trust items and also by the lower rates of responders referring to feel some discomfort (awkwardness, anxiety, and being bothered) during TB data download and sharing. Considering this controversial issue, it is noticeable that only 1.5% of the patients always mind to show the TB data to his/her doctor; this result confirms the very small impact on the mutual trust between patients and physicians.

In our setting, some parents refused the TB monitoring by saying that they really trust their sons/daughters and hence do not need to monitor them, and therefore, the trust theme rises again but from another point of view. Despite these issues used to justify objective monitor

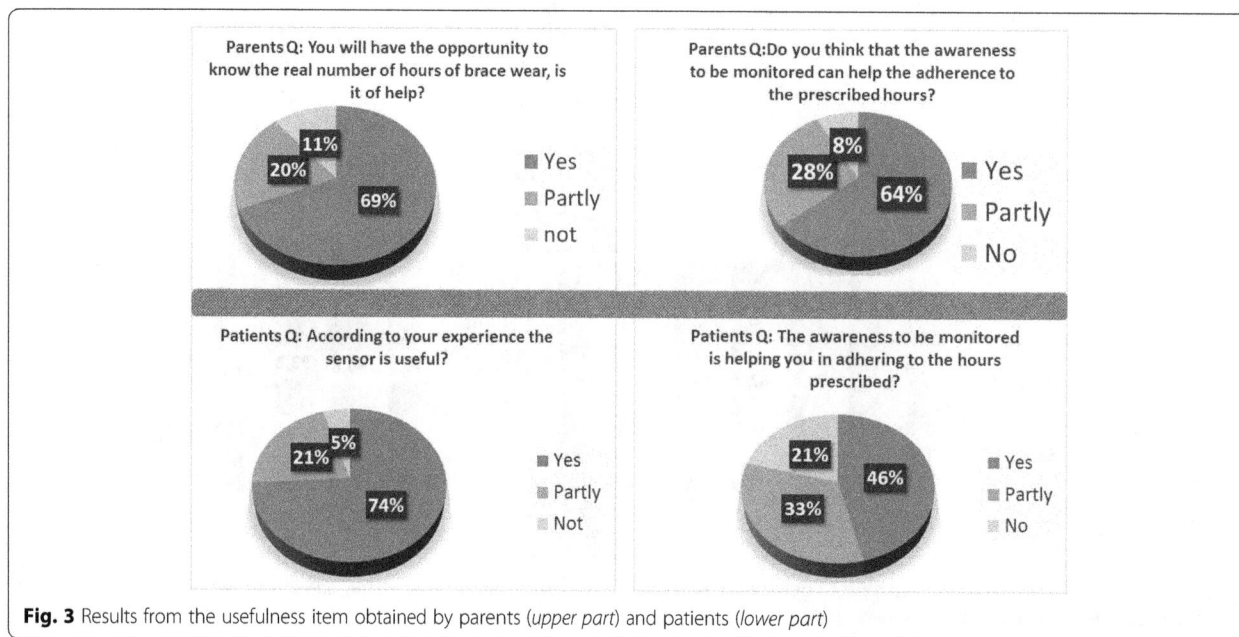

**Fig. 3** Results from the usefulness item obtained by parents (*upper part*) and patients (*lower part*)

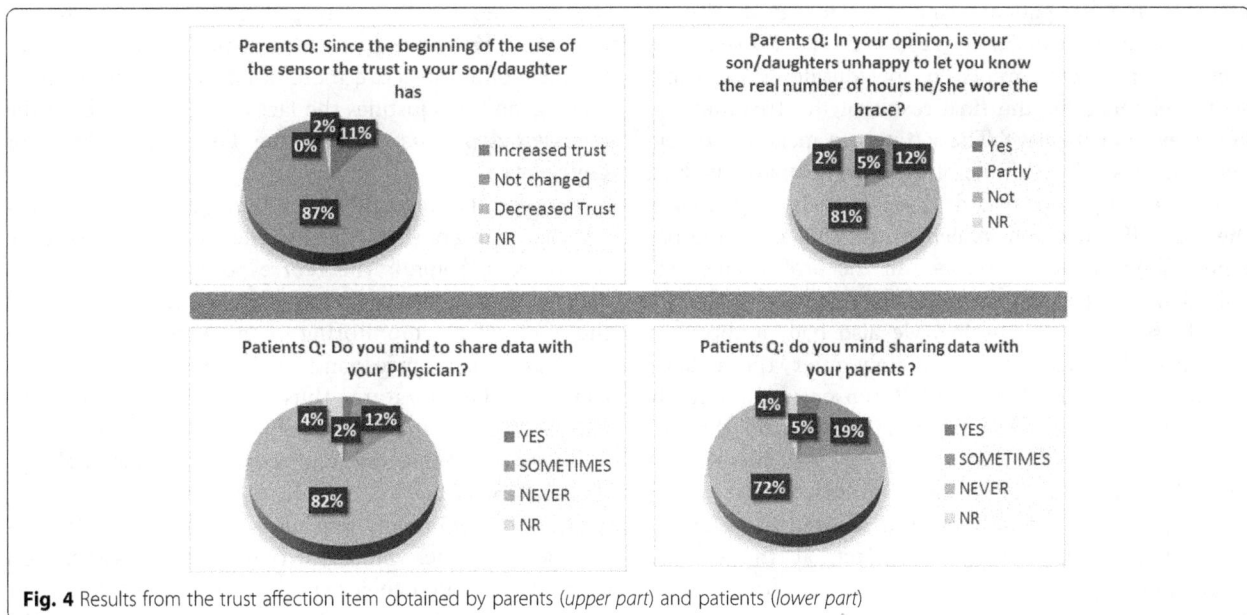

**Fig. 4** Results from the trust affection item obtained by parents (*upper part*) and patients (*lower part*)

avoidance, the results of the present survey subverted all these assumptions, as most of the parents after having experienced the TB monitoring state that the TB did not affect the trust in their children, and few of them states that the TB sensor increased their trust. Furthermore, we have to emphasize that according to this point of view, only 4.6% of the interviewed patients declare that they always mind to share the data with their parents.

Other reasons related to the difficulties in the spreading of compliance monitor in clinical practice are the economic issues; in fact, the families have to buy this device, even though it is not very expensive. The cost issue

is not only related to the cost itself but it also depends on what kind of expenses the families are used to face for treatment. For example, in Italy, braces are provided entirely by the National Health System; in our setting, a private practice facility, the medical visit and the physiotherapy treatment are paid by the patients, and only the brace is provided by the National Health System; therefore, the TB is an additional expense. When focusing on other settings, the economic issue arises again but it is influenced by different factors, for example, in the USA, the treatment costs, brace included, are covered by insurances, but the cost of the compliance monitors is not

**Table 1** Summary of the rate of responses related to the reliability of the TB sensor and the discomfort feelings related to the moment of data download of parents (upper part) and patients (lower part) (Additional file 1)

|  | Question number | Yes | Partly | No | I do not know | NR rate |
|---|---|---|---|---|---|---|
| Items/parents |  |  |  |  |  |  |
| TB reliability | 7 | 79.3% | 8.4% | 0.0% | 11.4% | 0.9% |
| Awkwardness | 8 | 4.8% | – | 94.3% | – | 0.9% |
| Anxiety | 9 | 6.9% | – | 92.5% | – | 0.6% |
| Surprise | 10 | 0.051 | – | 0.943 | – | 0.006 |
| Being bothered | 11 | 1.8% |  | 98.2% |  | 0.0% |
| Items/patients |  |  |  |  |  |  |
| TB reliability | 5 | 69.9% | 11.6 | 0.9% | 17.6% | 0.0% |
| TB = SPY | 3 | 16.1% | 35.9% | 47.7% | – | 0.3% |
| TB = ALLY | 4 | 40.1% | 42.2% | 16.7% | – | 1.0% |
| Awkwardness | 7 | 14.3% | – | 85.7% | – | 0.0% |
| Anxiety | 8 | 32.5% | – | 67.5% | – | 0.0% |
| Surprise | 10 | 12.8% | – | 86.6% | – | 0.60% |
| Bothering | 11 | 8.2% |  | 91.8% |  | 0.0% |

*NR* non-responder

included and the patient's family has to pay it with an additional burden of family expenses. The TB sensor is quite cheap, but if parents do not consider it as an essential element for the final result of the treatment, it becomes too expensive. The setting can make the difference, but also the attitude of the professionals involved in the treating team towards this new technology makes the real difference and influences the choices of the patients' families. In our setting, all the professionals involved in the treating team strongly believe in the TB usefulness. At the beginning, we also had doubts, but this attitude changed immediately after the experimental period in which the TB sensor was gradually introduced in clinical practice, starting from the patients at their first brace prescription, and involving a second time with the patients already under treatment. The use of the TB monitor showed to be useful for clinical decision-making; in fact, at the end of each follow-up visit, the physician is able to prescribe brace wear regimen, by taking into account the results obtained with the real-time brace wear. Dosage adjustments are related to risk factors for scoliosis progression and to the results already obtained. The physiotherapists check the TB data and together with the patients discuss the encountered difficulties in brace wear, to find together possible solutions and advise them to increase their adherence to the prescribed regimen: all our practitioners are fully convinced that all our patients can comply with full time prescription, and we transfer to them this conviction in all the visits. During brace weaning, it is very important to decrease the dosage gradually to avoid correction loss; therefore, the more we are precise in decreasing the time of brace wear, the best are our final results [15, 17, 22]. Globally, we can state that the TB contributes positively to the final results of the treatment [15]. The attitude towards the TB of the professionals involved in the treating team in our specific setting plays a major role in determining the acceptance of the TB by our patients and their families. In fact, among the patients followed in all our facilities around Italy, in the last year, 822 patients accepted to be monitored by the TB and 89 refused it (9.8%); if we consider only the main center in the North of Italy (Milan), last year, 251 patients accepted the TB and 18 refused (6.7%).

One of the reasons for such a low rate of refusals is within the results of the usefulness items of the survey presented in this research study. Most of the parents understand very well how the TB works and what it is aimed to. This is due to the wide explanations provided by the physicians at the moment of brace prescription and due to the team work: all the members of the treating team spread the same message to the patients and their families: the TB can help them in improving results [23, 24]. The treating physician explains always the importance of an objective monitoring for clinical decision-making, and this justifies the fact that the majority of the interviewed parents consider the TB mainly helpful for physicians.

Most of the responders in both groups of parents and patients consider the knowledge of the real-time brace wear helpful; this corresponds to the professionals' feeling about those who already experienced the effect of the monitoring of the adherence to brace wear and also corresponds to what is already published in the literature, thus confirming the positive effects on adherence of the objective monitoring combined with counseling and cognitive behavioral approach [16, 17].

The perception of reliability declared by the responders, together with the very high level of satisfaction of the parents after their experience with the TB monitor and the fact that most of them strongly recommend the use of the TB monitor to other patients, corroborates the perception which generated the idea of developing a survey to investigate the attitude of the patients and the family towards the TB temperature adherence monitor.

One of the main limits of the present study is the anonymous completion which increased the rate of responders at a very high level but on the other hand limits the possibility to correlate the clinical data to the results of the survey. In future research, it would be interesting to evaluate if the attitude towards the TB is influenced by the severity of the disease. While considering the very large sample surveyed and the very high rates of responders with a positive attitude and acceptance of the device, it is not possible to hypothesize if there is a significant correlation with clinical data.

## Conclusions

The results from the present innovative survey confirm that the experience with objective monitoring gives satisfaction not only to the professionals involved, in addition to their everyday clinical activity, but also to the patients and their families. Indeed, the TB sensor is widely accepted and perceived as very useful for treatment adherence, without affecting either the patient-parent or the patient-physician relationship. The high percentage of parents recommending the use of TB sensor to others can only endorse these findings.

In the light of the present results, we hope and we expect that a popularization of this technology will be encouraged, considering the various advantages which can be shared by all the professionals involved in the treating team.

## Abbreviations
NR: Non-responders; TB: Thermobrace

## Acknowledgements
All the authors appreciated the help of Dr. James Wynne who kindly helped us with the English translation of the survey.

## Funding
For this research, the authors received funding from the European community.

## Authors' contributions
SD created the survey, helped in data collection management and data analysis, and wrote the final manuscript. FZ helped collecting the data and edited the final version of the manuscript. FD helped in manuscript writing and data collection. GM contribute to data analysis and manuscript writing. AN managed the entire study, collected and summarized the data, and revised the manuscript. SN created the survey, helped in trial management, collected the data, and supervised the analysis of the data and manuscript writing. All authors read and approved the final manuscript.

## Competing interests
No competing interests to be declared by the authors, except for SN and AN who have some ISICO stocks.

## Author details
[1]ISICO, Via R Bellarmino 13/1, 20141, Milan, Italy. [2]ISICO, Barcelona, Spain. [3]University of Brescia, Don Gnocchi Foundation, Milan, Italy.

## References
1. Osterberg L, Blaschke T. Adherence to medication. N Engl J Med. 2005; 353(5):487–97.
2. Caronni A, Zaina F, Negrini S. Improving the measurement of health-related quality of life in adolescent with idiopathic scoliosis: the SRS-7, a Rasch-developed short form of the SRS-22 questionnaire. Res Dev Disabil. 2014; 35(4):784–99.
3. Aulisa AG, Guzzanti V, Perisano C, Marzetti E, Specchia A, Galli M, et al. Determination of quality of life in adolescents with idiopathic scoliosis subjected to conservative treatment. Scoliosis. 2010;5:21.
4. Brox JI, Lange JE, Gunderson RB, Steen H. Good brace compliance reduced curve progression and surgical rates in patients with idiopathic scoliosis. Eur Spine J. 2012;21(10):1957–63.
5. Morton A, Riddle R, Buchanan R, Katz D, Birch J. Accuracy in the prediction and estimation of adherence to bracewear before and during treatment of adolescent idiopathic scoliosis. J Pediatr Orthop. 2008;28(3):336–41.
6. Havey R, Gavin T, Patwardhan A, Pawelczak S, Ibrahim K, Andersson GBJ, et al. A reliable and accurate method for measuring orthosis wearing time. Spine. 2002;27(2):211–4.
7. Wiley JW, Thomson JD, Mitchell TM, Smith BG, Banta JV. Effectiveness of the Boston brace in treatment of large curves in adolescent idiopathic scoliosis. Spine. 2000;25(18):2326–32.
8. Vandal S, Rivard CH, Bradet R. Measuring the compliance behavior of adolescents wearing orthopedic braces. Issues Compr Pediatr Nurs. 1999; 22(2-3):59–73.
9. Rahman T, Borkhuu B, Littleton AG, Sample W, Moran E, Campbell S, et al. Electronic monitoring of scoliosis brace wear compliance. J Child Orthop. 2010;4(4):343–7.
10. Takemitsu M, Bowen JR, Rahman T, Glutting JJ, Scott CB. Compliance monitoring of brace treatment for patients with idiopathic scoliosis. Spine. 2004;29(18):2070–4. discussion 2074.
11. Dolan LA, Wright JG, Weinstein SL. Effects of bracing in adolescents with idiopathic scoliosis. N Engl J Med. 2014;370(7):681.
12. Weinstein SL, Dolan LA, Wright JG, Dobbs MB. Design of the Bracing in Adolescent Idiopathic Scoliosis Trial (BrAIST). Spine. 2013;38(21):1832–41.
13. Katz DE, Herring JA, Browne RH, Kelly DM, Birch JG. Brace wear control of curve progression in adolescent idiopathic scoliosis. J Bone Joint Surg Am. 2010;92(6):1343–52.
14. Landauer F, Wimmer C, Behensky H. Estimating the final outcome of brace treatment for idiopathic thoracic scoliosis at 6-month follow-up. Pediatr Rehabil. 2003;6(3-4):201–7.
15. Donzelli S, Zaina F, Negrini S. In defense of adolescents: they really do use braces for the hours prescribed, if good help is provided. Results from a prospective everyday clinic cohort using thermobrace. Scoliosis. 2012;7(1):12.
16. Reinker KA. Compliance counseling improves outcomes of bracing for patients with idiopathic scoliosis: commentary on an article by Lori A. Karol, MD, et al.: "Effect of compliance counseling on brace use and success in patients with adolescent idiopathic scoliosis". J Bone Joint Surg Am. 2016;98(1):e4.
17. Negrini A, Donzelli S, Lusini M, Minnella S, Zaina F, Negrini S. A cognitive behavioral approach allows improving brace wearing compliance: an observational controlled retrospective study with thermobrace. Scoliosis. 2014;9 Suppl 1:O79.
18. Negrini S, Hresko TM, O'Brien JP, Price N, SOSORT Boards, SRS Non-Operative Committee. Recommendations for research studies on treatment of idiopathic scoliosis: consensus 2014 between SOSORT and SRS non-operative management committee. Scoliosis. 2015;10:8.
19. Benish BM, Smith KJ, Schwartz MH. Validation of a miniature thermochron for monitoring thoracolumbosacral orthosis wear time. Spine. 2012;37(4):309–15.
20. Rahman T, Sample W, Yorgova P, Neiss G, Rogers K, Shah S, et al. Electronic monitoring of orthopedic brace compliance. J Child Orthop. 2015;28:1–5.
21. Donzelli S, Zaina F, Negrini S. Compliance monitor for scoliosis braces in clinical practice. J Child Orthop. 2015;9(6):507–8.
22. Negrini S, Fusco C, Romano M, Zaina F, Atanasio S. Clinical and postural behaviour of scoliosis during daily brace weaning hours. Stud Health Technol Inform. 2008;140:303–6.
23. Tavernaro M, Pellegrini A, Tessadri F, Zaina F, Zonta A, Negrini S. Team care to cure adolescents with braces (avoiding low quality of life, pain and bad compliance): a case-control retrospective study. 2011 SOSORT Award winner. Scoliosis. 2012;7(1):17.
24. Negrini S, Aulisa AG, Aulisa L, Circo AB, de Mauroy JC, Durmala J, et al. 2011 SOSORT guidelines: orthopaedic and rehabilitation treatment of idiopathic scoliosis during growth. Scoliosis. 2012;7(1):3.

# 5

# Neck and back problems in adults with idiopathic scoliosis diagnosed in youth: an observational study of prevalence, change over a mean four year time period and comparison with a control group

Christos Topalis[1,5*], Anna Grauers[1,2], Elias Diarbakerli[1,3], Aina Danielsson[4] and Paul Gerdhem[1,3]

**Abstract**

**Background:** The knowledge is sparse concerning neck problems in patients with idiopathic scoliosis. This is an observational study including a control group which aims to describe the prevalence of neck problems and the association with back problems among adult individuals with and without idiopathic scoliosis.

**Methods:** One thousand sixty-nine adults with a mean age of 40 years, diagnosed with idiopathic scoliosis in youth, answered a questionnaire on neck and back problems. Eight hundred seventy of these answered the same questionnaire at a second occasion in a mean of 4 years later. Comparisons were made with a cross-sectional population-based survey of 158 individuals. Statistical analyses were made with logistic regression or analysis of variance, adjusted for age, smoking status, and sex.

**Results:** Individuals with scoliosis were previously untreated ($n = 374$), brace treated ($n = 451$), or surgically treated ($n = 244$). Of the individuals with scoliosis, 42% ($n = 444$) had neck problems compared to 20% ($n = 32$) of the controls ($p = 0.001$). The prevalence of neck problems was not affected by the type of treatment ($p = 0.67$) or onset of scoliosis; juvenile ($n = 159$) or adolescent ($n = 910$; $p = 0.68$). Neck and/or back problems were experienced by 72% of the individuals with scoliosis and 37% of the controls ($p < 0.001$). Of the individuals with scoliosis having neck problems, 81% also reported back problems, compared to 59% of the individuals in the control group ($p < 0.001$). The prevalence of neck and back problems was similar at the second survey.

**Conclusions:** Neck problems are more prevalent and more often coexist with back problems in individuals with idiopathic scoliosis than in controls. The majority of individuals have persisting problems over time.

**Keywords:** Idiopathic scoliosis, Neck pain, Back pain, Quality of life, Long-term outcome

**Level of evidence:** 2

* Correspondence: christos.topalis@ki.se
[1]Department of Clinical Science, Intervention and Technology (CLINTEC), Karolinska Institutet, Stockholm, Sweden
[5]Department of Clinical Science, Intervention and Technology, Karolinska Institutet, K54, Karolinska University Hospital, SE-141 86 Stockholm, Sweden
Full list of author information is available at the end of the article

# Background

Idiopathic scoliosis is a three dimensional deformity of the spinal column that presents in otherwise healthy individuals. The prevalence of back problems as well as quality of life among adults with idiopathic scoliosis has been well described both in mid-term and long-term studies [1–5]. To the best of our knowledge, neck problems have not yet been under the focus in any study of idiopathic scoliosis. The prevalence of neck problems or pain has been described in a few studies. All have had some limitations, such as lack of a control group [6–8], or using a combined question for neck and back pain [9]. The relationship between regional cervical sagittal alignment and health-related quality of life in surgically treated individuals with adult spinal deformity has recently been reported, but the frequency of neck problems or pain was not described [6]. In addition, none of the previous studies have reported data for subgroups of idiopathic scoliosis patients such as men and individuals with a juvenile onset.

Hence, the aims of this study were to describe (i) the prevalence of neck problems in adults with and without idiopathic scoliosis diagnosed in youth and (ii) the relationship between neck and back problems, (iii) to analyze the effect of occupational strain and smoking habits on neck and back problems, and, finally, (iv) to describe any changes in the prevalence of neck problems over time in individuals with scoliosis.

# Methods

This is a multi-center observational study in adults diagnosed with either juvenile or adolescent idiopathic scoliosis, including comparisons with a cross-sectional population-based control group.

## Idiopathic scoliosis cohort

Individuals with juvenile idiopathic scoliosis (onset 4 to 9 years of age) or adolescent idiopathic scoliosis (onset 10 to 20 years of age), with a Cobb angle equal or greater than 10° were invited to take part in this survey [3, 10]. Age of scoliosis onset was based on self-reported data (in 94%) or according to the date of the first available radiograph which was confirmative for scoliosis (in 6%).

Recruitment took place from those currently under treatment or follow-up at the Karolinska University Hospital, Stockholm; the Skåne University Hospital, Malmö; and the Sundsvall and Härnösand County Hospital, Sundsvall, or from registers containing previously treated individuals at any of the three mentioned hospitals and from the Sahlgrenska University Hospital, Gothenburg. In this specific study, individuals under the age of 20 years or treated over the age of 20 years were excluded. A flow chart of the study is shown in Fig. 1.

In all, 1069 individuals with scoliosis completed the study. After a mean of 4 years (range 1–7) all individuals were asked to participate in a second survey, in which 870 (81%) individuals took part.

## Treatment

The individuals with scoliosis had been treated according to the general guidelines at the time of their treatment. Bracing was recommended at curves 24° to 50° in the 1960s and 1970s, except in lumbar curves, which were braced when Cobb angles were between 24° and 60°. For patients treated later, brace treatment was indicated in scoliosis curves between 25° and 45° in case of remaining growth. Larger curves after growth cessation resorted to surgery.

## Radiology and medical records

The radiological information was collected from the regular care of the individuals with scoliosis. The last radiograph was defined as the radiograph taken before the age of 27, since it was expected that all regular follow-ups had terminated at this age at all participating departments [3, 10].

## Individuals without scoliosis

A reference population was created by the Swedish Tax Agency by randomly selecting individuals from the Swedish population. Identical questionnaires as used for the patients, were mailed to 421 individuals, with up to three reminders, and 202 accepted to participate. After exclusion, 158 remained (Fig. 1). No clinical examination was done on the control cohort.

## Questionnaire

Identical questions regarding neck problems, back problems, work status, occupational strain, and smoking were used in both cohorts and at both surveys. The questions are listed in Appendix 1 [11].

## Statistics

Descriptive data are depicted as mean (SD) or number (%). Logistic regression or analysis of variance were used for statistical analyses and adjusted for age (20–44 vs. 45 years and older), smoking status, and sex (with the exception of analyses stratified on sex). The occupational strain data were dichotomized into two groups: sedentary/light and moderate/heavy occupational strain. Statistical software was IBM SPSS version 22. A $p$ value less than 0.05 was considered statistically significant.

# Results

## Results of the first survey

Descriptive data for the 1069 individuals with scoliosis and the 158 controls are shown in Table 1.

The prevalence of neck problems, back problems and the co-existence of neck and back problems were more

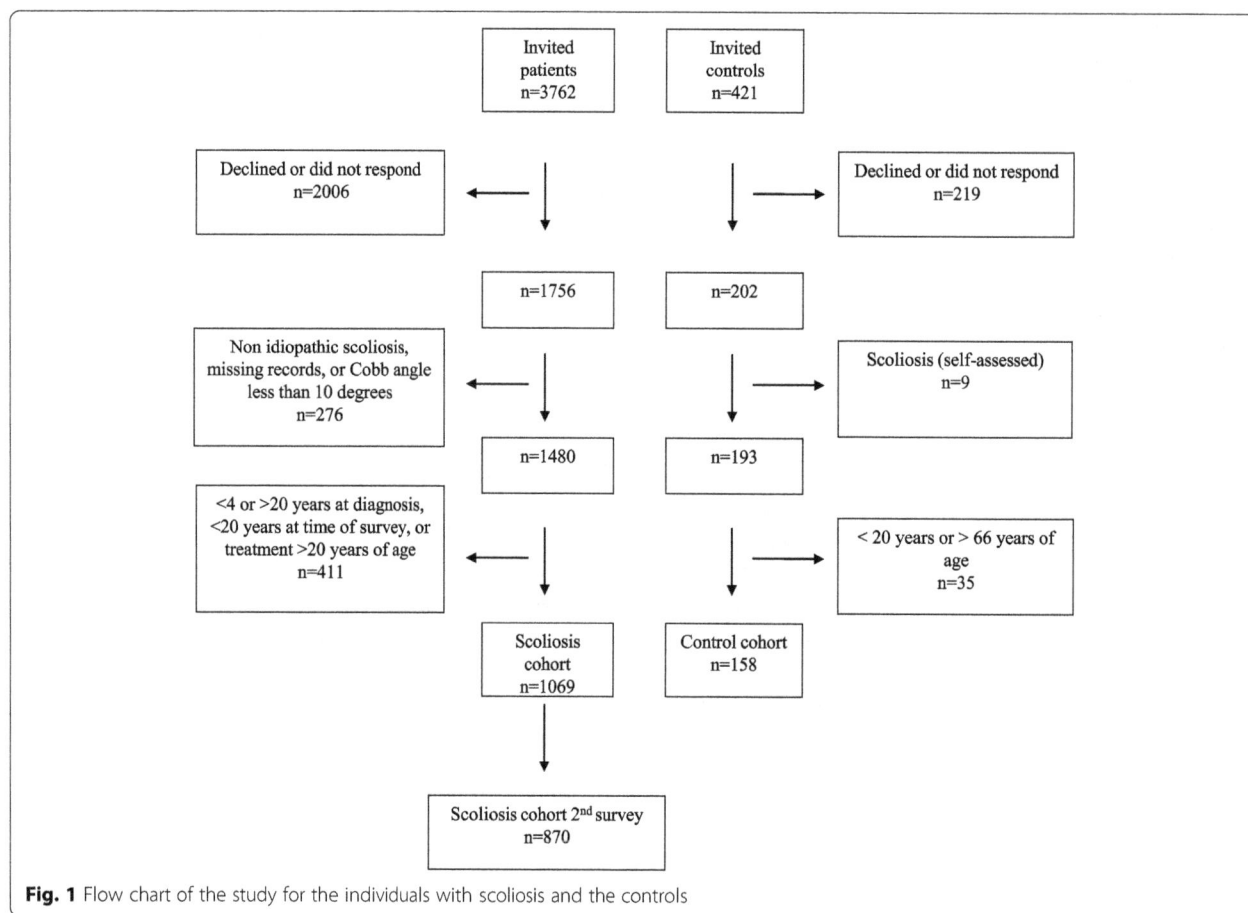

**Fig. 1** Flow chart of the study for the individuals with scoliosis and the controls

frequent among individuals with scoliosis than in those without (Table 2).

Neck problems compromising the level of activity were more frequent in the scoliosis population, but the difference did not reach statistical significance (Table 2).

Neither the prevalence of neck and/or back problems nor the prevalence of neck problems compromising the activity level were affected by the type of previously performed treatment for the scoliosis curve (no treatment/bracing/surgery) (Table 3).

**Table 1** Descriptive data of the cohorts shown as number (%) or mean (SD). The scoliosis cohort is also divided into the different treatment groups

| | Scoliosis | | | | Controls |
|---|---|---|---|---|---|
| Variable | All (*n* = 1069) | Untreated (*n* = 374) | Brace treated (*n* = 451) | Surgically treated (*n* = 244) | (*n* = 158) |
| Age, years, first survey | 41 (9) | 40 (10) | 40 (8) | 43 (10) | 45 (14) |
| Age, years, second survey[a] | 45 (9) | 44 (9) | 45 (8) | 46 (10) | – |
| Curve size, (°)[b] | 28 (14) | 23 (14) | 30 (12) | 30 (15) | – |
| Females | 946 (88%) | 320 (86%) | 411 (91%) | 215 (88%) | 83 (53%) |
| Smokers | 122 (11%) | 53 (14%) | 37 (8%) | 32 (13%) | 18 (11%) |
| Gainfully employed | 931 (87%) | 322 (86%) | 404 (90%) | 205 (84%) | 124 (78%) |
| Moderate or heavy occupational strain[c] | 246 (27%) | 98 (31%) | 91 (23%) | 57 (28%) | 42 (34%) |

[a]Based on the 870 individuals with idiopathic scoliosis that answered to the second survey
[b]Curve size is defined as the Cobb angle of the largest curve, determined from the last available radiological follow-up before the age of 27. The curve size for men was 28° (17) and for women 27° (13), and for individuals with juvenile scoliosis 28° (14) and for patients with an adolescent scoliosis 28° (13). Curve apex was thoracic in 562, thoracolumbar in 172, lumbar in 105, and double primary in 230 cases. In the surgically treated, Harrington rods had been used in 213, segmental fixation in 28, and non-instrumented fusion in situ in 3 cases. A posterior approach had been used in 232 cases
[c]Answered by 924 individuals in the scoliosis group (321 untreated, 401 brace treated, and 202 surgically treated) and 124 individuals in the control group

**Table 2** Prevalence of neck problems and back problems in the 1069 individuals with idiopathic scoliosis and the 158 controls. Data is presented as number (%). The p-value shown is for the comparison between the two groups, adjusted for age (20–44 or 45 years and older), smoking, and sex. The −2 log likelihood and Nagelkerke's $R^2$ for the model are shown

| Variable | Scoliosis ($n = 1069$) | Controls ($n = 158$) | −2 log likelihood | Nagelkerke's $R^2$ | p value |
|---|---|---|---|---|---|
| Neck problems | 444 (42%) | 32 (20%) | 1590 | 0.05 | <0.001 |
| Neck problems compromising the level of activity[a] | 187 (42%) | 9 (28%) | 631 | 0.04 | 0.11 |
| Back problems | 688 (64%) | 46 (29%) | 1560 | 0.10 | <0.001 |
| Neck and back problems | 362 (34%) | 19 (12%) | 1460 | 0.07 | <0.001 |
| Neck or back problems | 770 (72%) | 59 (37%) | 1453 | 0.10 | <0.001 |

[a]Answered by 444 individuals in the scoliosis group and 32 in the non-scoliosis group

In the surgically treated individuals, neck problems and activity level were not related to the cranial fusion level (Fig. 2).

Forty-three percent of the women in the scoliosis group had neck problems compared to 22% of the women in the non-scoliosis group ($p < 0.001$). Corresponding figures for men were 32% and 19% ($p = 0.029$). Women with scoliosis had a higher prevalence of neck problems than men with scoliosis (43% vs. 32%, $p = 0.030$).

Comparisons between patients with adolescent ($n = 910$) and juvenile onset ($n = 159$) scoliosis showed no differences for the prevalence of neck problems in general or for neck problems compromising the activity level ($p = 0.68$ and $p = 0.34$, respectively).

In the scoliosis group, those with moderate and heavy occupational strain had a higher prevalence of neck problems compromising the activity level than those with sedentary and light work ($p = 0.047$), while no differences were found within the control group ($p \geq 0.10$).

There were also significantly more smokers in the group with scoliosis who had neck problems (54%) compared to the non-smokers (40%) ($p = 0.004$). Corresponding figures for the non-scoliosis group was 4 out of 18 (22%) and 28 out of 140 (20%) ($p = 0.72$).

**Results of the second survey**

Out of the 870 individuals with scoliosis that answered the second questionnaire, 367 (42%) of these reported neck problems. Of these 367 individuals, 267 (73%) had

reported neck problems also at the first survey. Back problems were reported by 524 (60%) of the 870 individuals that answered the second questionnaire. Of these 524 individuals, 460 (88%) reported back problems also at the first survey.

**Non-response analysis**

We compared the 199 individuals with scoliosis that did not respond to the second survey with the 870 individuals who did respond. There were no differences in the prevalence of back problems ($p = 0.4$) or neck problems ($p = 0.5$) in the first survey between the 199 non-responders and the 870 responders. Differences were seen for age, sex, and smoking; the mean age among responders was 41 years, compared to 39 years among non-responders ($p = 0.003$); 89% of the responders were females, compared to 84% of the non-responders ($p = 0.046$); and 90% of the responders were non-smokers, compared to 81% of the non-responders ($p = 0.001$).

**Discussion**

In summary, neck problems are more common and more often coexist with back problems in individuals with idiopathic scoliosis than in the general population.

Previous studies on neck problems in idiopathic scoliosis patients show contradictory results. In a follow-up 27 years after non-instrumented fusion for idiopathic scoliosis, 14 out of 22 (64%) patients complained of neck pain [7]. Another study reported significantly less neck pain but more

**Table 3** There were no differences in the prevalence of neck and/or back problems between untreated, brace-treated, or surgically treated individuals. Data are shown as numbers (%). P-values are shown for the comparison between the three groups, adjusted for age (20–44 and 45 years and older), smoking, and sex. The F test and $R^2$ for the model are shown

| Variable | Scoliosis | | | F | $R^2$ | p value |
|---|---|---|---|---|---|---|
| | Untreated ($n = 374$) | Brace treated ($n = 451$) | Surgically treated ($n = 244$) | | | |
| Neck problems | 150 (40%) | 193 (42%) | 101 (41%) | 3.7 | 0.02 | 0.67 |
| Neck problems compromising the level of activity[a] | 67 (45%) | 75 (39%) | 45 (45%) | 2.7 | 0.03 | 0.78 |
| Back problems | 258 (69%) | 274 (61%) | 156 (64%) | 6.5 | 0.03 | 0.06 |
| Neck and back problems | 133 (36%) | 146 (32%) | 83 (34%) | 5.0 | 0.02 | 0.67 |
| Neck or back problems | 275 (73%) | 321 (71%) | 174 (71%) | 4.9 | 0.02 | 0.61 |

[a]Answered by 150 individuals in the untreated group, 193 in the brace-treated group and 101 in the surgically treated group

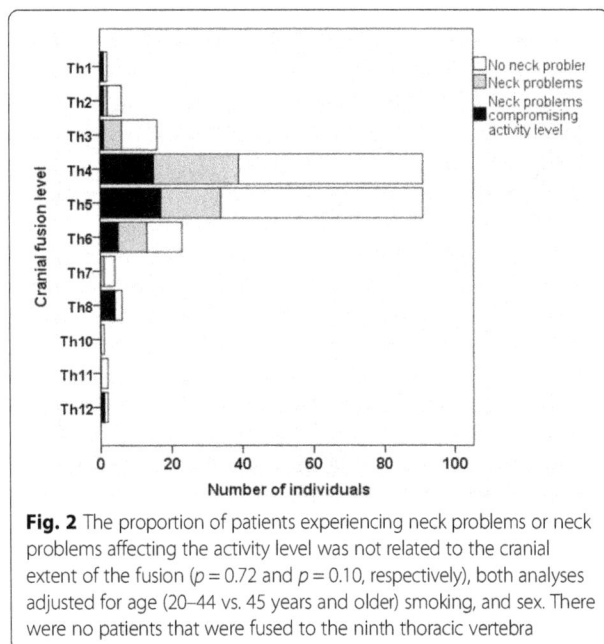

**Fig. 2** The proportion of patients experiencing neck problems or neck problems affecting the activity level was not related to the cranial extent of the fusion ($p = 0.72$ and $p = 0.10$, respectively), both analyses adjusted for age (20–44 vs. 45 years and older) smoking, and sex. There were no patients that were fused to the ninth thoracic vertebra

generalized back pain in adult subjects with idiopathic scoliosis noted after age nine who were non-operated than in controls [9]. However, the participants in that study had a limited amount of answer alternatives and had to choose between neck pain, upper back pain, lower back pain, or generalized pain only, leading perhaps to some uncertainty about the true prevalence of neck pain alone or combined with other regions in the spinal column.

Edgar and Mehta found that cervicodorsal pain was more common after non-instrumented fusion for idiopathic scoliosis than after conservative treatment about 15 years after reaching skeletal maturity [8]. In more recent studies on both braced and operated patients with adolescent idiopathic scoliosis, neck pain was not significantly more common among the scoliosis patients than in a matched control group, 17% of the braced and 27% of the operated patients compared to 17% of the controls [1, 2]. It was also found that neck pain was significantly less usual in patients that were fused more cranially, 14% of those fused to the T4 or above admitted neck pain compared to 35% in those fused to the T5 only or below.

In this study, we could not confirm that surgical treatment was associated with more neck problems. A distinct favor of the current study is its size, which is considerably larger than previous studies, giving better precision of estimates.

The caudal fusion level may affect activity level [3]. We therefore analyzed whether the cranial fusion level had the same effect on neck activity. No such association could be found. Therefore, the choice of the upper level of the thoracic fusion does not seem to affect the activity level.

We could not find any differences related to juvenile or adolescent onset, similar to previous reports on back problems [3, 12]. It seems evident that at least for individuals that are treated according to the general guidelines, age of diagnosis is not important for the long-term outcome concerning neck or back problems. That women experience slightly more neck problems than men seems to be consistent with previous reports [13].

The co-existence of chronic neck and back pain is common [14, 15]. Population-based data from Sweden, with individuals of similar ages as in this study, show similar prevalence of chronic neck pain [16] and co-existence of neck and back pain as in our data of neck and back problems in the controls [15].

Smokers more often reported neck problems than non-smokers in the scoliosis group, but this was not seen in the control group. This comparison is somewhat hampered by the low amount of smokers and the group size of the controls. The relationship between smoking and neck pain and problems is conflicting [13, 16].

The study design has advantages such as a sufficient group size enabling comparisons between treatment groups, individuals with juvenile and adolescent onset, and males and females. It also includes a prospective observation indicating changes over time. In addition, the inclusion of a control group increases the validity of the findings.

One might argue that physical activity can compensate pain issues and problems in general in scoliosis patients. However, data based on the same individuals as in this study indicate that self-reported physical activity does not seem to differ between individuals with and without scoliosis [17] despite the apparent differences in the prevalence of neck and back problems.

However, this study also has some limitations that have to be discussed. The main limitations include the response rate and the use of non-validated questions, including the use of the term neck problems rather than neck pain. Moreover, extra radiographic surveillance at the time of the study was not available; thus, any association between coronal and sagittal plane parameters and the questionnaire data could therefore not be determined.

A major limitation of this study is the response rate, 47% in the scoliosis patients and 48% in the controls. We have no information on the initial non-responders and cannot be certain on the representativeness of the available sample. However, representativeness is not necessary when interpreting the relationships between neck problems and other variables [18]. Another major limitation is the lack of information on whether the neck pain was acute, sub-acute, or chronic, which may have different impacts on quality of life and lead to different therapeutic approaches. The higher prevalence of neck problems in the scoliosis group does not seem to have an impact on the strain and ability to work [3].

For the second survey in the scoliosis cohort, a non-response analysis indicated that the prevalence of neck and back problems did not differ between responders and non-responders, and the differences in other descriptive variables were small.

The today widely used and validated Scoliosis Research Society (SRS)-questionnaire was not available in Swedish at the time of the study start [19], and anyhow, it does not address neck problems. Questionnaires specifically studying neck pain in scoliosis patients are not available, but others such as the Neck Disability Index would have been an option [20]. Nevertheless, the questions used were simple and straightforward and both the scoliosis group and the controls answered to exactly the same questions, to some extent making up for the use of previously non-validated questions.

We deliberately chose the term neck problems, embracing pain and signs and symptoms manifesting in the cervical area such as discomfort, stiffness, soreness, and numbness, giving a wider view of any problem in the neck. The study design was influenced by the fact that studies focused on neck pain or other neck problems did not exist for idiopathic scoliosis patients. To date, this study is the only one that elucidates these problems to such an extent. It includes an adult population with a span of 20 to 65 years of age, all treated before the age of 20, indicating the long-term results and the natural history of neck problems in the idiopathic scoliosis population.

There were some differences in age and sex distribution between the scoliosis and control groups. The control group was deliberately sampled with a similar proportion of men and women to be able to study men separately with a smaller control group, than if sex had been matched to equal proportions with the scoliosis cohort. Age spans in the groups were identical and mean ages differed only slightly. Both sex and age differences were accounted for in the calculations. It is possible that other unmeasured confounders could have a role.

The controls answered only once to the survey, and therefore lacking prospective data. However, other studies indicate that the prognosis of neck problems in the scoliosis population does not diverge from the expected in the general population [13].

## Conclusions

The current study and a recent increase in the interest of the cervical spine and its relation to health-related quality of life [6] may intensify further studies in this area.

In summary, neck problems are more prevalent and more often coexist with back problems in individuals with idiopathic scoliosis than in controls. The majority of individuals seem to have similar problems some years later.

### Acknowledgements
There was no such acknowledgment for this study.
The manuscript submitted does not contain information about medical device(s)/drug(s).

### Funding
This study was financially supported by funds from the Swedish Research Council (number K-2013-52X-22198-01-3), the regional agreement on medical training and clinical research (ALF) between the Stockholm County Council and Karolinska Institutet, the Karolinska Institutet research funds, the Research and Development Council of Region Skåne, the Swedish Society of Spinal Surgeons, and the Alfred Österlund Foundation.

### Authors' contributions
CT participated at the drafting of the manuscript; and analysis, acquisition and interpretation of data; performance of the statistical analysis; and writing of the article. AG contributed to the conception and design of the study as well as to the acquisition of the data and the critical revision of the manuscript. ED participated in the acquisition of the data, drafting of the manuscript, and the revision of the article. AD participated in the acquisition of data and revised the manuscript critically. PG participated in the conception and design of the study, acquisition of the data, drafting of the manuscript, interpretation of the statistical analysis, and finally revised the manuscript. All authors read and approved the final manuscript.

### Competing interests
The authors declare that they have no competing interests.

### Author details
[1]Department of Clinical Science, Intervention and Technology (CLINTEC), Karolinska Institutet, Stockholm, Sweden. [2]Department of Orthopaedics, Sundsvall and Härnösand County Hospital, Sundsvall, Sweden. [3]Department of Orthopaedics, Karolinska University Hospital, Stockholm, Sweden. [4]Department of Orthopaedics, Sahlgrenska University Hospital, Gothenburg, Sweden. [5]Department of Clinical Science, Intervention and Technology, Karolinska Institutet, K54, Karolinska University Hospital, SE-141 86 Stockholm, Sweden.

## References

1. Danielsson AJ, Nachemson AL. Back pain and function 22 years after brace treatment for adolescent idiopathic scoliosis: a case–control study-part I. Spine (Phila Pa 1976). 2003;28:2078–85. discussion 2086.

2. Danielsson AJ, Nachemson AL. Back pain and function 23 years after fusion for adolescent idiopathic scoliosis: a case–control study-part II. Spine (Phila Pa 1976). 2003;28:E373–383.

3. Grauers A, Topalis C, Möller H, Normelli H, Karlsson M, Danielsson A, Gerdhem P. Prevalence of back problems in 1069 adults with idiopathic scoliosis and 158 adults without scoliosis. Spine (Phila Pa 1976). 2014;39:pp 886-892.

4. Akazawa T, Minami S, Kotani T, Nemoto T, Koshi T, Takahashi K. Long-term clinical outcomes of surgery for adolescent idiopathic scoliosis 21 to 41 years later. Spine (Phila Pa 1976). 2012;37:402–5.

5. Danielsson AJ. What impact does spinal deformity correction for adolescent idiopathic scoliosis make on quality of life? Spine (Phila Pa 1976). 2007;32:S101–108.

6. Protopsaltis TS, Scheer JK, Terran JS, Smith JS, Hamilton DK, Kim HJ, Mundis GM, Hart RA, McCarthy IM, Klineberg E, et al. How the neck affects the back: changes in regional cervical sagittal alignment correlate to HRQOL improvement in adult thoracolumbar deformity patients at 2-year follow-up. J Neurosurg Spine. 2015;23:153–8.

7. Moskowitz A, Moe JH, Winter RB, Binner H. Long-term follow-up of scoliosis fusion. J Bone Joint Surg Am. 1980;62:364–76.

8. Edgar MA, Mehta MH. Long-term follow-up of fused and unfused idiopathic scoliosis. J Bone Joint Surg Br. 1988;70:712–6.

9. Mayo NE, Goldberg MS, Poitras B, Scott S, Hanley J. The Ste-Justine Adolescent Idiopathic Scoliosis Cohort Study. Part III: back pain. Spine (Phila Pa 1976). 1994;19:1573–81.

10. Grauers A, Danielsson A, Karlsson M, Ohlin A, Gerdhem P. Family history and its association to curve size and treatment in 1,463 patients with idiopathic scoliosis. Eur Spine J. 2013;22:2421–6.

11. Saltin B, Grimby G. Physiological analysis of middle-aged and old former athletes. Comparison with still active athletes of the same ages. Circulation. 1968;38:1104–15.

12. Lange JE, Steen H, Gunderson R, Brox JI. Long-term results after Boston brace treatment in late-onset juvenile and adolescent idiopathic scoliosis. Scoliosis. 2011;6:18.

13. Carroll LJ, Hogg-Johnson S, van der Velde G, Haldeman S, Holm LW, Carragee EJ, Hurwitz EL, Côté P, Nordin M, Peloso PM, et al. Course and prognostic factors for neck pain in the general population: results of the Bone and Joint Decade 2000–2010 Task Force on Neck Pain and Its Associated Disorders. Spine (Phila Pa 1976). 2008;33:S75–82.

14. Nyman T, Mulder M, Iliadou A, Svartengren M, Wiktorin C. High heritability for concurrent low back and neck-shoulder pain: a study of twins. Spine (Phila Pa 1976). 2011;36:E1469–1476.

15. Guez M, Hildingsson C, Nasic S, Toolanen G. Chronic low back pain in individuals with chronic neck pain of traumatic and non-traumatic origin: a population-based study. Acta Orthop. 2006;77:132–7.

16. Guez M, Hildingsson C, Stegmayr B, Toolanen G. Chronic neck pain of traumatic and non-traumatic origin: a population-based study. Acta Orthop Scand. 2003;74:576–9.

17. Diarbakerli E, Grauers A, Danielsson A, Gerdhem P. Adults with idiopathic scoliosis diagnosed at youth experience similar physical activity and fracture rate as controls. Spine (Phila Pa 1976). 2017;42:E404-10.

18. Rothman KJ, Gallacher JE, Hatch EE. Why representativeness should be avoided. Int J Epidemiol. 2013;42:1012–4.

19. Asher MA, Lai SM, Glattes RC, Burton DC, Alanay A, Bago J. Refinement of the SRS-22 health-related quality of life questionnaire function domain. Spine (Phila Pa 1976). 2006;31:593–7.

20. Vernon H, Mior S. The Neck Disability Index: a study of reliability and validity. J Manipulative Physiol Ther. 1991;14:409–15.

# 6

# Upright, prone, and supine spinal morphology and alignment in adolescent idiopathic scoliosis

Rob C. Brink[1*], Dino Colo[1], Tom P. C. Schlösser[1], Koen L. Vincken[2], Marijn van Stralen[3], Steve C. N. Hui[4], Lin Shi[5], Winnie C. W. Chu[4], Jack C. Y. Cheng[6] and René M. Castelein[1]

## Abstract

**Background:** Patients with adolescent idiopathic scoliosis (AIS) are usually investigated by serial imaging studies during the course of treatment, some imaging involves ionizing radiation, and the radiation doses are cumulative. Few studies have addressed the correlation of spinal deformity captured by these different imaging modalities, for which patient positioning are different. To the best of our knowledge, this is the first study to compare the coronal, axial, and sagittal morphology of the scoliotic spine in three different body positions (upright, prone, and supine) and between three different imaging modalities (X-ray, CT, and MRI).

**Methods:** Sixty-two AIS patients scheduled for scoliosis surgery, and having undergone standard pre-operative work-up, were included. This work-up included upright full-spine radiographs, supine bending radiographs, supine MRI, and prone CT as is the routine in one of our institutions. In all three positions, Cobb angles, thoracic kyphosis (TK), lumbar lordosis (LL), and vertebral rotation were determined. The relationship among three positions (upright X-ray, prone CT, and supine MRI) was investigated according to the Bland-Altman test, whereas the correlation was described by the intraclass correlation coefficient (ICC).

**Results:** Thoracic and lumbar Cobb angles correlated significantly between conventional radiographs (68° ± 15° and 44° ± 17°), prone CT (54° ± 15° and 33° ± 15°), and supine MRI (57° ± 14° and 35° ± 16°; ICC ≥0.96; $P < 0.001$). The thoracic and lumbar apical vertebral rotation showed a good correlation among three positions (upright, 22° ± 12° and 11° ± 13°; prone, 20° ± 9° and 8° ± 11°; supine, 16° ± 11° and 6° ± 14°; ICC ≥0.82; $P < 0.001$). The TK and LL correlated well among three different positions (TK 26° ± 11°, 22° ± 12°, and 17° ± 10°; $P ≤ 0.004$; LL 49° ± 12°, 45° ± 11°, and 44° ± 12°; $P < 0.006$; ICC 0.87 and 0.85).

**Conclusions:** Although there is a generalized underestimation of morphological parameters of the scoliotic deformity in the supine and prone positions as compared to the upright position, a significant correlation of these parameters is still evident among different body positions by different imaging modalities. Findings of this study suggest that severity of scoliotic deformity in AIS patients can be largely represented by different imaging modalities despite the difference in body positioning.

**Keywords:** Adolescent idiopathic scoliosis, Three-dimensional morphology, Body positioning, Upright radiographs, Computed tomography, Magnetic resonance imaging

* Correspondence: R.C.Brink@umcutrecht.nl
[1]Department of Orthopaedic Surgery, University Medical Center Utrecht, P.O. Box 85500, 3508 GA Utrecht, The Netherlands
Full list of author information is available at the end of the article

## Background

Adolescent idiopathic scoliosis (AIS) is a complex three-dimensional (3-D) deformity of the spine, with a prevalence of 1.5–3% within the general population, that normally develops in the beginning of the growth spurt of previously healthy adolescents [1, 2]. For diagnosis, monitoring of progression, and clinical decision-making, periodical radiographic follow-up is traditionally performed using posterior-anterior and lateral upright radiographs. The Scoliosis Research Society defines scoliosis as a lateral curvature of the spine of more than 10° in the coronal plane on upright radiographs, also emphasizing the importance of radiography [3]. In addition, supine or prone magnetic resonance imaging (MRI) and computed tomography (CT) are frequently used to obtain more in-depth information about neuroaxis and bony architecture abnormalities. Some imaging involves ionizing radiation, and the radiation doses are cumulative, resulting in 9 to 10 times more radiation exposure and a 17 times higher incidence of cancer in the AIS cohort as compared to the general population [4, 5]. The importance of the 3-D character of the scoliotic deformity has long been recognized, and the upright X-ray, the gold standard, is not able to accurately represent the true 3-D deformity [6–9]. CT scanning can obtain accurate 3-D information of bony structures but relies on radiation and is not obtained upright [10]. An important step in attempts to visualize this 3-D character has been the development of low-dose upright imaging modalities that allow for 3-D reconstruction such as the EOS apparatus. Alternatively, MRI utilizes no harmful radiation but is considered inferior in visualizing the bone and is usually also not obtained upright. This study was designed to compare the morphology of the scoliotic spine on conventional radiographs in the upright position to those on MRI and CT obtained in supine and prone positions, respectively.

## Methods

### Study population

A subsequent series of AIS patients of ten or more years of age scheduled for scoliosis surgery in one of our centers between 2011 and 2014 and had complete standard pre-operative work-up were included in this study. Complete work-up consisted of posterior-anterior and lateral upright radiographs of the spine, supine bending X-rays, T2-weighted MRI (3.0-T MR scanner (Achieva TX; Philips Healthcare, Best, The Netherlands)) of the spinal cord for exclusion of neural axis abnormalities obtained in a supine position, and high-resolution CT (64 Slice Multi-detector CT scanner, GE Healthcare, Chalfont, St. Giles, UK, slice thickness 0.625 mm), obtained in a prone position. The CT scans were made for navigation purposes according to protocol in one of our

institutions, in a position mimicking the position at surgery as closely as possible. Children with other spinal pathology than AIS, early onset scoliosis, previous spinal surgery, neurological symptoms or neural axis abnormalities, syndromes associated with disorders of growth, or atypical left convex thoracic curves or right convex (thoraco)lumbar curves were excluded to obtain an as homogeneous a population as possible. Moreover, cases that had undergone the different imaging methods with an interval of more than 6 months in between imaging were also excluded. Curve characteristics (curve type according to the Lenke classification, Cobb end vertebrae, and apical levels) were determined on the conventional radiographs [11, 12].

## Outcome parameters

The conventional radiographs were analyzed for main thoracic and (thoraco)lumbar Cobb angle, apical rotation (using Perdriolle's method [13]), thoracic kyphosis (TK; superior endplate T4–inferior endplate T12), and lumbar lordosis (LL; superior endplate L1–sacral plate), using our picture archiving and communications system (PACS) workstation (Carestream solution working station, Carestream Health, Version 11.0, Rochester, NY, USA).

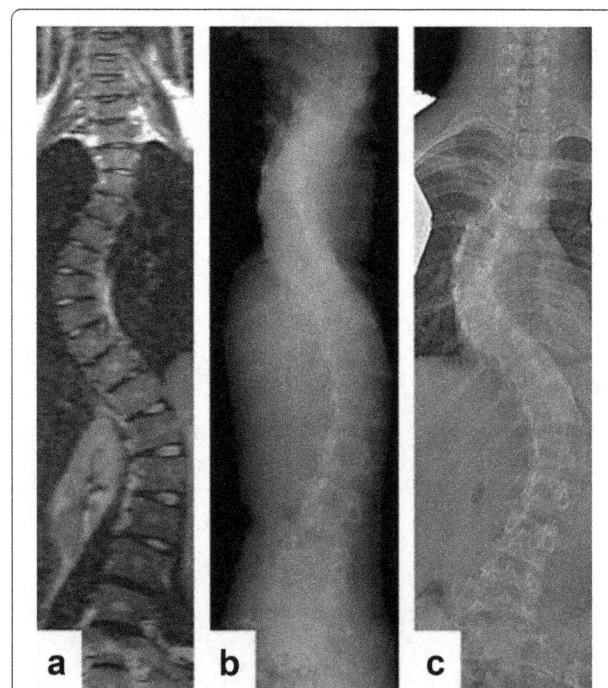

**Fig. 1** On the MRI and CT images, the main thoracic and (thoraco)lumbar Cobb angle, thoracic kyphosis, and lumbar lordosis were measured using the same technique as for the conventional radiographs on the image where the curve and endplates were best visible by using the multiplanar reconstruction (MPR, **a**) for the MRI and the digitally reconstructed radiograph (**b**) for the CT scan. **c** The conventional X-ray

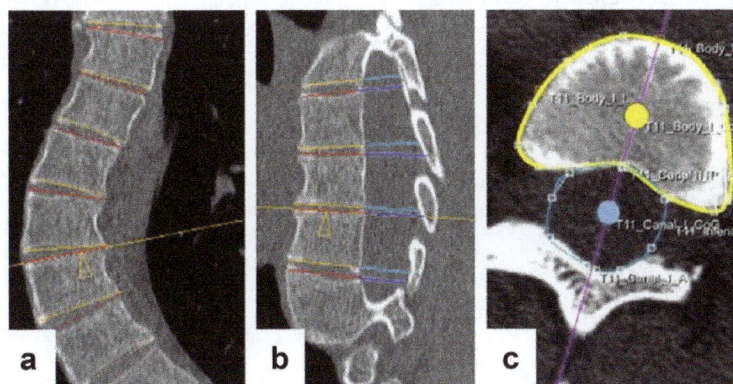

**Fig. 2** The orientation of the upper and lower endplates of each individual vertebra of the computed tomography scans was determined by using the semi-automatic software, correcting for coronal and sagittal (**a** and **b**) tilt, to reconstruct the true transverse sections. The observer drew a contour around the vertebral body (*yellow line* in **c**) and spinal canal (*blue line* in **c**). The software calculated a center of gravity of the vertebral body (*yellow dot* in **c**) and spinal canal (*blue dot* in **c**). For each endplate, its longitudinal axis was calculated as the line between those two points (*purple line* in **c**). The rotation of this axis minus the rotation of the neutral sacral plate represents the rotation of the endplate

On the MRI and CT images, the main thoracic and (thoraco)lumbar Cobb angle, TK, and LL were measured using the same technique as for the conventional radiographs, by using multiplanar reconstruction technique through the midsection of each vertebral body for the MRI and the digital reconstructed radiograph (DRR) for the CT scan (Fig. 1). The same levels were used for each patient on the three different imaging methods. Cobb end vertebrae were selected on the radiographs and applied to the other imaging modalities [14]. For measurement of apical rotation on the MRI and CT scans, complete 3-D reconstructions were acquired using semi-automatic analysis software (ScoliosisAnalysis 4.1, Imaging Division, Utrecht, The Netherlands) and a previously validated imaging method [15]. The observer selected the upper and lower endplates of the vertebral body. Then, the observer used the sagittal and coronal orientation of the endplates to correct for coronal and sagittal tilt. Thus, each vertebral level was manually positioned in the true transverse plane as accurately as possible. Subsequently, for each endplate, its longitudinal axis was calculated automatically after manual segmentation of the vertebral body and spinal canal. The rotation was defined as the rotation of this axis minus the rotation of the neutral sacral plate (Fig. 2).

Intra- and interobserver reliability for measurement of apical rotation using this method was tested in a previous study; intraclass correlation coefficients were 0.92 (95% confidence interval, 0.82–0.97) and 0.89 (0.74–0.95) on the 3-D scans [9]. In this study, the intra- and interobserver reliability analysis of the rest of the outcome parameters (Cobb angles, TK, and LL on all the three modalities and the vertebral rotation on the X-rays) was studied. Two observers independently analyzed a randomly selected subset of ten X-rays, CT scans, and MRI scans of the subjects.

**Table 1** Demographics are shown for all included AIS patients and controls. Also, the excluded patients are shown

| Demographic parameter | | $n = 62$ |
|---|---|---|
| Age at radiograph (years) | Range | 10–23 |
| | Mean ± sd | 15.6 ± 2.5 |
| Girls, $n$ (%) | | 56 (90.3%) |
| Right convexity of main thoracic curve, $n$ (%) | Right convex | 62 (100%) |
| Interval CT–radiograph (days) | Range | −7 to 130 |
| | Mean ± sd | 2.98 ± 17.2 |
| Interval radiograph–MRI (days) | Range | −46 to 181 |
| | Mean ± sd | 81.3 ± 51.4 |
| Interval CT–MRI (days) | Range | −26 to 181 |
| | Mean ± sd | 84.2 ± 47.1 |
| Lenke curve type | | |
| I | | 26 |
| II | | 12 |
| III | | 6 |
| IV | | 4 |
| V | | 5 |
| VI | | 9 |
| Exclusion criteria | | n |
| Scan interval >6 months | | 38 |
| No MRI available | | 14 |
| No CT scan available | | 10 |
| Incomplete radiologic work-up | | 1 |
| Associated congenital or neuromuscular pathologies | | 12 |
| Left convex main thoracic curve | | 4 |
| Prior spinal surgery | | 1 |

*sd* standard deviation

**Table 2** Differences (mean ± standard deviation) between upright (X), prone (CT), and supine (MRI) positions for Cobb angle, thoracic kyphosis, lumbar lordosis, and apical vertebral rotation in the thoracic as well as lumbar curves. According to the Bland-Altman plot, the *P* value showed if there is agreement by using the *t* test. If this test showed no significant different (*P* > 0.05), a regression analysis was performed to see is if there is agreement, written in brackets

|  | Upright | Prone | Supine | P value | | |
|  |  |  |  | X vs. CT | X vs. MRI | CT vs. MRI |
|---|---|---|---|---|---|---|
| Thoracic |  |  |  |  |  |  |
|   Cobb (°) | 68.2 ± 15.4 | 53.9 ± 14.8 | 56.7 ± 13.5 | <0.001 | <0.001 | <0.001 |
|   Kyphosis (°) | 25.8 ± 11.4 | 22.4 ± 11.6 | 17.3 ± 9.8 | 0.004 | <0.001 | <0.001 |
|   Vertebral rotation (°) | 21.6 ± 11.7 | 19.9 ± 8.9 | 16.3 ± 10.8 | 0.161 (0.007) | 0.001 | 0.002 |
| Lumbar |  |  |  |  |  |  |
|   Cobb (°) | 44.3 ± 16.8 | 33.1 ± 15.0 | 35.2 ± 15.9 | <0.001 | <0.001 | 0.018 |
|   Lordosis (°) | 48.8 ± 12.0 | 45.4 ± 10.8 | 43.7 ± 12.4 | 0.006 | <0.001 | 0.341 (0.620)[a] |
|   Vertebral rotation (°) | 10.7 ± 12.8 | 7.5 ± 11.4 | 6.2 ± 13.7 | 0.428 (<0.001) | 0.663 (0.129)[a] | 0.679 (0.006) |

[a]Agreement according to the Bland-Altman plot

## Statistical analysis

Statistical analyses were performed using SPSS 22.0 for Windows (SPSS Inc., Chicago, IL, USA). Descriptive statistics were computed providing means, ranges, and standard deviations. Potential outliers were identified. The agreement between the three positions was tested according to the Bland-Altman plot; first, the one-sample *t* test showed if there was a significant difference between the measurements; second, if there was no significant difference, the regression analysis showed if there was agreement between the measurements [16]. The two-way mixed intraclass correlation coefficient (ICC) was used to evaluate the correlation between the parameters in different body positions. The intra- and interobserver reliability were obtained as intraclass correlation coefficients. The statistical significance level was set at 0.05 for all analyses.

## Results

### Population

A total of 142 subjects underwent surgery for AIS during the study period. Eighty subjects had to be excluded for several reasons, as shown in Table 1. Ultimately, 62 AIS patients with full documentation were left for the purpose of this study. On average, the subjects were 15.6 ± 2.5 years of age, 56 (90%) were girls, and most of the curves were classified as type Lenke 1 of these moderate to severe AIS patients (thoracic Cobb angle 37°–110°, lumbar Cobb angle 18°–82°; Table 1).th=tlb=

### Coronal parameters

In the coronal plane, the main thoracic Cobb angle was on average 68° ± 15°, 54° ± 15°, and 57° ± 14° on the upright radiographs, prone CT, and supine MRI, respectively, and differed significantly between all the three positions (*P* < 0.001; Table 2). The average (thoraco)lumbar Cobb angle on the conventional upright radiograph was 44° ± 17° as compared to those on the prone CT (33° ± 15°) and supine MRI (35° ± 16°) (*P* ≤ 0.018, between the three positions). Although the upright angles were larger, the Cobb angles correlated very well between the three positions (ICC: thoracic 0.97 and lumbar 0.96; Table 3; Fig. 3). Significant linear correlations were found, indicating that with increasing Cobb angle, differences between the body positions increased simultaneously. The conversion equations that resulted from the correlation analyses of the different parameters between the upright X-ray, prone CT scan, and supine MRI could be used for conversion purposes (Table 4).

### Axial rotation

Parallel to the coronal Cobb angles, in both the thoracic curve and the (thoraco)lumbar curve, the mean apical vertebral rotation was larger in the upright position (Table 2). Significant correlations, however, were observed between the apical rotation as measured using the Perdriolle method on upright radiographs and the rotation on the prone CT and supine MRI (ICC: thoracic 0.82 and lumbar 0.90; Tables 3 and 4).

**Table 3** Two-way mixed intraclass correlation coefficient (ICC) and 95% confidence interval (CI) between upright, prone, and supine positions

|  | ICC (95% CI) | P value |
|---|---|---|
| Thoracic Cobb angle | 0.967 (0.950–0.979) | <0.001 |
| Lumbar Cobb angle | 0.964 (0.945–0.977) | <0.001 |
| Thoracic kyphosis | 0.873 (0.806–0.919) | <0.001 |
| Lumbar lordosis | 0.854 (0.777–0.907) | <0.001 |
| Thoracic apical rotation | 0.815 (0.718–0.882) | <0.001 |
| Lumbar apical rotation | 0.900 (0.848–0.937) | <0.001 |

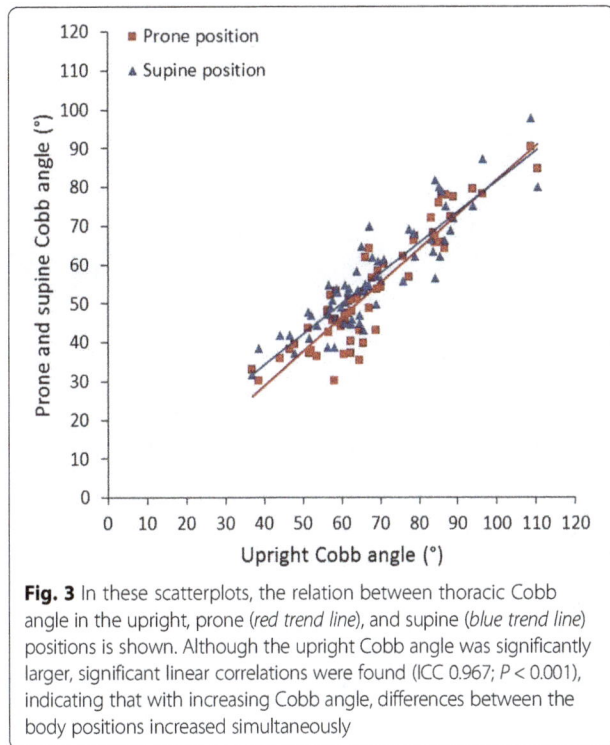

**Fig. 3** In these scatterplots, the relation between thoracic Cobb angle in the upright, prone (*red trend line*), and supine (*blue trend line*) positions is shown. Although the upright Cobb angle was significantly larger, significant linear correlations were found (ICC 0.967; $P < 0.001$), indicating that with increasing Cobb angle, differences between the body positions increased simultaneously

## Sagittal parameters

Also in the sagittal plane, the TK in the upright position ($26° \pm 11°$) was significantly larger as compared to that in the prone ($22° \pm 12°$) and supine ($17° \pm 10°$; $P \leq 0.004$) positions. The upright LL ($49° \pm 12°$) was significantly higher as compared to the prone LL ($45° \pm 11°$) and supine LL ($44° \pm 12°$; $P \leq 0.006$). According to the Bland-Altman method, there was agreement between the LL in the supine and prone positions. The TK and the LL correlated well between all the positions (ICC 0.87 and 0.85; Tables 3 and 4).

## Reliability

The ICCs for intra- and interobserver reliabilities of the Cobb angles, TK, LL, and vertebral rotation on the three

modalities were all excellent (>0.93 and >0.74, respectively; Table 5).

## Discussion

X-rays for scoliosis are, by convention, obtained in an upright position, allowing gravity to have its influence on the morphology of the spine. The drawbacks of this X-ray imaging in analyzing the deformity as well as planning treatment are becoming increasingly clear: the deformity has a complex 3-D nature that is hardly appreciated on plain films, and radiation exposure, even with modern day equipment, is becoming a serious concern. Although the use of ultrasound for diagnosis and follow-up of spinal deformities has been explored and seems promising, this technique gives little detail of the anatomy and needs further evaluation [17–19]. Additional imaging studies are frequently obtained in scoliosis; CT scanning is still considered the gold standard for providing accurate and detailed information on bony anatomy (for instance, in cases where congenital malformations are suspected) and can give accurate 3-D reconstructions of complex deformities [10]. However, CT carries even more radiation exposure and is performed non-weight bearing [10]. MRI is safe, provides accurate information on the spinal cord and other soft tissues, but is also (usually) performed in a non-weight-bearing manner, and is known to show less detail of bony structures. Therefore, it is important to define where these techniques overlap, in order to reduce costs and radiation exposure. Previous studies have already described the differences in morphology of the spine in AIS between different imaging methods and between different body positions [20–26]. This study is, however, to the best of our knowledge, the first to look into the relationship between the three different positions in all three planes of the body to visualize the scoliotic spine.

In this study, we observed that there is underestimation of the deformation of the spine in the supine and prone positions as compared to that in the upright position, which is overall more pronounced in the thoracic

**Table 4** For translational purposes, the conversion equations that resulted from the linear correlation analyses of the different parameters between the upright X-ray, prone CT scan, and supine MRI are provided for the thoracic (Th) and lumbar (L) Cobb angles

| | | Cobb angle | | |
| --- | --- | --- | --- | --- |
| | | Upright X-ray | Prone CT scan | Supine MRI |
| Cobb angle | Upright X-ray | – | Th: CT (°) = −6.2 + 0.88 * X-ray (°)<br>L: CT (°) = −2.7 + 0.81 * X-ray (°) | Th: MRI (°) = 2.9 + 0.79 * X-ray (°)<br>L: MRI (°) = −2.1 + 0.85 * X-ray (°) |
| | Prone CT | Th: X-ray (°) = 16.6 + 0.96 * CT (°)<br>L: X-ray (°) = 11.1 + 1.00 * CT (°) | – | Th: MRI (°) = 11.0 + 0.85 * CT (°)<br>L: MRI (°) = 4.9 + 0.92 * CT (°) |
| | Supine MRI | Th: X-ray (°) = 10.8 + 1.01 * MRI (°)<br>L: X-ray (°) = 9.5 + 0.98 * MRI (°) | Th: CT (°) = −2.8 + 1.00 * MRI (°)<br>L: CT (°) = 2.6 + 0.86 * MRI (°) | – |

**Table 5** Intra- and interobserver reliability analysis and 95% confidence interval

| | X-ray | | CT scan | | MRI scan | |
|---|---|---|---|---|---|---|
| | Intra | Inter | Intra | Inter | Intra | Inter |
| Thoracic Cobb | 0.993 (0.971–0.998) | 0.972 (0.888–0.993) | 0.997 (0.988–0.999) | 0.995 (0.980–0.999) | 0.995 (0.982–0.999) | 0.974 (0.896–0.994) |
| Lumbar Cobb | 0.999 (0.996–1.00) | 0.995 (0.980–0.999) | 0.999 (0.996–1.00) | 0.995 (0.981–0.999) | 0.997 (0.990–0.999) | 0.986 (0.945–0.997) |
| Thoracic kyphosis | 0.989 (0.954–0.997) | 0.922 (0.610–0.984) | 0.931 (0.722–0.983) | 0.864 (0.454–0.966) | 0.992 (0.967–0.998) | 0.940 (0.759–0.985) |
| Lumbar lordosis | 0.986 (0.944–0.997) | 0.989 (0.956–0.997) | 0.995 (0.980–0.999) | 0.973 (0.890–0.993) | 0.995 (0.981–0.999) | 0.971 (0.884–0.993) |
| Thoracic rotation | 0.979 (0.915–0.995) | 0.977 (0.906–0.994) | [a] | [a] | 0.939 (0.756–0.985) | 0.744 (0.409–0.964) |
| Lumbar rotation | 0.975 (0.899–0.994) | 0.996 (0.985–0.999) | [a] | [a] | 0.906 (0.620–0.977) | 0.885 (0.539–0.972) |

[a]Intra- and interobserver reliability for the rotation on 3-D scans; this method was tested previously (ICC 0.92 and 0.89) [9]

curves as compared to the (thoraco)lumbar curves. The lying positions underestimated the thoracic and (thoraco)lumbar Cobb angles for 12°–14° and 9°–11°, respectively; the TK and LL for 3°–9° and 3°–5°, respectively; and the thoracic and lumbar apical vertebral rotations for 2°–5° and 3°–5°, respectively. Therefore, the parameters on supine and prone scans could not directly be compared to the upright radiographs. However, good and excellent linear correlations were observed for the morphological parameters in the coronal (ICC ≥0.964), sagittal (ICC ≥0.854), and axial (ICC ≥0.815) planes between X-ray, CT, and MRI. This implies that reliable conversion of the parameters between the different positions is possible. A limitation of this study is the population that only includes relatively severe curves. From our results, the reliability of conversion of parameters between different positions for patients with mild AIS curves cannot be derived. Shi et al. described the correlation of the coronal Cobb angle between upright and supine positions in mild, moderate, and severe AIS patients and concluded that the correlation coefficients were more reliable in the severe group, probably due to the reduced curve flexibility in the severe group [26, 27]. As we demonstrated before, evaluation of the true sagittal plane in scoliosis on plain X-rays is notoriously unreliable and differs greatly from the true sagittal plane as may be analyzed more accurately on both CT and MRI [28].

## Conclusions

There is a good to excellent correlation of the morphology of the scoliotic spine in all three planes between standard upright X-ray, MRI, and CT scan in these moderate to severe AIS patients. Apparently, at least part of the information obtained by these different modalities overlaps. Findings of this study suggest that severity of scoliotic deformity in AIS patients can be largely represented by different imaging modalities despite the differences in body position. Future longitudinal studies to demonstrate the practical implications of these findings are planned.

## Abbreviations

3-D: Three-dimensional; AIS: Adolescent idiopathic scoliosis; CI: Confidence interval; CT: Computed tomography; DRR: Digital reconstructed radiograph; ICC: Intraclass correlation coefficient; LL: Lumbar lordosis; MRI: Magnetic resonance imaging; PACS: Picture archiving and communications system; sd: Standard deviation; TK: Thoracic kyphosis

## Acknowledgements
None.

## Funding
Rob C. Brink received funding from the Alexandre Suerman, MD/Ph.D. program, and René M. Castelein from a Medtronic research grant and a K2M research grant.

## Authors' contributions
RCB handled the conception and design, acquisition of the data, analysis and interpretation of the data, drafting of the manuscript, statistical analysis, and obtaining funding. DC handled the acquisition of the data, analysis and interpretation of the data, drafting of the manuscript, and supervision. TPCS handled the conception and design, acquisition of the data, analysis and interpretation of the data, critical revision of the manuscript for important intellectual content, statistical analysis, and supervision. KLV handled the acquisition of the data, analysis and interpretation of the data, and technical and material support. MvS handled the acquisition of the data, analysis and interpretation of the data, and technical and material support. SCNH handled the acquisition of the data and technical and material support. SL handled the acquisition of the data, analysis and interpretation of the data, critical revision of the manuscript for important intellectual content, and technical and material support. WCWC handled the Acquisition of the data, analysis and interpretation of the data, critical revision of the manuscript for important intellectual content, and supervision. JCY handled the acquisition of the data, analysis and interpretation of the data, and critical revision of the manuscript for important intellectual content and supervision. RMC handled the conception and design, analysis and interpretation of the data, critical revision of the manuscript for important intellectual content, obtaining funding, and supervision. All authors read and approved the final manuscript.

## Competing interests
The authors declare that they have no competing interests.

## Author details
[1]Department of Orthopaedic Surgery, University Medical Center Utrecht, P.O. Box 85500, 3508 GA Utrecht, The Netherlands. [2]Image Sciences Institute, University Medical Center Utrecht, Utrecht, The Netherlands. [3]Imaging Division, University Medical Center Utrecht, Utrecht, The Netherlands. [4]Department of Imaging and Interventional Radiology, Prince of Wales Hospital, The Chinese University of Hong Kong, Shatin, Hong Kong. [5]Department of Diagnostic Radiology and Organ Imaging, Prince of Wales Hospital, The Chinese University of Hong Kong, Shatin, Hong Kong. [6]Department of Orthopaedics and Traumatology, Prince of Wales Hospital, The Chinese University of Hong Kong, Shatin, Hong Kong.

## References
1. Lonstein JE. Adolescent idiopathic scoliosis. Lancet. 1994;344(8934):1407–12.
2. Schlosser TP, van der Heijden GJ, Versteeg AL, Castelein RM. How 'idiopathic' is adolescent idiopathic scoliosis? A systematic review on associated abnormalities. PLoS One. 2014;9(5):e97461.
3. Brooks HL, Azen SP, Gerberg E, Brooks R, Chan L. Scoliosis: a prospective epidemiological study. J Bone Joint Surg Am. 1975;57(7):968–72.
4. Simony A, Christensen SB, Jensen KE, Carreon LY, Andersen MO. Incidence of cancer and infertility, in patients treated for adolescent idiopathic scoliosis 25 years prior. Eur Spine J. 2015;24(6):S740.
5. Presciutti SM, Karukanda T, Lee M. Management decisions for adolescent idiopathic scoliosis significantly affect patient radiation exposure. Spine J. 2014;14(9):1984–90.
6. Nicoladoni C. Anatomie und mechanismus der skoliose. In: Kocher, König, Von Mikulicz, eds. Bibliotheca medica. Stuttgart, Germany: Verlag von erwin nagele. 1904
7. Von Meyer H. Die mechanik der skoliose. Archiv für pathologische Anatomie und Physiologie und für klinische Medicin. 1866;35:225–53.
8. Bernstein P, Hentschel S, Platzek I, et al. The assessment of the postoperative spinal alignment: MRI adds up on accuracy. Eur Spine J. 2012;21(4):733–8.
9. Schlosser TP, van Stralen M, Brink RC, et al. Three-dimensional characterization of torsion and asymmetry of the intervertebral discs versus vertebral bodies in adolescent idiopathic scoliosis. Spine (Phila Pa 1976). 2014;39:E1159–66.
10. Glaser DA, Doan J, Newton PO. Comparison of 3-dimensional spinal reconstruction accuracy: biplanar radiographs with EOS versus computed tomography. Spine (Phila Pa 1976). 2012;37(16):1391–7.
11. Lenke LG, Edwards 2nd CC, Bridwell KH. The Lenke classification of adolescent idiopathic scoliosis: how it organizes curve patterns as a

template to perform selective fusions of the spine. Spine (Phila Pa 1976). 2003;28(20):S199–207.

12. Cobb J. Outline for the study of scoliosis. The American Academy of Orthopaedic Surgeons (2nd edn), Instructional Course Lectures. 1948;5:261

13. Perdriolle R, Vidal J. Thoracic idiopathic scoliosis curve evolution and prognosis. Spine (Phila Pa 1976). 1985;10(9):785–91.

14. Keenan BE, Izatt MT, Askin GN, Labrom RD, Pearcy MJ, Adam CJ. Supine to standing Cobb angle change in idiopathic scoliosis: the effect of endplate pre-selection. Scoliosis. 2014;9:16. 7161-9-16.

15. Kouwenhoven JW, Vincken KL, Bartels LW, Castelein RM. Analysis of preexistent vertebral rotation in the normal spine. Spine (Phila Pa 1976). 2006;31(13):1467–72.

16. Altman DG, Bland JM. Measurement in medicine: the analysis of method comparison studies. The Statistician. 1983;32(3):307–17.

17. Suzuku S, Yamamuro T, Shikata J, Shimizu K, Iida H. Ultrasound measurement of vertebral rotation in idiopathic scoliosis. J Bone Joint Surg Br. 1989;71-B:252-5.

18. Chen W, Lou EH, Zhang PQ, Le LH, Hill D. Reliability of assessing the coronal curvature of children with scoliosis by using ultrasound images. J Child Orthop. 2013;7(6):521–9.

19. Young M, Hill DL, Zheng R, Lou E. Reliability and accuracy of ultrasound measurements with and without the aid of previous radiographs in adolescent idiopathic scoliosis (AIS). Eur Spine J. 2015;24:1427–33.

20. Al-Aubaidi Z, Lebel D, Oudjhane K, Zeller R. Three-dimensional imaging of the spine using the EOS system: is it reliable? A comparative study using computed tomography imaging. J Pediatr Orthop B. 2013;22(5):409–12.

21. Yazici M, Acaroglu ER, Alanay A, Deviren V, Cila A, Surat A. Measurement of vertebral rotation in standing versus supine position in adolescent idiopathic scoliosis. J Pediatr Orthop. 2001;21(2):252–6.

22. Lee MC, Solomito M, Patel A. Supine magnetic resonance imaging Cobb measurements for idiopathic scoliosis are linearly related to measurements from standing plain radiographs. Spine (Phila Pa 1976). 2013;38(11):E656–61.

23. Wessberg P, Danielson BI, Willen J. Comparison of Cobb angles in idiopathic scoliosis on standing radiographs and supine axially loaded MRI. Spine (Phila Pa 1976). 2006;31(26):3039–44.

24. Harmouche R, Cheriet F, Labelle H, Dansereau J. 3D registration of MR and X-ray spine images using an articulated model. Comput Med Imaging Graph. 2012;36(5):410–8.

25. Schmitz A, Jaeger UE, Koenig R, et al. A new MRI technique for imaging scoliosis in the sagittal plane. Eur Spine J. 2001;10(2):114–7.

26. Shi B, Mao S, Wang Z, et al. How does the supine MRI correlate with standing x-ray of different curve severity in adolescent idiopathic scoliosis? Spine (Phila Pa 1976). 2015;40(15):1206–1212.

27. Deviren V, Berven S, Kleinstueck F, Antinnes J, Smith JA, Hu SS. Predictors of flexibility and pain patterns in thoracolumbar and lumbar idiopathic scoliosis. Spine (Phila Pa 1976). 2002;27(21):2346–9.

28. Schlosser TP, van Stralen M, Chu WC, et al. Anterior overgrowth in primary curves, compensatory curves and junctional segments in adolescent idiopathic scoliosis. PLoS One. 2016;11(7).

# 7

# Results of ultrasound-assisted brace casting for adolescent idiopathic scoliosis

Edmond H. Lou[1,2*], Doug L. Hill[1,2†], Andreas Donauer[3†], Melissa Tilburn[3†], Douglas Hedden[1†] and Marc Moreau[1†]

## Abstract

**Background:** Four factors have been reported to affect brace treatment outcome: (1) growth or curve based risk, (2) the in-brace correction, (3) the brace wear quantity, and (4) the brace wear quality. The quality of brace design affects the in-brace correction and comfort which indirectly affects the brace wear quantity and quality. This paper reported the immediate benefits and results on using ultrasound (US) to aid orthotists to design braces for the treatment of scoliosis.

**Methods:** Thirty-four AIS subjects participated in this study with 17 (2 males, 15 females) in the control group and 17 (2 males, 15 females) in the intervention (US) group. All participants were prescribed full time TLSO, constructed by either of the 2 orthotists in fabrication of spinal braces. For the control group, the Providence brace design system was adopted to design full time braces. For the intervention group, the custom standing Providence brace design system, plus a medical ultrasound system, a custom pressure measurement system and an in-house software were used to assist brace casting.

**Results:** In the control group, 8 of 17 (47%) subjects needed a total of 11 brace adjustments after initial fabrication requiring a total of 28 in-brace radiographs. Three subjects (18%) required a second adjustment. For the US group, only 1 subject (6%) required adjustment. The total number of in-brace radiographs was 18. The $p$ value of the chi-square for requiring brace adjustment was 0.006 which was a statistically significant difference between the two groups. In the intervention group, the immediate in-brace correction as measured from radiographs was $48 \pm 17\%$, and in the control group the first and second in-brace correction was $33 \pm 19\%$ and $40 \pm 20\%$, respectively. The unpaired 2 sided Student's $t$ test of the in-brace correction was significantly different between the US and the first follow-up of the control group ($p = 0.02$), but was not significant after the second brace adjustment ($p = 0.22$).

**Conclusions:** The use of the 3D ultrasound system provided a radiation-free method to determine the optimum pressure level and location to assist brace design, resulting in decreased radiation exposure during follow-up brace evaluation, increased the in-brace correction, reduced the patients' visits to both brace adjustment and scoliosis clinics. However, the final outcomes could not be reported yet as some of patients are still under brace treatment.

**Keywords:** Adolescent idiopathic scoliosis, 3D ultrasound imaging, Brace treatment, Brace design, Optimum brace pressure

* Correspondence: elou@ualberta.ca
†Equal contributors
¹Department of Surgery, University of Alberta, 6-110F, Clinical Science Building, 8440-112 Street, Edmonton, Alberta T6G 2B7, Canada
²Department of Research and Innovation Development, Glenrose Rehabilitation Hospital, Edmonton, Alberta T5G 0B7, Canada
Full list of author information is available at the end of the article

## Background

Adolescent idiopathic scoliosis (AIS) is a three-dimensional deformity of the spine associated with vertebral rotation due to an unknown cause. It is a chronic and a potentially progressive spinal deformity affecting 2–3% of the population [1]. Girls tend to progress more often than boys [2]. Although scoliosis is rarely life threatening, the long-term impact of untreated scoliosis is still controversial [3–8]. Patients with untreated curves usually have more back pain [2, 5], loss of function, external deformity, poor self-image, and in more severe cases, can impair respiratory capacity later in their life. Bracing is typically prescribed either based on guidelines set by the Scoliosis Research Society [9] or by the Society on Scoliosis Orthopaedic and Rehabilitation Treatment (SOSORT) [10], in which the Cobb angle is greater than 20° with considerable growth remaining or show at least 5° of Cobb angle increase between consecutive clinic visits. Recent scientific evidence has shown that brace treatment is effective [11–14], and a pilot study from a single centre has shown a predicted success rates of 95%, when brace wear quantity combined with the brace wear quality is over 43% of the prescribed dosage [15]. A combined value of brace wear quantity and quality can be achieved in many different ways by trading off wear time and wear tightness; a subject can wear the brace 43% of prescribed time (9.9 h/day) and 100% of time at the prescribed tightness level. Similarly, when a subject wears a brace 100% of prescribed time (23 h/day), but only 43% of time at the prescribed level, the subject may get a similar result. Besides these two factors, the (a) growth or curve based risk and (b) the in-brace correction [16, 17] also affect brace treatment outcomes. The curve-based risk is estimated by physical maturity, gender, the severity and location of the curve, and the spinal balance. The in-brace correction may be affected by the brace design and spinal flexibility.

A typical spinal brace is a hard plastic shell with pads installed inside the liner to concentrate and direct the corrective pressure to oppose the spinal curvature. However, the locations of pads are set empirically based on guidelines for the type of the brace or knowledge derived from orthotists' experiences. Suboptimal pad placement and applied pressure will reduce the in-brace correction which is typically reviewed 6 weeks after the brace has been initiated. If the in-brace correction is not deemed to be satisfactory by the treating orthopedic surgeon, the patient returns to the orthotist for readjustment. This adjustment is required because there is no real time feedback provided to the orthotist during the brace design and construction stage. The standard of care requires the use of radiographs to check the in-brace correction. Radiographs are not taken during brace design and construction to minimize radiation exposure to

growing children because of the increased risk of cancer. Unfortunately, after the adjustment, the in-brace correction examination is often required again which increases cumulative radiation exposure and shortens effective brace usage.

Although finite element (FE) models have been developed to determine optimal orientations and load magnitudes of pressure pads for brace design [18, 19], these still have practical limitations [20] with evaluation of the brace correction not available until the in-brace follow-up clinic. Recently, ultrasound (US) imaging, a real-time non-invasive and non-ionizing method, was demonstrated to be successful in measuring proxy Cobb angles, vertebral rotation, and flexibility [21–27]. The proxy Cobb angles which use vertebrae lamina positions rather than end plates, measured from ultrasound images have high intra- and inter-reliability as well as correlate well with radiographic measurements [22, 26]. Furthermore, there were studies applying ultrasound to determine the optimum location of the major brace pad [28, 29], but their approach did not provide real-time feedback nor determine the optimum pad pressure. Their ultrasound data were processed between the time the patient had their brace fitting and were returned to receive the modified brace. Researchers were also able to use ultrasound to investigate the time lag between application of spinal orthosis and its effect on scoliotic curvature [30]. Therefore, a clinical trial using ultrasound to assist orthotists to determine optimum pad pressure level and location during the brace design stage was conducted. This paper reports the immediate results obtained from this clinical trial.

## Methods

### Patients

Seventeen consecutive AIS subjects (2 males, 15 females; age $13.2 \pm 1.5$ years, Cobb $32 \pm 9°$), with retrospectively collected data who were prescribed a new full time TLSO between January and June 2013 and met the inclusion criteria, served as the control group to match the intervention group recruitment. The distribution of the primary curve of the control group was 7 major thoracic, 6 thoracolumbar, and 4 lumbar curves. Another 17 new AIS subjects (2 male, 15 female; age $13.2 \pm 1.4$ years, Cobb $35 \pm 8°$), who were prescribed a TLSO were prospectively recruited between January 2014 and April 2015 into the intervention group. There was no significant difference of the Cobb angle between groups. The distribution of the primary curve of the intervention group was 6 major thoracic, 6 thoracolumbar, and 5 lumbar curves. Local ethics approval (Pro00028133) was granted by the local institution ethics board and all subjects signed consent forms before participation. The inclusion criteria followed the guidelines set by the non-operational management committee of the Scoliosis Research Society [9] (a) age 10 years or older when brace is prescribed, (b) Risser 0–2, (c) primary curve angles 20°–45°, (d) no prior treatment, and (e) if female, either pre-menarchal or less than 1 year post-menarchal. Both participating orthotists are aligned with the same pediatric scoliosis program and worked together using the same methodology to design spinal brace for over 10 years. There was no change on the X-ray system and the clinical protocol during the entire recruitment period (January 2013–April 2015).

## Control group protocol

For the control group, the traditional plaster cast and molded method with the assistance of the Providence brace system to design spinal braces was used. The orthotist first reviewed the standing posteranterior pre-brace radiograph to identify the location of the apices. He/she then applied a plaster rigid wrap to the AIS body while the subject is standing and instructed the subject to lay upon the Providence brace system. The orthotist used the bolsters to apply pressures and adjusted the pressure level based on the location of the curve apex and his/her experience. After the plaster hardened, the subject stood up again to remove the hardened cast. Reflective markers were then placed around the cast and then scanned by a handheld laser scanner to create a 3D casting image file. The 3D file was then imported into software that was linked to a carving machine. Some minor adjustment was done at this stage to smooth the surface. A 3D body mold was then carved using foam material. After subjective modifications for improved fitting and comfort on the foam positive mold, a brace was fabricated. Subjects typically returned to the orthotist to fit the brace and make the final adjustments within a

week. After that, the subject would use the brace for about 6 weeks, slowly building up their wear time, and returned to the scoliosis clinic to evaluate the design of the brace primarily based on wearability and the correction obtained from the in-brace radiograph.

## Intervention group protocol

A custom Providence brace standing frame, a medical ultrasound (US) system, a custom pressure measurement system, and in-house US measurement software were used to assist brace casting for the intervention group. A 14 cm × 50 cm opening was cut at the middle of the Providence frame to allow for the ultrasound scanning probe. Figure 1 shows the back of the frame and the custom Providence brace design set up with a subject. The subject wore a gown and stood against the standing frame. An operator with several years US scanning experience scanned the subject using the US system. It took approximately 1.5 min to acquire, process, and display the image. The pre-brace X-ray and the standing pre-pressure US spinal image were displayed side-by-side to assist the orthotist to decide on pressure pads locations. The orthotist used the custom standing Providence brace design system to secure bolsters with subjectively determined applied pressure levels against the patient's torso to simulate in-brace correction. At each bolster, an air bag was attached on the surface to measure the interface pressure applied between the bolster and body. The simulated in-brace US scan was then acquired. A real-time US spinal image was displayed and the proxy Cobb angles were measured using in-house developed software. This process took less than 2 min. The difference of the ultrasound measurements compared to the corresponding radiographic measurements was 2–3° with good consistency [22]. The orthotist then

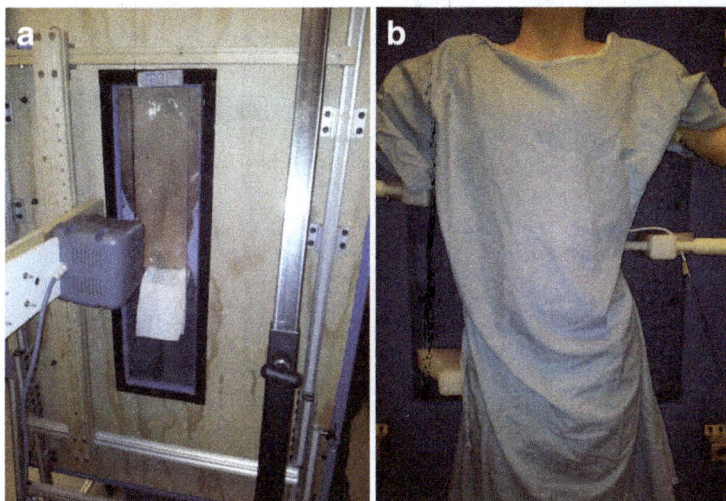

**Fig. 1 a** The opening at the back of the frame, and **b** a subject stands on a frame with a custom Providence brace design system

decided if altering bolster locations and pressure levels might improve correction. Another US scan was taken if the bolster positions were altered. The procedures were repeated until the orthotist attained the best simulated in-brace correction configuration. The target goal was still to try to get at least 50% correction. During scanning, the pressure levels at each bolster were recorded. Figure 2 shows (a) the pre-brace standing X-ray with a right thoracic curve of 37° between T8 and T12, (b) the standing baseline US image with proxy Cobb angle 35°, (c) the first US scan with axilla, thoracic, and lumbar pads pressure levels at 60, 75, and 75 mmHg, respectively, at which the Cobb angle is 25°, (d) the second US scan with axilla, thoracic, and lumbar pads pressure levels at 60, 90, and 90 mmHg, respectively at which the Cobb angle was 23°. The location of each bolster relative to the waist level was recorded. The orthotist then applied a plaster rigid wrap and identical pressure levels to the subject to the best stimulated in-brace correction configuration on a supine position with the Providence system. The pads' positions and pressure levels recorded from the standing frame were applied. After the plaster hardened and was removed, the cast was scanned by a handheld laser scanner to create a positive mold which was used for brace fabrication. Figure 3 shows the US second trial image overlapped with the in-brace radiograph at which the Cobb angle from the in-brace radiograph was 21°.

### First follow-up clinic
Approximately, 6 weeks after braces initiation, all subjects returned to scoliosis clinics to inspect the effectiveness of the brace based on the in-brace correction. The treating orthopedic surgeons used the target threshold of in-brace Cobb correction of 50%. They also used their clinical experience to consider whether the in-brace correction was optimal because the target threshold may not be attainable for rigid curves. If the surgeon was not satisfied with the in-brace correction, the subject would return to the orthotist for adjustments. Ultrasound was not used to assist in the adjustment for either group. Additional follow-up clinic visits with radiographs occurred approximately 2 months after adjustments.

### Results
In the 17 control subjects, the major pre-brace Cobb angle was $32° ± 9°$. Eight of these required brace adjustment (47%) and 3 of these adjusted subjects (38%) requiring a second adjustment. A total of 11 brace adjustments were needed and 28 in-brace radiographs were taken (average 1.6 radiographs per subject). The average in-brace major Cobb angle correction at the first in-brace follow-up clinic and at the final accepted follow-up clinic were $33 ± 19\%$ and $40 ± 20\%$, respectively.

For the intervention group, the major pre-brace Cobb angle from the radiographs prior to bracing was $35° ± 8°$. Only 1 subject (6%) required adjustment. A total of 18 in-brace radiographs were taken (average 1.1 radiographs per subject). The orthotist was satisfied with the first attempt with the US information in 8 out of 17 cases. With 9 subjects, the location and pressure level of the bolsters were altered one time. Among these 9

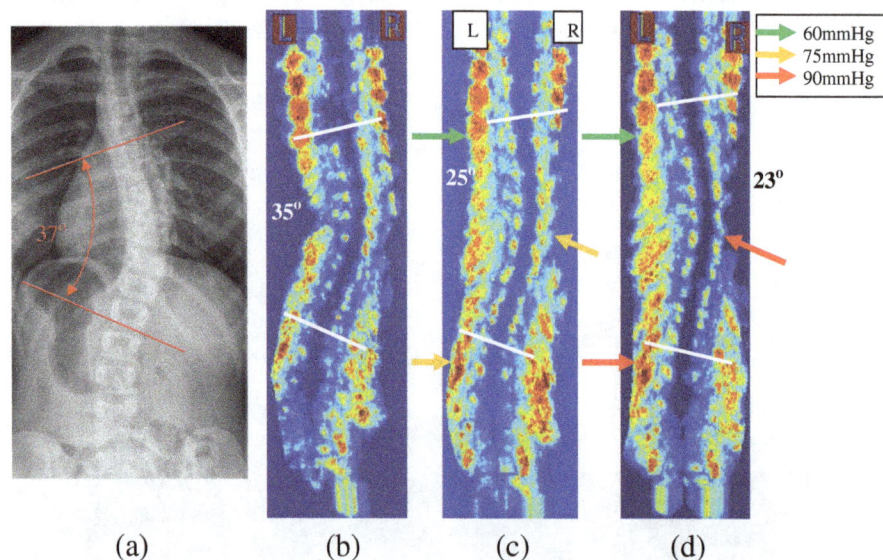

(a) (b) (c) (d)

**Fig. 2 a** The standing pre-brace X-ray with Cobb angle 37°. **b** The baseline US scan (Cobb angle 35°). **c** The first trial US scan (Cobb angle 25°). **d** The 2nd trial US scan (Cobb angle 23°)

The $p$ value of the chi-square for requiring brace adjustment between the control and the intervention groups was 0.0065 which was a statistically significant difference. The $p$ values of the unpaired two sided Student's $t$ test of the in-brace correction between the two groups were 0.02 and 0.22 between the first and second time of adjustment, respectively. It showed statistically significant difference between the US and the first time for the control group, but no statistically significant difference between the US and the second time of the control group. The reduction of the number of in-brace radiographs was large, 18 in-brace radiographs from the US group versus 28 in-brace radiographs from the control group, a saving of 10 radiographs in 17 subjects. Table 1 also shows the comparison of the health system time to cast and make the brace adjustment between the control and the intervention groups; on average an extra 1 h/per subject was needed in the control group. Furthermore, the time that the control and the intervention group received their optimum designed brace after prescription averaged $3.5 \pm 1.9$ months compared to $2.1 \pm 0.5$ months. There was a significant delay to start the effective brace treatment between the two groups.

## Discussion

Brace treatment is now generally accepted as a proven effective method to stop the progression of AIS. Besides compliance, a good brace design is vitally important. In current practice, the skill and experience of the orthotist are the major factors which affect the design of the brace. The pressure pads' levels, locations, and directions are subjectively selected by the orthotist. Without real-time feedback, trial and error in brace design is used. Lack of acceptable in-brace correction may trigger brace adjustment. Even though Li et al. [28, 29] applied the ultrasound method to assist brace fitting by investigating the locations of pressure pads, they did not provide the real-time feedback to the orthotist. They processed the data later to determine the optimum pad location and required patients to have an extra visit to receive the final brace. In this study, the intervention group has 7/17 (42%) that benefitted from having a brace adjustment after the initial setting of the pad placements. Those 7 cases which included 3 thoracic, 2 thoracolumbar, and 2 lumbar cases, did not indicate this

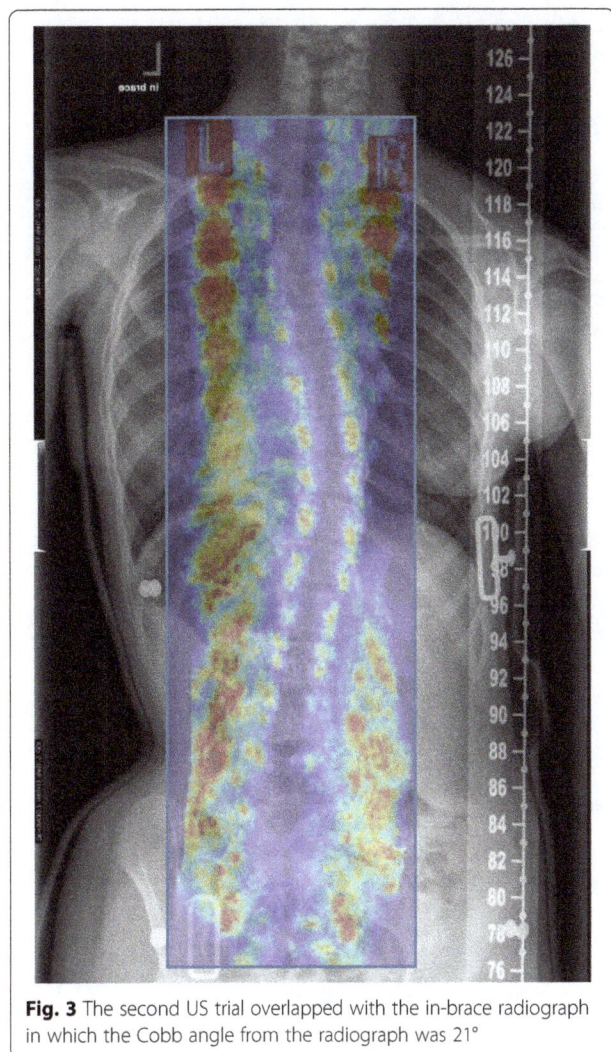

**Fig. 3** The second US trial overlapped with the in-brace radiograph in which the Cobb angle from the radiograph was 21°

revised cases, 7 showed better stimulated in-brace corrections, 1 had no change, and 1 got worse. The intervention resulted in 7 out of 17 subjects (42%) having their brace designed using an improved pressure level and/or pad placement. For the 7 improved cases, the in-brace Cobb correction from the US measurements in the first and second trials were $29 \pm 11\%$ and $42 \pm 14\%$, respectively. For the intervention group as a whole, the average final in-brace Cobb angle was $19° \pm 8°$ which was $48 \pm 17\%$ in-brace correction, which was slightly higher than the simulated US in-brace correction.

**Table 1** Comparison of the casting and the brace adjustment time per subject

|  | Control group | Intervention group |
| --- | --- | --- |
| Casting time | 17 h (1 h per subject) | 20.4 h (1.2 h per subject) |
| Brace adjustment time | 11 h (1 h per adjustment) | 1 h |
| Extra scoliosis clinic | 11 h | 1 h |
| Total time | 39 h | 22.4 h |
| Health system time per subject | 2.3 h | 1.3 h |

method was only beneficial for specific types of curves. However, since the number of cases is still limited, no conclusive statement can be made. The advantage with the intervention group was that the adjustment was made prior to brace fabrication rather than after the first follow-up visit. The compromise between the comfort and treatment outcomes is influenced by how aggressively the orthotist designs the brace. With the immediate feedback, 7 out of 9 cases (80%) showed the revised bolster placements or pressure alterations resulted in better correction than the first trial. This demonstrates how importantly the pressure pads location affects the effectiveness of the brace treatment. The subjects are able to report their pressure tolerance level that they feel in real-time. Requiring brace adjustment increases not only the number of radiographs and the cost of the health care system (orthotists', surgeons' and clinics time), but also the burden for the families that they need to travel to both brace adjustment and extra follow-up clinics. Furthermore, the benefits of getting the best designed brace in the shortest time may improve the overall effectiveness of the brace treatment because the patient will be using the brace most effectively sooner, during the most beneficial period of rapid adolescent growth. More clinical data are required to truly answer the total benefits of using ultrasound to assist brace casting. The limitation of this method is an experienced ultrasound technician is required during the brace casting to acquire and analyze the data. To overcome this, an automatic ultrasound machine which can scan the back automatically is being considered for future improvements. Also, the custom software developed for the ultrasound imaging measurement needs to be enhanced so that 3D information and automatic measurements can be obtained without requiring significant operator experience.

## Conclusions

The use of the ultrasound system provided a radiation-free method to determine the optimum pressure level and location to obtain the best stimulated in-brace correction during brace casting. Although the long-term results have not yet known the immediate benefits of reduced cost, radiation exposure, and patient impact have merit. The number of radiograph taken per subject was reduced, and the acceptable in-brace correction was attained sooner in the intervention group with less burden on the families and patients.

### Abbreviations
3D: Three dimensional; AIS: Adolescent idiopathic scoliosis; F: Female; M: Male; T: Thoracic; TLSO: Thoraco-lumbo-sacral orthosis; US: Ultrasound

### Acknowledgements
Special thanks to Dr. Rui Zheng who assisted on acquisition of ultrasound data.

### Funding
Edmond Lou, Doug Hill, Douglas Hedden, and Marc Moreau received funding from the Glenrose Rehabilitation Hospital Foundation. Edmond Lou also received the grant from the Natural Sciences and Engineering Council of Canada (RGPIN-2015-04176).

### Authors' contributions
EL participated in the conception, design and coordination, and to analysis and interpretation of data and prepared the manuscript. DLH is involved in the conception, design and coordination, and editing the manuscript. AD conceived of the study and participated to the acquisition of data. MT conceived of the study and participated to the acquisition of data. DH and MM were the attending orthopedic surgeons for the study; they are also involved in the conception, design, and coordination. All authors read and approved the final manuscript.

### Competing interests
The authors declare that they have no competing interests.

### Author details
[1]Department of Surgery, University of Alberta, 6-110F, Clinical Science Building, 8440-112 Street, Edmonton, Alberta T6G 2B7, Canada. [2]Department of Research and Innovation Development, Glenrose Rehabilitation Hospital, Edmonton, Alberta T5G 0B7, Canada. [3]Department of Prosthetics and Orthotics, Glenrose Rehabilitation Hospital, Edmonton, Alberta T5G 0B7, Canada.

### References
1.  Lonstein JE, Carlson JM. The Prediction of curve progression in untreated idiopathic scoliosis during growth. J Bone Joint Surg. 1984;66A:1061–71.
2.  Lonstein JE. Adolescent Idiopathic Scoliosis. Lancet. 1994;344:1407–12.
3.  James JIP. Idiopathic Scoliosis. The prognoses, diagnosis, and operative indications related to curve patterns and the age at onset. J Bone Joint Surg. 1954;36B:36–49.
4.  Nachemson A. A long term follow-up study of non-treated scoliosis. Acta Orthop Scand. 1968;39(4):446–76.
5.  Weinstein SL, Zavala DC, Ponseti IV. Idiopathic scoliosis: long term follow-up and prognosis in untreated patients. J Bone Joint Surg. 1981;63-A(5):702–12.
6.  Weinstein SL, Ponseti IV. Curve progression in idiopathic scoliosis. J Bone Joint Surg. 1983;65-A:447–55.
7.  Edgar MA, Mehta MH. Long-term follow-up of fused and unfused idiopathic scoliosis. J Bone Joint Surg. 1988;70(5):712–6.
8.  Dickson JH, Mirkovic S, Noble PC, Nalty T, Erwin RW. Results of operative treatment of idiopathic scoliosis in adults. J Bone Joint Surg. 1995;77(4):513–23.
9.  Richards BS, Bernstein RM, D'Amato CR, Thompson GH. Standardization of criteria for adolescent idiopathic scoliosis brace studies: SRS Committee on Bracing and Nonoperative Management. Spine. 2005;30:2068–75.
10. Stefano N, Aulisa AG, Lorenzo A, et al. 2011 SOSORT guidelines: Orthopaedic and Rehabilitation treatment of idiopathic scoliosis during growth. Scoliosis. 2012;7:3.
11. Dolan LA, Wright JG, Weinstein SL. Effects of bracing in adolescents with idiopathic scoliosis. N Engl J Med. 2014;370(7):681. Feb 13.
12. Aulisa AG, Guzzanti V, Galli M, Perisano C, Falciglia F, Aulisa L. Treatment of thoraco-lumbar curves in adolescent females affected by idiopathic scoliosis with a progressive action short brace (PASB): assessment of results according to the SRS committee on bracing and nonoperative management standardization criteria. Scoliosis. 2009;4:21.
13. Negrini S, Minozzi S, Bettany-Saltikov J, Zaina F, Chockalingam N, Grivas TB, Kotwicki T, Maruyama T, Romano M, Vasiliadis ES. Braces for idiopathic scoliosis in adolescents. Spine (Phila Pa 1976). 2010;35:1285–93.
14. Aulisa AG, Guzzanti V, Perisano C, Marzetti E, Falciglia F, Aulisa L. Treatment of lumbar curves in scoliotic adolescent females with progressive action short brace: a case series based on the Scoliosis Research Society Committee Criteria. Spine (Phila Pa 1976). 2012;37(13):E786–91.
15. Lou E, Moreau M, Mahood JK, Hedden DM, Hill D, Raso JV. How Quantity and Quality of Brace Wear Affect the Brace Treatment Outcomes for AIS Patients. J Eur Spine. 2016;25(2):495–9. doi:10.1007/s00586-015-4233-22015.

16. Lou E, Hill DL, Parent E, Raso VJ, Moreau MJ, Mahood JK, Hedden D. Prediction of Brace Treatment Outcomes. In: Proceeding of SOSORT 2009 The 6th International Conference on Conservative Management of Spinal Deformities. 2009. p. 2192.

17. Lou E, Chan A, Donauer A, Tilburn M, Hill D. Ultrasound assisted brace casting for adolescent idiopathic scoliosis, IRSSD Best Research Paper 2014. Scoliosis. 2015;10:13. doi:10.1186/s13013-015-0037-8.

18. Cheng FH, Shih SL, Chou WK, et al. Finite element analysis of the scoliotic spine under different loading conditions. Biomed Mater Eng. 2010;20:251–9.

19. Clin J, Aubin CE, Parent S, Sangole A, et al. Correlation between immediate in-brace correction and biomechanical effectiveness of brace treatment in adolescent idiopathic scoliosis. Spine. 2010;35(18):1706–13.

20. Clin J, Aubin CE, Parent S, Sangole A, Labelle H. Comparison of the biomechanical 3D efficiency of different brace designs for the treatment of scoliosis using a finite element model. Eur Spine J. 2010;19:1169–78.

21. Chen W, Lou E, Le LH. Reliability of the axial vertebral rotation measurements of adolescent idiopathic scoliosis using the center of lamina method on ultrasound images: in-vitro and in-vivo study. J Eur Spine. 2016. doi: 10.1007/s00586-016-4492-6.

22. Zheng R, Young M, Hill D, Le L, Moreau M, Mahood JK, Hedden D, Southon S, Lou E. Improvement on the Accuracy and Reliability of Ultrasound Coronal Curvature Measurement on AIS with the Aid of Previous Radiographs. Spine. 2016;41(5):404–11. doi:10.1097/BRS.0000000000001244.

23. Wang Q, Li M, Lou E, Wong MS. Reliability and Validity Study of Clinical Ultrasound Imaging on Lateral Curvature of Adolescent Idiopathic Scoliosis. PLOS ONE. 2015. doi:10.1371/journal.pone.0135264.

24. Young M, Hill D, Zheng R, Lou E. Reliability and Accuracy of Ultrasound Measurements With and Without the Aid of Previous Radiographs in Adolescent Idiopathic Scoliosis. J Eur Spine. 2015;24(7):1427–33. doi:10.1007/s00586-015-3855-8.

25. Zheng R, Chan A, Chen W, Hill D, Le LH, Moreau M, Mahood JK, Hedden D, Southon S, Lou E. Intra- and Inter-rater Reliability of coronal curvature measurement for AIS using ultrasonic imaging method. J Spine Deform. 2015;3(2):151–8. doi:10.1016/j.jspd.2014.08.008.

26. Lou E, Zhang R, Donauer A, Tilburn M, Hill D, Raso J. Can ultrasound imaging be used to determine curve flexibility when designing spinal orthoses? Scoliosis Spinal Disord. 2016;11(Suppl 1):23. Published online 2016 Aug 23. doi:10.1186/s13013-016-0077-8.

27. Zheng YP, Lee T, Lai K, Yin B, Zhou GQ, Jiang WW, Cheung J, Wong MS, Ng B, Cheng J, Lam TP. A reliability and validity study for Scolioscan: a radiation-free scoliosis assessment system using 3D ultrasound imaging. Scoliosis Spinal Disord. 2016;11:13.

28. Li M, Cheng J, Ying M, Ng B, Zheng YP, Lam TP, Wong WY, Wong MS. Application of 3-D ultrasound in assisting the fitting procedure of spinal orthosis to patients with adolescent idiopathic scoliosis. Stud Health Technol Inform. 2010;158:34–7.

29. Li M, Cheng J, Ng KW, Lam TP, Zheng YP, Ying M, Wong MS. Could clinical ultrasound improve the fitting of spinal orthosis for the patients with AIS? Eur Spine J. 2012;21:1926–35.

30. Li M, Wong MS, Luk KD, Wong KW, Cheung KM. Time-dependent response of scoliotic curvature to orthotic intervention: when should a radiograph be obtained after putting on or taking off a spinal orthosis. Spine. 2014;39:1408–16.

# 8

# Low back pain in older adults: risk factors, management options and future directions

Arnold YL Wong[1]*[iD], Jaro Karppinen[2,3] and Dino Samartzis[4]

## Abstract

Low back pain (LBP) is one of the major disabling health conditions among older adults aged 60 years or older. While most causes of LBP among older adults are non-specific and self-limiting, seniors are prone to develop certain LBP pathologies and/or chronic LBP given their age-related physical and psychosocial changes. Unfortunately, no review has previously summarized/discussed various factors that may affect the effective LBP management among older adults. Accordingly, the objectives of the current narrative review were to comprehensively summarize common causes and risk factors (modifiable and non-modifiable) of developing severe/chronic LBP in older adults, to highlight specific issues in assessing and treating seniors with LBP, and to discuss future research directions. Existing evidence suggests that prevalence rates of severe and chronic LBP increase with older age. As compared to working-age adults, older adults are more likely to develop certain LBP pathologies (e.g., osteoporotic vertebral fractures, tumors, spinal infection, and lumbar spinal stenosis). Importantly, various age-related physical, psychological, and mental changes (e.g., spinal degeneration, comorbidities, physical inactivity, age-related changes in central pain processing, and dementia), as well as multiple risk factors (e.g., genetic, gender, and ethnicity), may affect the prognosis and management of LBP in older adults. Collectively, by understanding the impacts of various factors on the assessment and treatment of older adults with LBP, both clinicians and researchers can work toward the direction of more cost-effective and personalized LBP management for older people.

**Keywords:** Risk factors, Spine, Disc degeneration, Management, Low back pain, Elderly, Genetics, Falls, Brain, Pain assessment

## Background

The average lifespan of humans has dramatically increased in the last decade due to the advance in medicine [1]. According to the United Nations, the world population of individuals aged 60 years or above will triple by 2050 [2]. In the UK alone, approximately 22% of the population will be 65 years or older by 2031, exceeding the number of those aged less than 25 years [3]. However, the fast-growing aging population also increases the likelihood of non-communicable diseases (e.g., musculoskeletal complaints). Studies have suggested that the prevalence of musculoskeletal pain in older adults ranges from 65 to 85% [4, 5], with 36 to 70% of them suffering from back pain [5, 6].

Low back pain (LBP) is the most common health problem among older adults that results in pain and disability [4, 7–10]. Older adults, aged 65 years or above, are the second most common age group to visit physicians for LBP [11]. Earlier research suggests that LBP prevalence progressively increases from teenage [12] to 60 years of age and then declines [13–16], which may be ascribed to occupational exposure among working-age adults [17, 18], or age-related changes in pain perception or stoicism [19]. However, recent studies have revealed that LBP remains ubiquitous among older adults at their retirement ages [20, 21]. In population-based studies, the 1-year prevalence of LBP in community-dwelling seniors ranged from 13 to 50% across the world [4, 13, 22–24]. Similarly, while up to 80% of older residents in long-term care facility experience substantial musculoskeletal pain [25–27] and one-third of these cases are LBP [28], often older residents' pain is underreported and inadequately treated [25–27].

* Correspondence: arnold.wong@polyu.edu.hk
[1]Department of Rehabilitation Sciences, Faculty of Health and Social Sciences, The Hong Kong Polytechnic University, Hung Hom, Hong Kong, SAR, China
Full list of author information is available at the end of the article

It is noteworthy that both the incidence and prevalence of severe and chronic LBP increase with older age [13, 29, 30]. Docking et al. [17] reported that the 1-month prevalence of disabling back pain (pain that affected daily activities within the past month) increased from 3.8% among people aged between 77 and 79 years to 9.7% among those aged between 90 and 100 years. Williams and coworkers [31] also found that individuals aged 80 years or above were three times more likely to experience severe LBP than those aged between 50 and 59 years. Because severe LBP usually results in poor treatment outcomes and functional disability [17, 32], timely LBP management of older adults is crucial. Importantly, compared to working-age adults, older adults aged 65 years or above are more likely to develop chronic LBP that lasts for more than 3 months [13, 33]. A Spanish study found that the prevalence rates of chronic LBP among females and males aged 65 years or older were 24.2 and 12.3%, respectively [34], while an Israeli study documented that the prevalence of chronic LBP in people aged 77 years was as high as 58% [35].

Notwithstanding the high prevalence of LBP among older adults, their pain is usually undertreated. A recent study showed approximately 25% of senior nursing home residents with chronic pain did not receive analgesics, and only 50% of all analgesics were prescribed as standing orders at suboptimal doses, which did not follow geriatric clinical guidelines [36, 37]. According to those guidelines, older patients with chronic pain should receive analgesics as a standing dose rather than on an as-needed basis in order to ensure adequate concentration of analgesic in serum for continuous pain relief [36, 38]. Standing-dose analgesics are particularly important for people with cognitive impairment because they cannot appropriately request medication.

While undertreatment of LBP in older adults may be ascribed to the avoidance of high-dose analgesics (e.g., opioid) prescription, it may also be attributed to the difficulty in identifying the presence or causes of LBP. Research has shown that less than 50% of primary care physicians have strong confidence in diagnosing the causes of chronic LBP in older adults [32]. Consequently, this may result in over-reliance on medical imaging or improper LBP management (e.g., undertreatment). Imperatively, untreating or undertreating older adults with LBP may result in sleep disturbances, withdrawal from social and recreational activities, psychological distress, impeded cognition, malnutrition, rapid deterioration of functional ability, and falls [39]. These LBP-related consequences may compromise their quality of life and increase their long-term health care expenses [40].

Although various medical associations have published clinical guidelines on conservative management of chronic pain in older adults [37, 41, 42], there is paucity of literature summarizing various causes or risk factors of developing severe/chronic LBP among older adults. Since a better understanding of these factors can improve LBP management, the objectives of the current narrative review were to summarize potential causes of LBP, risk factors for chronic LBP, special consideration for LBP management (e.g., pain evaluations among patients with dementia) in older people aged 60 years or older, and future research directions.

## Search strategies and selection criteria

Potential articles were identified for review through PubMed from January 1, 1990, to November 30, 2016. Search terms included keywords and medical subject headings related to "low back pain," "LBP," "older adult*," "senior*," "elderly," "cognitive impairment," "dementia," "nonverbal," "community-dwelling," "nursing home," "long-term care facilities," "risk factor*," "brain," "genetics," "assessment*," and "intervention*." Various Boolean terms were used in conjunction with various search terms. Articles were selected based on the relevance of topic and restricted to the English language. The reference lists of relevant articles were also included for review. A total of 2182 citations were identified from the search. Of them, information from 320 articles was used in the current review.

## Potential causes of low back pain
### Non-specific or mechanical low back pain

Like among young adults, the majority of LBP among older adults has no definite pathology (e.g., fracture or inflammation) and is diagnosed as non-specific LBP. These patients experience LBP that is altered by posture, activity, or time of the day. Non-specific LBP may originate from different pain sources [43]. Disc degeneration on magnetic resonance imaging (MRI) is more prevalent with age progression and as such in older adults; however, it is less likely to be the pain source as compared to young adults [44]. Conversely, facet joint pain in seniors may present as localized LBP with or without posterior thigh pain during walking. The pain may be aggravated during trunk extension, ipsilateral lateral flexion, and/or rotation [45]. Lumbar degenerative spondylolisthesis (defined as forward or backward slippage of a cephalic vertebra over a caudal one secondary to a degenerated disc and altered facet joint alignment) is common among women aged 60 years or older and is usually associated with facet hypertrophy [46]. The presence of degenerative spondylolisthesis alongside facet hypertrophy and thickening of ligamentum flavum may results in pain, spinal stenosis, and neurological deficits in older adults [46, 47]. Although spinal degenerative changes may induce LBP, not all anomalies on lumbar medical imaging are related to LBP because abnormal imaging phenotypes are ubiquitous among asymptomatic older adults [44, 48–50].

Additionally, non-specific LBP may originate from structures other than the lumbar spine. Many older patients with chronic LBP display physical findings comparable to sacroiliac joint pain (83.6%) and myofascial pain (95.5%) [51]. Symptoms of sacroiliac joint disorders are similar to facet joint pain, which includes localized LBP with or without posterior thigh pain that can be alleviated by lying [52]. Myofascial pain is a localized palpable tenderness and tightness within a muscle that resists passive stretching and reproduces predictable referred pain pattern on palpation [53]. Myofascial pain in lumbar muscles or piriformis are common among seniors. Collectively, it is difficult to identify the sources of non-specific LBP because its causes are usually multifactorial. Various factors (e.g., anxiety, depression, coping strategies, and pain genes) can modify the severity and chronicity of LBP [31, 35, 50].

### Radiculopathy

While non-specific LBP is usually localized at the lumbar region and/or thigh, the compression of nerve roots or spinal meninges by degenerated spinal structures (e.g., herniated discs, facet joints, and/or epidural fat) [54] may lead to radiculopathy that radiates distal to the knee. The clinical presentation of radiculopathy depends on the location of neural tissue compression. Lumbar spinal stenosis (LSS) secondary to degenerative changes (e.g., osteophytes and hypertrophic ligamentum flavum) at a single or multiple level(s) may lead to unilateral or bilateral radiculopathy and neurogenic claudication with or without LBP [55–57]. Neurogenic claudication is characterized by numbness and heaviness of legs after prolonged walking, which can be eased by a flexed position (e.g., forward leaning or sitting) [58–60]. On the contrary, the presence of osteophyte/narrowing in the lateral recess or in the vertebral foramen may result in radicular leg pain without LBP [61]. Research on asymptomatic or some clinical populations have suggested that the prevalence of degenerative LSS ranged from 6 to 13.1% [62, 63] and the rate increases with age [64]. A population-based imaging study found that the prevalence of degenerative LSS (i.e., ≤10-mm anteroposterior diameter of spinal canal) in young (<40 years) and older adults (>60 years) were 4.0 and 14.3%, respectively [64].

### Osteoporotic vertebral fractures

Given the hormonal changes following menopause, women are more susceptible to osteoporotic fracture and related LBP [65, 66]. Approximately 25% of all postmenopausal women suffer from vertebral compression fracture and the prevalence of this condition increases with age [65]. It is estimated that the prevalence of vertebral compression fracture in women aged 80 years or above can be as high as 40% [65]. As compared to patients with non-specific LBP, patients with vertebral fractures experience more disability [67]. Unfortunately, only one third of the cases are correctly diagnosed because many seniors assume bone and joint pain as part of the aging process [68]. As such, physicians should pay more attention to examine seniors with acute onset of localized LBP that may or may not present with paraspinal muscle spasm. A recent systematic review suggests that older age, corticosteroid use, and significant trauma are the risk factors for vertebral fractures [69]. The common site of compression fractures occur at the thoracolumbar region [70–72]. Depending on the mechanism of fractures, some vertebral compression fracture may result in radiculopathy. The most common fracture mechanism is due to a flexion movement or trauma that causes an anterior wedge fracture [73]. Since the posterior vertebral body remains intact and the collapsed anterior vertebra heals without regaining height, it will result in a kyphotic deformity without compromising the spinal cord [73]. Another type of vertebral compression fracture involves the center part of the vertebral body without affecting the anterior or posterior wall. This type of fracture does not affect the spinal cord. A less common osteoporotic vertebral fracture involves the axial compression of the entire vertebral body or the posterior portions of the vertebra that may compress the spinal canal and results in neurological deficit [71–73].

### De novo degenerative lumbar scoliosis

De novo degenerative lumbar scoliosis (DNDLS) is a spinal deformity in older adults that results in disabling LBP/leg pain and suboptimal quality of life. [74–76]. DNDLS is defined as a lumbar scoliotic curve with a Cobb angle ≥10° in the coronal plane that develops after 50 years of age in people without a history of adolescent idiopathic scoliosis. [77]. The reported prevalence of DNDLS in the adult population has ranged from 8.3 to 13.3% [78–80], while that in adults older than 60 years was as high as 68% [81]. Multifactorial causes have been suggested for DNDLS, including intervertebral disc degeneration and genetic predisposition [82–84]. It is believed that the asymmetrical biomechanical load on the vertebral endplate on the concave side of the curve may cause inflammatory responses in the endplate and adjacent bone marrow of the vertebral body, which may result in LBP. [85–87]. This premise has been substantiated by a recent study that found (1) bone marrow edema in DNDLS was more prevalent in older adults with LBP than those without LBP, (2) bone marrow edema was more frequent on the concave side of the DNDLS curve, and (3) the location of bone marrow edema on MRI was closely associated with local lumbar tenderness [87]. However, no significant relation between Cobb angle and LBP symptoms in older adults has been reported [81]. Interestingly, the curve progression rate of DNDLS is higher than that of adolescent idiopathic scoliosis [77]. Three radiological variables (i.e., increased intervertebral disc degeneration, an intercrest line passing through the L5 level (not L4 or higher), and apical lateral vertebral translation for at least 6 mm)) have been identified as predictors of DNDLS curve progression [77].

### Tumors/cancers

The incidence rates for all neoplasms exponentially increase with age [88] although only less than 1% of the causes of LBP presented to primary care physicians are attributed to spinal tumors [89]. A majority of these tumors are related to metastasis and only a handful of them are primary tumors [90–95]. The common metastatic sources of LBP are prostate and kidney although primary malignant tumors (e.g., chordoma, plasmacytoma, or lymphoma) are also be found in older adults [90]. Unlike young adults, seniors are unlikely to have primary benign tumors (e.g., osteoblastoma, osteochondroma, osteoma, eosinophilic granuloma, and aneurysmal bone cysts). Clinically, typical symptom of spinal tumors is progressive, unremitting, localized, or radiating pain that are aggravated by movement, worse at night, and cannot be eased by rest. In addition, patients may experience weakness and feel the presence of a lump [96].

### Spinal infection

Vertebral osteomyelitis (VO) is a life-threatening infectious musculoskeletal disease in older people caused by an infection of vertebral bones [97]. Given the growing aging population, the incidence of VO is increasing [98–100]. Although the reported incidence rate of VO in the general population only ranges from 2.5 cases to 7 cases per 100,000 people-years [99, 101], the mortality of these patients can be as high as 12% [99, 102]. Four causes of VO have been suggested. First, pathogenic bacteria may be disseminated hematogenously from a distant infected source and multiply at the metaphyseal arterioles of vertebral bone that causes microabscess formation, bone necrosis, and fistula within bone [103]. *Staphylococcus aureus* is the most common pathogen. Second, tubercular VO may occur in seniors who have contracted tuberculous infection at young age. *Mycobacterium tuberculosis* may be transmitted to and remains in the vertebral bone. Age-related deterioration of the host's immunity or certain incidences (e.g., osteoporosis, trauma, or non-myobacterial infections) may reactivate *M. tuberculosis* in the bone that causes osteomyelitis. Third, aerobic gram-negative bacilli in older men with urinary tract infection may rarely reach the lumbar spine through Batson's plexus and cause VO [97]. Fourth, iatrogenic infection following spinal surgeries or injections may cause vertebral osteomyelitis. Clinically, patients with VO may present with fever, elevated C-reactive protein, paraspinal muscle spasm, LBP, neurological deficits, and epidural abscess. Additionally, patients with tuberculous osteomyelitis may have a groin mass because of the presence of abscess in psoas muscle [97]. Taken together, greater age and certain comorbidities (e.g., diabetes, hemodialysis usage, liver cirrhosis, malignancy, and infectious endocarditis) are known to increase inpatient mortality of VO [99]. Clinicians should be suspicious of VO if older patients with the abovementioned comorbidities demonstrate unidentified fever and/or LBP [99]. Clinical findings, laboratory results, bone scintigraphy, and/or spinal biopsy are usually used to make differential diagnosis of VO.

Similarly, older people are more prone to develop pyogenic spondylodiscitis, which involves the infection of disc and adjacent vertebral bones. It has been estimated that the incidence rate of non-tuberculous or non-postoperative spondylodiscitis in the general population is approximately 0.2 to 2.4 cases per 100,000 people-years [101, 104–106], while that for people over 65 years old is as high as 9.8 cases per 100,000 person-years [107]. A recent population-based study reported that males aged 70 years or older displayed six times higher incidence rate of pyogenic non-tuberculosis spondylodiscitis than males under 70 years old. Likewise, females aged 70 years or above were three times more likely to exhibit pyogenic non-tuberculosis spondylodiscitis than younger counterparts [98]. Clinical presentations of spondylodiscitis are comparable VO. *S. aureus* is the major cause of pyogenic spondylodiscitis [108], while other bacteria (e.g., Streptococcus and Pneumococcus) may also cause the disease [98]. Magnetic resonance imaging is the gold standard for imaging pyogenic spondylodiscitis, which is visualized as reduced signal intensity of the affected disc and adjacent vertebral bodies with unclear endplates definition on T1-weighted images and enhanced signal intensity on T2-weighted images [109].

### Visceral diseases

Since it is not uncommon for seniors to have comorbidities, it is important to consider other non-spinal pathologies that usually present as chronic LBP. Several visceral diseases (e.g., dissecting abdominal aortic aneurysm, cholecystolithiasis, nephrolithiasis, prostatitis, urinary tract infection, and pelvic inflammatory disease) have known to generate symptoms comparable to chronic LBP [110].

### Cauda equina syndrome

This syndrome is ascribed to the compression of multiple lumbar and sacral nerve roots in the spinal canal that lead to bowel, bladder, and/or sexual dysfunction, as well as perianal region numbness [111]. Depending on the location of nerve roots compression, patients with cauda equina syndrome may or may not experience sciatica. Potential causes of this syndrome include central disc herniation or spondylolisthesis at the lower lumber levels, spinal tumors, dislocated fracture, and abscess within the spinal canals [111]. Additionally, this syndrome may be secondary to some rare iatrogenic causes (e.g., spinal anesthesia or postoperative hematoma).

### Risk factors of developing severe/chronic low back pain in older adults

Although most LBP is self-limiting and begins to improve after a few days and resolves within a month [110], some patients are susceptible to chronic LBP that lead to significant disability. While age is a well-known risk factor for chronic LBP [112], other factors may perpetuate LBP in older adults (Fig. 1). The understanding of these factors can help identify high-risk patients and improve their LBP management. Since older adults usually face both age-related physical and psychosocial issues, comprehensive assessments and treatments are needed to effectively manage LBP in seniors.

### Non-modifiable risk factors
#### Altered supraspinal pain processing

Recent evidence suggests that normal aging may be associated with alterations in pain perception [113, 114] central pain processing [114] and/or neuroplastic changes to pain responses [115]. Both experimental pain and functional neuroimaging studies have found that older people display age-related increase in the heat pain threshold [116] and reduced responses in middle insular and primary somatosensory cortices toward a 44 °C heat stimulus [117]. These age-related neuropsychological changes in pain processing may reduce older peoples' awareness and reporting of pain that may lead to undiagnosed health problems/injuries.

Conversely, some psychophysical studies reported that older adults displayed lower tolerance to various types of pain stimuli (e.g., ischaemic, mechanical, electrical, heat, or cold) [113, 114, 118] decreased pain thresholds for mechanical pressure [114, 116] or ischemic pain stimuli [119] and higher pain rating for noxious stimuli as

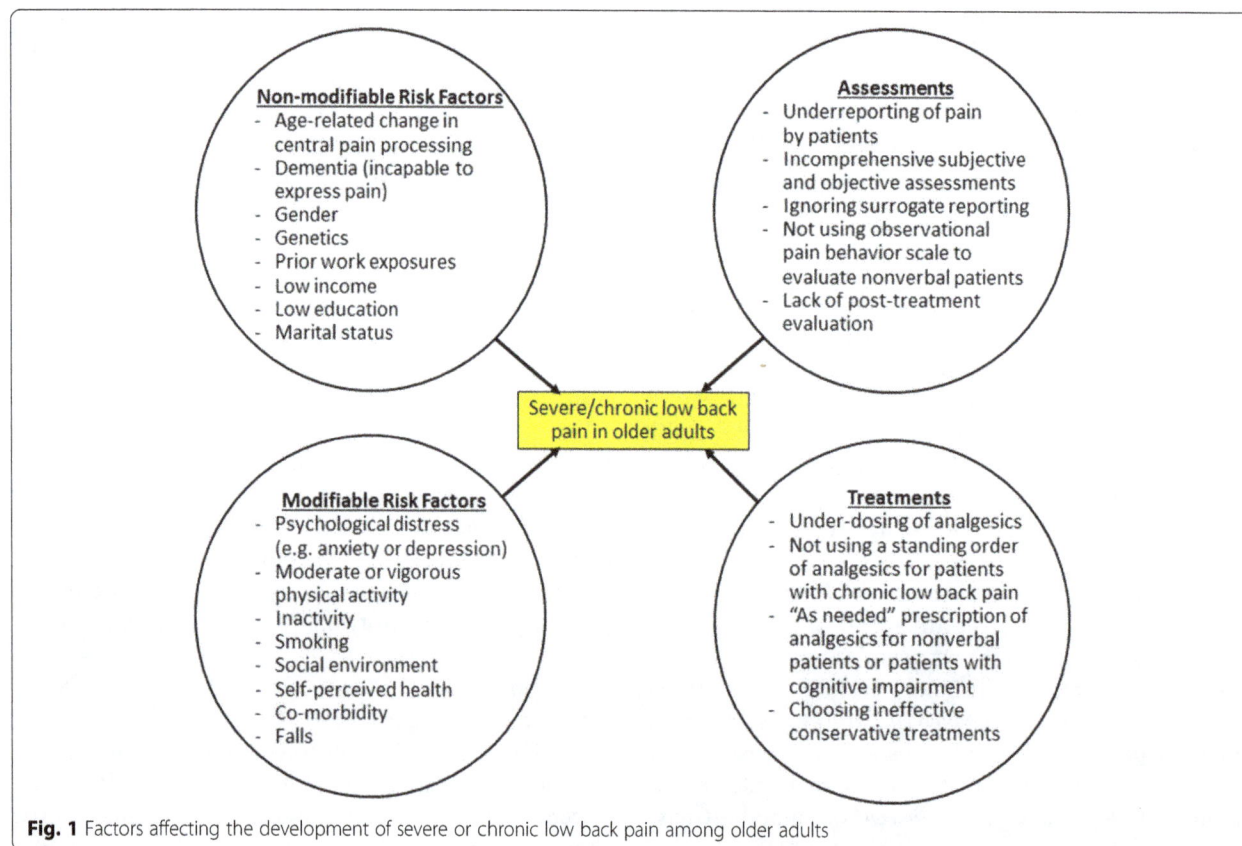

**Fig. 1** Factors affecting the development of severe or chronic low back pain among older adults

compared to young adults [120]. Although speculative, the increased pain sensitivity in older adults may be attributed to diminished descending pain inhibition in older adults. Neuroimaging studies have shown that the volumes of brain regions responsible for pain processing (i.e., the cingulate, insula, striatum, hippocampus, cerebellum, and prefrontal cortex) significantly reduce as people age [121–126]. These findings may indicate age-related reduction in perceptual motor processing, diminished coordination of inhibitory motor response to noxious stimuli, and/or impaired descending endogenous pain inhibitory modulation [127–130]. Since patients with fibromyalgia are known to have significantly less striatal release of dopamine in response to experimental muscle pain [131] and people with chronic LBP are characterized by regional decreases in gray matter density in bilateral striatum (especially nucleus accumbens, putamen, and caudate) [132], the reduced pain-related striatal activity in seniors may indicate age-related impairment in endogenous pain modulation [127–129].

Additionally, age-related changes in neuroplasticity may decrease the pain tolerance in older adults. Compared to younger individuals, older people tend to show more rapid temporal summation of noxious heat stimuli in their central nervous system [116, 133–135]. Similarly, older adults display a prolonged period of capsaicin-induced hyperalgesia that may lead to relentless pain sensitization and sluggish resolution of neuroplastic change [115]. Importantly, the central pain processing can be further complicated by dementia-related neurodegeneration [113, 136]. Depending on the severity, locations or types of neurodegenerative changes, seniors with dementia or Alzheimer's disease have demonstrated increased pain threshold and tolerance [137] or decreased pain threshold [138, 139]/pain tolerance [140]. Taken together, age-related changes in central pain processing of older adults may contribute to severe or chronic LBP in seniors.

Importantly, people with chronic back pain suffer from global and regional changes in functional connectivity and/or gray matter density in the brain that may perpetuate persistent pain [132, 141]. Human resting-state functional MRI research has revealed that, as compared to asymptomatic individuals, patients with chronic pain (i.e., back pain, osteoarthritis, and complex pain regional syndrome) demonstrate significantly decreased functional connectivity of the whole-brain and diminished regional connectivity in specific brain regions (e.g., supplementary motor cortex, mid-anterior cingulate cortex, superior parietal lobe, and part of the somatosensory network) but enhanced connectivity in thalamus and hippocampus [141]. These patients also display changes in allegiance of insula nodes or some lateral parietal

nodes to certain brain modules (e.g., the sensorimotor brain module, default–mode network module, and attention module) [141]. These findings indicate that chronic pain is associated with decreased motor planning (supplementary motor cortex) and attention (superior parietal lobe) but increased somatosensory inputs to the cortex (thalamus) and chronification (hippocampus) [142, 143]. Similarly, a 1-year longitudinal study showed that people who experienced persistent back pain during the study period demonstrated significant decreases in global gray matter density as compared to healthy controls and patients who recovered during the period [132]. The same study found that patients with persistent back pain had significant regional decreases in gray matter density at bilateral nucleus accumbens (a key mesolimbic region), insula (pain perception cortex) [144–146], and left primary sensorimotor cortex, yet reduced negative functional connectivity between insula and precuneus/dorsolateral prefrontal cortex, and diminished functional connectivity of primary sensorimotor cortex [132]. The consistent findings of various studies suggest that chronic pain may lead to global and/or regional disruption of functional connectivity and structures of the brain that may hinder the treatment effectiveness for people with a history of recurrent or chronic pain [141].

### Gender

Females are more susceptible to chronic LBP than males regardless of age [20, 31, 34, 112]. Jimenez-Sanchez and coworkers [34] estimated that women were two times more likely to develop chronic LBP than men. The higher prevalence of chronic pain in females may be attributed to complex biopsychosocial mechanisms (e.g., less efficient pain, habituation or diffuse noxious inhibitory control [147], genetic sensitivity, pain coping [148], and a higher vulnerability to develop temporal summation of chemically [149] or mechanically evoked pain) [150]. Further, women commonly have a higher number of concomitant chronic diseases (e.g., osteoporosis, osteopenia, and osteoarthritis), which are known to be risk factors for developing chronic LBP and psychological distress in older adults [34, 112].

### Genetic influences

Recent research has highlighted that genetic factors play an imperative role in modulating pain sensitivity, responses to analgesics, and vulnerability to chronic pain development [50]. Some genetic factors not only predispose people to spinal disorders (e.g., scoliosis [151] and intervertebral disc degeneration [152, 153]) but also alter brain structures [154, 155] that may modify central pain processing and perception [156]. For instance, polymorphisms of the catechol-O-methyltransferase gene are known to affect the cognitive and emotion processing of pain in the brain [156]. While variations in some gene expression (e.g., val[158]met single-nucleotide polymorphism (SNP)) may modulate temporal summation of pain [157], other SNPs (e.g., catechol-O-methyltransferase gene, interleukin-6 GGGA haplotype or SCN9A gene, or hereditary sensory neuropathy type II gene) may alter pain sensitivity through different mechanisms (e.g., affecting voltage-gated sodium channels, altering myelination of nerve fibers, or modulating anabolism/catabolism of catecholamine neurotransmitters) [158–163]. Collectively, some people (including seniors) may be more susceptible to develop chronic LBP because of their genetic makeup. Future studies are warranted to examine if age may modify the expression of pain genes in older adults.

Additionally, genetic variations may influence the analgesic requirement or treatment responses to opioid analgesics [164]. A recent meta-analysis underscores that SNP A118G (a genetic variant of $\mu$-opioid receptors, OPRM1) can modify postoperative opioid requirement and analgesic responses [165]. Notably, while Asians with minor G allele require more postoperative opioid analgesics, Caucasian counterparts do not display increased opioid analgesic requirements. This discrepancy highlights the genetic differences between the two ethnic groups and/or distinct interactions between A118G SNP and environmental influences [165]. Interestingly, the OPRM1 A118G SNP has significant influence only on the treatment responses of patients receiving morphine but not fentanyl [165]. The divergent pharmacogenetic responses indicate that different opioids may have different ligand-receptor dynamics [166]. Importantly, the expression of other pain genes (e.g., COMT or beta-2 adrenergic receptor alleles) [158, 167, 168] and other polymorphisms in the OPRM1 gene locus [169] can interact with A118G SNP and environment to cause differential pain sensitivity and opioid treatment responses in different races and gender [164, 170]. As such, it highlights that individual treatment responses of patients with LBP may be related to different pharmacogenetic variations.

### Prior work exposures

While occupational exposures to whole-body vibrations, lifting, bending, twisting, stooping, have been identified as potential risk factors for LBP in the working-age group [171], increasing evidence suggests that previous occupational exposure to physically strenuous work increases the risks of LBP in retired seniors [172, 173]. A prospective study involving more than 1500 individuals showed that previous occupational biomechanical exposure to bending/twisting or driving for at least 10 years increased the odds of having persistent LBP in retired

adults aged 58 to 67 years after adjusting for body mass index and psychological disorders [172]. Likewise, retired post office workers aged 70 to 75 years with LBP were characterized by more than 20 years of work-related regular lifting of heavy weights [173].

### Demographic factors

Lower education levels, lower income, and smoking are related to higher propensity of LBP in older people [20, 21, 31, 112]. It is suggested that more educated individuals experience less LBP symptoms because they have a better understanding of pain, a better compliance to treatment, and a strong willingness to adopt a healthy lifestyle [174]. Conversely, people with poor economic status may have difficulty in accessing healthcare in certain places [175]. Patients with limited resources may delay seeking healthcare until their symptoms are intolerable, which in turn increases the chronicity/severity of LBP across the life course [176]. A multinational study has shown that people in the poorest socioeconomic quintile were 1.4 times more likely to have LBP with reference to the highest quintile [31]. Interestingly, compared to those older adults who have never married, those divorced, married, separated, and widowed have at least 1.5 times odds to experience LBP [31].

### Modifiable risk factors
### Yellow flags

Psychological distress (e.g., anxiety or depression) is a risk factor for persistent or debilitating LBP in older adults [34]. A longitudinal study showed that older persons with a high depressive symptom score at baseline were two times more likely to have LBP at the 4-year follow-up [17]. Similarly, Reid et al. [177] found that depression was significantly correlated to disabling LBP in seniors aged 70 years or above. Importantly, since persistent LBP can also be a predictor of depression and anxiety [178], psychological assessments should be incorporated in the examination of older patients with chronic LBP.

Multiple studies have found that fear-avoidance beliefs (FAB) are closely related to chronic LBP in older people [179–181]. A cross-sectional study consisting of 103 older patients with chronic LBP (65 years or older) and 59-age-matched asymptomatic controls showed that higher FAB as measured by a questionnaire, older age, and higher LBP intensity predicted poorer self-reported functional capacity [179]. Another study on 200 older adults with chronic LBP revealed that higher physical activity subscale scores of the FAB questionnaire were related to higher Roland Morris Disability Questionnaire scores and slower gait speed [180]. Similarly, a population-based survey study found that increased FAB were related to higher self-reported LBP-related disability, poorer physical health, and higher risk of falls in older people (62 years or older) with LBP [181]. Vincent et al. also found that kinesiophobia was related to chronic LBP-related disability in obese older adults [182]. These consistent findings suggest that FAB are important therapeutic target to address among older people with chronic LBP.

Conversely, some studies reported inconsistent findings regarding the relation between other yellow flags (e.g., kinesiophobia and pain catastrophizing) and functional capacity or LBP-related disability [182–184]. A recent randomized controlled trial among 49 obese, older adults with chronic LBP demonstrated that reduction in pain catastrophizing following 4-month resistance exercise was related to decreased self-reported LBP-related disability [184]. However, Ledoux and co-workers found that kinesiophobia, pain catastrophizing, and depression were unrelated to the functional capacity among older adults with chronic LBP [185]. Kovac and colleagues also found that FAB and pain catastrophizing had only a minimal clinically significant effect on self-reported LBP-related disability of community-dwelling older (above 60 years) adults with LBP [183]. This discrepancy may be attributed to differences in study designs, cultures, living environment, or age-related changes in the relative influence of FAB on LBP-related disability level [183]. Given that multiple psychological factors (e.g., anxiety, depression, FAB, and coping strategy) may have different interactions among themselves and other age-related physical and social factors in influencing the genesis and persistence of chronic LBP, future studies should clarify the effect of individual yellow flags on LBP progression among older adults. The findings may help develop optimal multimodal treatment approaches for older adults with LBP [186].

### Physical activity

Different types and amounts of physical activity are related to persistent LBP in older adults [112]. Generally, moderate or vigorous physical activity heightens the risk of LBP regardless of age [112, 171]. A population-based study found that moderate (at least 30 min of moderate intensity activity on five or more days per week) and vigorous (at least 20 min of vigorous activity on three or more days per week) physical activity were significantly associated with increased risk of persistent LBP among women aged greater than or equal to 65 years, while walking for 30 min on five or more days a week and strength exercises on two or more days per week lowered the risk of persistent LBP after adjusting for age and body mass index (BMI) [112]. Similarly, the study identified that strength exercises lowered the risk of LBP among men aged greater than or equal to 65 years after

accounting for age and BMI [112]. As such, clinicians should evaluate the activity level of patients and provide recommendations accordingly.

### Smoking

Like in other age groups, smokers are more likely to experience LBP. It is thought that smokers may have different pain perception as compared to non-smoker although the effect of smoking on pain perception remains unclear [187]. However, animal and human studies have shown that smoking may induce degenerative changes in spinal structures, such as intervertebral discs [188–191]. As such, these degenerative changes may compress the neural structures and cause neuropathic LBP.

### Social factors

Social factors may affect the genesis and persistence of LBP [192]. It is well known that social factors (e.g., the social environment or groups that individuals live, grow up, or belong) can influence the onset and progression of diseases or disability (including widespread pain) [193, 194], especially among older adults [195, 196]. Because social conditions can induce social stressors (e.g., poor housing, crime, and poor living environment), affect risk exposure (e.g., poor eating habit leading to obesity), influence psychology and emotion (e.g., social pressure and sense of inequalities), and compromise access to health services (e.g., health-care education or use of healthcare) [192]. Health-care stakeholders should recognize and address various social factors that can impact older adults with LBP. For example, since older adults with less social ties are more likely to experience disabling pain because of depression [192], proper public health programs and resource allocation (e.g., social work counseling services and health education) may target these vulnerable seniors (e.g., oldest old or seniors with depression). Importantly, residents with LBP living in long-term care facilities may rely on nursing home staff (e.g., nursing assistants) to provide medications or personal care. The attentiveness and responsiveness of nursing home staff will affect the recovery and persistency of LBP in these residents.

### Self-perceived health

Seniors with poor self-perceived health status are more likely to experience severe LBP. A cross-sectional study on adults aged between 70 to 102 years found that poor self-rated health was strongly associated with LBP [197]. Similarly, a longitudinal study revealed that people with poor self-reported health were four times more likely to report LBP at the 4-year follow-up than those reporting very good health [17]. The same study also found that those who required health or social services (e.g., meals on wheels or home help) at baseline had a significantly higher risk of reporting LBP at follow-up [17].

### Comorbidity

Research has shown that comorbidities are related to chronic LBP in seniors. Jacobs et al. [35] found that females, hypertension, joint pain, pre-existing LBP, and loneliness, were predictors for developing persistent LBP in individuals aged 70 years. Another study revealed that comorbid chronic conditions were positively related to at least one LBP episode in the last month in low- and middle-income countries [31]. Specifically, the odds of LBP were 2.7 times higher among seniors with one chronic comorbid condition, compared to seniors without comorbidities, while the odds ratio was 4.8 for people with two or more comorbidities [31]. As mentioned above, patients with Parkinson's disease may experience hypersensitivity of pain due to the decrease in striatal dopaminergic function [198, 199]. However, such pain can be alleviated by the administration of L-dopa [200].

### Special considerations for low back pain management of seniors

While comprehensive history taking, self-reports of pain characteristics and pain-related disability, as well as proper physical examination all are necessary for differential diagnosis among older adults with LBP [201], attention should be also given to assessment and

treatment of seniors with LBP so as to optimize pain management (Fig. 1).

### Self-reported pain assessments

While patients with mild-to-moderate dementia can reliably report pain intensity using traditional visual analog scale or Numeric Rating Scale (NRS) [202, 203], other self-reported pain assessment tools have been developed and validated in the older population to improve pain evaluation (Table 1). The 11-point NRS is commonly used in clinical settings, where 0 means no pain and 10 means the worst pain imaginable [204]. Faces Pain Scale and Revised Faces Pain Scale (FPS) comprise different facial expressions indicating different severity of pain experienced by patients [205]. They have been validated among different older populations [168, 204, 206–208] and were rated as preferred tools over the NRS by Chinese [209] and African-Americans [210]. The Iowa Pain Thermometer (IPT) is a descriptor scale presented alongside a thermometer to help patients conceptualize pain intensity as temperature levels [204]. Compared to the FPS, Verbal Descriptor Scale, and visual analog scale, the IPT is deemed to be the most preferred scale among older adults [204].

### Observational pain assessments

Although self-reported pain assessment is the gold standard, clinicians need to validate the self-reported pain with observed pain behavior during physical

**Table 1** Self-reported pain assessment tools for older adults with cognitive impairment

| Scale | Description | Psychometric properties |
|---|---|---|
| Numeric Rating Scale (NRS) [204] | A line with numbers 0 to 10 displayed at equal intervals, where 0 means no pain and 10 means the worst pain imaginable. | NRS has been validated among older adults [300, 311, 312]. The completion rate was high for people with cognitive impairment. The completion rate decreased in people with mild (76%) to moderate (58%) cognitive impairment [313]. |
| Faces Pain Scale (FPS) Revised Faces Pain Scale (FPS-R) [206, 207] | Consists of different facial expressions to indicate different severity of pain experienced by patients. | Both are reliable and valid in older people with cognitive impairments and with different cultural background [204, 209, 210, 314, 315] For patients with deficits in facial recognition, the results should be interpreted with care [316]. |
| Iowa Pain Thermometer (IPT) [204] | A descriptor scale presented with a graphic thermometer showing a color gradient from white to red in order to help patients rate their pain intensity as temperature. Additional choices between words are available to improve the sensitivity of the scale. | Older adults with cognitive impairment are more likely to correctly complete IPT as compared to NRS, Verbal Descriptor Scale, FPS, and visual analog scale [204]. IPT is the most preferred scale by both young and older adults (with osteoarthritic pain) [204]. |
| Verbal Descriptor Scale (VDS) [317] | Consists of seven verbal descriptions to indicate different severity of pain ranging from 0 to 6, where 0 means "no pain" and 6 means "pain as bad as it could be." | VDS score agrees with the ratings of FPS or NRS but their associations are not linearly related [317]. The majority (90%) of people with moderate cognitive impairment can accurately use VDS [313]. A simplified version has been developed for people with severe dementia [318] |
| Visual Analog Scale (VAS) [319] | A 10-cm line with 0 means no pain and 10 means the worst possible pain. | VAS has significantly higher error (approximately 20%) among older adults as compared to NRS and VDS [203, 320, 321]. |

examination. While some seniors with cognitive impairment may report exaggerated pain without coherent pain behavior due to perseveration [211–214], others (e.g., with severe dementia or poststroke aphasia) may have difficulty in communicating pain intensity or pain-related disability [215] that may lead to insufficient/inappropriate treatment [216]. Currently, there is no consented guideline regarding the relation between the trustworthiness of self-reported pain and cognitive functioning [217]. Therefore, healthcare providers (e.g., physicians or nursing home nurses) should identify people with potential cognitive impairment and modify their pain assessment and treatment in order to effectively manage cognitively impaired patients with LBP. It has been suggested that clinicians should consider assessing the cognitive function of older adults with LBP if patients have a known history of dementia, self or family report of memory loss, difficulty in providing details of LBP history that requires supplementary input from caregivers, age above 85 years, or inconsistency between observed pain behaviors and self-reported pain [212, 213, 218]. Some dementia screening tools (e.g., Montreal Cognitive Assessment [219], Mini-Cog [220, 221], and Saint Louis University mental status examination [222]) have been recommended based on their psychometric properties, ease of use, and accuracy in identifying people with dementia [223]. Patients with positive screening results should be referred to subspecialty dementia experts (e.g., neurologists, geriatricians, or geriatric psychiatrists) for formal dementia evaluation in addition to LBP treatment. Collectively, early identification of cognitive impairment and psychiatric comorbidity (e.g., depression) in older adults with LBP can optimize the pain management plan (e.g., assistance from caregivers and prescription of psychiatric medications).

Since people with moderate to severe dementia may display agitation, anxiety, or nonverbal pain behaviors (e.g., grimacing, yelling, hitting, or bracing), failure to detect pain as a potential cause of agitation may result in unnecessary prescription of anxiolytics or antipsychotics [224]. As such, proper procedures for evaluating nonverbal dementia patients should include: using a validated observational assessment tool to evaluate pain behaviors during rest and painful conditions/procedures, seeking surrogate report of pain behaviors, and monitoring responses following an analgesic trial [223]. Since the prevalence of dementia in people aged 85 or older can be as high as 50% [218], family members or informants are recommended to accompany these patients to meet health-care providers so as to provide detailed pain information [223]. Several recent reviews have identified at least 24 observational pain assessment instruments for estimating pain in nonverbal patients [225–227]. Table 2 describes six commonly used assessment instruments. Unfortunately, since many of

them only detect the presence/absence of pain, rather than quantify the pain severity [217, 228], these tools may be better used to monitor longitudinal changes in pain (e.g., increases/decreases in pain behavior) or treatment responses. Regardless, if the observational pain behavior assessment indicates the presence of significant pain in patients, the sources of pain should be identified through physical examination and proper treatment should be given. If inconsistency occurs between the observational assessment and self-report of pain, other causes (e.g., fear of pain and depression) should be identified and managed. If comprehensive evaluations and an analgesic trial cannot identify any sources of pain experienced by patients with dementia, the persistent pain complaint may be attributed to pain perseveration, which is the repetitive reporting of pain without actual distress. Collectively, future studies should refine existing observational tools by identifying the most important behaviors for evaluating the presence and severity of pain (including LBP) in cognitively impaired patients.

It is noteworthy that although certain physiological parameters (e.g., increased heart rate, blood pressure, and perspiration) may indicate the presence of pain, these physiological indicators may be inaccurate among older adults with chronic pain [217]. Additionally, older adults with dementia may have diminished autonomic reactions to pain [229, 230]. Therefore, effective evaluation of pain behavior may be more relevant for older adults with severe dementia and pain.

### Fall assessment and prevention

Given that older people usually display reduced physical capacity [231], cardiac output [232], muscle mass and strength [233], and older adults with LBP are more likely to suffer from decreased mobility and functional deterioration than younger sufferers. In addition, older adults with musculoskeletal pain are more likely to experience fear of falling [234] and fall incidents [23]. Specifically, LBP is known to be an independent risk factor for repeated falls in older women [235]. A prospective study revealed that community-dwelling seniors with chronic LBP (more than 3 months) had a significantly higher risk of falls (adjusted OR for injurious falls ranged from 2.11 to 2.46) as compared to asymptomatic counterparts [236]. Likewise, seniors with LBP in the past 12 months are more likely to be recurrent fallers [23]. Since falls is the leading cause of persistent pain, disability, and mortality among seniors [36, 237], physicians and nursing home workers should assess fall risks of older adults with LBP [238] and refer them for fall prevention intervention, if necessary.

**Table 2** Six commonly used nonverbal pain tools for older adults with cognitive impairment

| Scale | Description | Psychometric Properties |
|---|---|---|
| Checklist of Nonverbal Pain Indicators (CNPI) [322] | An observational scale monitoring pain behaviors in 6 behavioral items (vocal complaints, nonverbal sound, facial grimace/winces, bracing, rubbing, and restlessness) at rest and during movement. An item is rated 0 or 1 based on the absence or presence of a pain behavior. The presence of any of the pain behavior indicates pain. There are no cutoff scores to represent pain severity. | Nursing home residents. Good internal consistency ($a = 0.92$ to 0.97 at rest; $a = 0.74$ to 0.90 during movement); Good construct validity but having a great floor effect at rest [323] Good construct validity against NOPPAIN, PACSLAC, and PAINAD ($r = 0.66$ to 0.71) [324] Interrater reliability for behaviors ($K$ ranged from 0.63 to 0.82) [322] moderate inter-rater reliability at rest ($K = 0.43$); Fair inter-rater reliability with movement ($K = 0.25$) [323] Test-retest reliability ranged from 0.44 to 0.56, inter-rater reliability ranged from 0.58 to 0.71, internal consistency $a$ ranged from 0.76 to 0.82, and factor analysis revealed that CNPI might have more than 1 factor [325]. Older patients with hip fracture in a surgical ward internal consistency ($a = 0.54$ at rest; $a = 0.64$ with movement) [322] |
| The Abbey Pain Scale (APS) [326] | For people with end-stage dementia. Comprises 6 questions regarding the facial expression, vocalization, change in body language, behavioral change, physiological change, and physical changes. Each question can be given a score from 0 to 3, where 0 means absence while 3 means severe. Higher total scores indicate higher pain intensity. | The Australian Pain Society has endorsed this scale for evaluating pain in older people with dementia [226]. Nursing home residents. A strong agreement (66.1 to 78.3%) between proxy-reported APS scores and presence of self-reported pain, moderate correlation between self-reported pain intensity and APS ($r = 0.56$; $p < 0.01$) residents with cognitive impairment; 25.4% above chance to correctly identify cognitively impaired patients with pain [300]. Concurrent validity between the APS and nurse's holistic pain assessment was acceptable (Gamma = 0.59; $p < 0.01$), internal reliability ($a = 0.74$–0.81), inter-rater reliability was modest (but no actual statistics) [326] Moderate to good construct validity against PACSLAC and PAINAD at rest and exercise ($r = 0.56$–0.85) [327] Test-retest reliability ($r = 0.62$–0.68), inter-rater reliability (ICC = 0.70–0.75), internal consistency ($a = 0.65$–0.80). Factor analysis only revealed 1 single factor [325]. Patients in Geriatric wards It has been translated into Danish and tested on severely demented and non-communicative older patients in geriatric wards. There was a poor agreement between APS and verbal rating scale ($k = 0.42$), interrater reliability was good (ICC = 0.84). Fair internal consistence (Cronbach's $a = 0.52$) [328]. |
| The Doloplus 2 [329] | 10-item scale evaluating three domains: (1) somatic, (2) psychomotor, and (3) psychosocial; Each item has four potential scores, where 0 means normal behavior and 3 indicates high levels of pain-related behavior. It is administered by a trained nurse. | It was originally developed in French but has been translated into English. Two systematic reviews rated Doloplus 2 as a scale with high-psychometric properties [226]. Nursing home residents. Internal consistency ($a = 0.82$–0.87) [325, 330]. Criterion validity between Doloplus-2 score rated by a geriatric expert nurse and pain evaluation conducted by a pain expert ($R2 = 0.54$); inter-rater reliability (ICC = 0.74–0.77). Small but significant correlation between the expert's pain in movement score and the Doloplus-2 item for protective body at rest score and for the expert's pain at rest score ($R2 = 0.12$; $p < 0.01$) and between Doloplus-2 item and pain complaints ($R2 = 0.13$; $p < 0.01$) [330]. Factor analysis only revealed one single factor [325]. Test-retest reliability ($r = 0.71$), inter-rater reliability (ICC = 0.73–0.81) [325]. |
| Noncommunicative Patient's Pain Assessment Instrument (NOPPAIN) [331] | A nursing assistant-administered observation tool for recognizing and rating of extent of pain behaviors. Contains four sections considering six pain behaviors (pain-related words, facial expression, pain noises, rubbing, bracing, and restlessness) during common care conditions (e.g., bathing). Each pain response can be rated from 0 to 5 on a surrogate Likert scale, where 0 indicates the lowest possible intensity and 5 means the highest possible intensity. | The National Nursing Home Pain Collaborative acknowledged the scale in evaluating pain behaviors but reported that the complexity of NOPPAIN might limit its clinical use [225]. It has to be validated in clinical setting. Nursing home setting. Excellent agreement ($k = 0.87$) for assessing video tape results [300]. Strong agreement (69.2 to 80.0%) between proxy-rated pain behaviors and self-reported presence of pain [300]. |

**Table 2** Six commonly used nonverbal pain tools for older adults with cognitive impairment *(Continued)*

| | | |
|---|---|---|
| | | Moderate correlation between self-reported pain intensity and NOPPAIN ($r = 0.68$; $p < 0.01$) in residents with cognitive impairment. There was 25.4% above chance to correctly identify cognitively impaired patients with pain [300]. Good construct validity against CNPI, PACSLAC, and PAINAD ($r = 0.71$–$0.78$) [324, 327]. High intra-rater reliability ($k = 0.70$–$0.86$), high inter-rater reliability ($k = 0.72$–$1.0$) [324, 331, 332]. |
| Pain Assessment Checklist for Seniors with Limited Ability to Communicate (PACSLAC) [333] | PACSLAC evaluates 60 pain behaviors classified into four subscales: (1) facial expression, (2) social behavior mood and personality, (3) physical activity and body movement, and (4) physiological changes, eating or sleeping changes, and vocal behaviors. PASCLAC-II consists of 31 items by removing items that may be mixed with signs of delirium [334]. | Both PACSLAC and PACSLAC-II cover all observational pain assessment domains recommended by the American Geriatrics Society Guideline [301, 335]. Two systematic reviews also suggest PACSLAC as one of the psychometrically strongest assessment tools [226, 227]. Nursing home settings. PACSLAC internal consistency ($a = 0.62$–$0.92$) [336, 337]. PACSLAC-II internal consistency ($a = 0.74$–$0.77$) [334]. Moderate correlations between PACSLAC scores and global pain intensity ratings ($r = 0.39$–$0.54$) [337]. Good correlation between PACSLAC scores and VDS ($r = 0.81$) and VAS ($0.72$–$0.86$) for unblended rating of acute influenza injection [336]. Both PACSLAC and PACSLAC-II have demonstrated good differentiation between painful and non-painful states in patients ($p < 0.01$) [324, 334]. Good construct validity against NOPPAIN and PAINAD ($r = 0.66$–$0.78$) [324]. Good construct validity against APS ($r = 0.79$) [327]. PACSLAC and PACSLAC-II have strong correlation ($r = 0.81$–$0.89$) and the NOPPAIN ($r = 0.73$) [334]. Inter-rater reliability at rest and during movement (ICC $\geq 0.76$) [299, 324, 327]. Inter-rater reliability ($k = 0.63$) for PACSLAC-II [334]. Excellent inter-rater reliability (ICC $= 0.93$–$0.96$); Intra-rater reliability (ICC $= 0.86$) for unblended rating of acute influenza vaccination [336]. |
| The Pain Assessment in Advanced Dementia (PAINAD) Scale [228, 338] | A 5-min observation during activity. It evaluates five behaviors (breathing, negative vocalization, facial expression, body language, and consolability) as five indicators of discomfort rated on three levels: 0=absent, 1=present but not constant or severe, 2=severe/constant. | The National Nursing Home Pain Collaborative recommended the PAINAD for clinical use [225]. It has been validated in acute care setting and nursing homes [339]. Nursing home settings. High internal consistency ($a > 0.70$) [323, 327]. It can detect the presence or absence of pain but not the severity of pain [340]. Strong agreement (66.1 to 73.3%) between PAINAD and proxy-rated pain behaviors or self-reported presence/absence. There was 19.2% above chance to correctly identify cognitively impaired patients with pain [300]. High correlation between PAINAD scores and nurses' pain reports (Kendall's $\tau = 0.84$) [341]. PAINAD scores decreased following administration of analgesics and changes with potentially painful activity [324, 336]. Good construct validity with CNPI, APS, NOPPAIN, and PACSLAC at rest and during exercise ($r = 0.56$–$0.90$) [324, 327] High inter-rater reliability ($r = 0.80$–$0.97$) and test-retest reliability ($r = 0.90$) [228, 342, 343]. |

### Pain medications

The American Geriatrics Society has published recommendations on pain management of geriatric patients with nonmalignant pain. In particular, a standing order of analgesic (e.g., acetaminophen) is recommended for older adults with chronic pain so that they can have a steady concentration of analgesic in the blood stream [239]. Tramadol is recommended to be prescribed with caution for patients with a known risk of seizure (e.g.,

stroke, epilepsy, and head injury) or for those taking medications that may lower seizure threshold (e.g., neuroleptics and tricyclics) [239]. In addition, the guideline also suggests that if acetaminophen cannot control pain, non-steroidal anti-inflammatory drugs (NSAIDs) (e.g., COX-2 therapy or non-acetylated salicylates) may be used as adjunct therapy [239]. However, since some traditional NSAIDs may cause gastrointestinal upset, clinicians are recommended to prescribe non-acetylated salicylates for older patients with peptic ulcer and gastrointestinal bleeding. Although there is no ideal dose for opioid prescription among older adults with LBP, the effective dose should be carefully titrated to fit individual needs. To attain better pain relief with minimal side effects secondary to a high dose of a single medication, it is recommended to concurrently use two or more pain medications with different mechanisms of action or different drug classes (e.g., opioid and non-opioid analgesics). It is noteworthy that opioid (e.g., codeine) may increase the risk of falls and other drug-related adverse effects (e.g., depression, nausea, tachycardia, seizure, or falls [240, 241]) in opioid-naïve older patients during the opioid initiation period (i.e., within the first 3 months) or during the use of long-acting opioids [242, 243]. Therefore, specific education and caution should be given to these patient groups.

In addition, because older patients with chronic LBP are commonly associated with depression or anxiety, it is not uncommon for them to take antidepressants (e.g., serotonin reuptake inhibitors) or benzodiazepines. Since some of these psychoactive drugs may compromise their memory, cognition, alertness and motor coordination [244, 245], special care should be given to these patients to minimize their risks of falls, hip fractures, or road traffic accidents [246]. For instance, concurrent prescription of tramadol and the selective serotonin reuptake inhibitor (an antidepressant) may increase the risk of serotonin syndrome (e.g., hyperthermia, agitation, diarrhea, tachycardia, and coma) that may lead to sudden death [247, 248]. If patients have an elevated risk of opioid overdose (e.g., alcoholism [249], a history of opioid overdose/drug abuse [250], concurrent consumption of benzodiazepine or sedative hypnotics [251], or poor compliance to opiate medications [252]), they should undergo an overdose risk assessment, a urine drug abuse screening prior to opioid prescription, an education on drug overdose, and frequent clinical follow-up so as to mitigate their risk [253]. Further, physicians can prescribe naloxone to these high-risk patients and teach them/their caregivers to use it at emergency. Naloxone is an opiate antidote for neutralizing the toxicity of opioid overdoses [253, 254]. For patients who are taking long-acting opioids (e.g., oxycodone or methadone) or having hepatic or renal dysfunction, they should be reassessed regularly in order to ensure timely tapering/discontinuing of opioids if necessary [253]. Collectively, existing medical guidelines generally recommend low-dose initiation and gradual titration of opioid therapy and constipation prophylaxis, increased awareness of potential interactions among concurrent medications, as well as close monitoring of treatment responses in patients. It is necessary to provide updated education to health-care

providers so as to optimize pain management for older patients with chronic pain.

### Other conservative treatments

Although analgesics are the first line treatment for older people with LBP, older people with LBP (especially those with a prolonged history of LBP) may require other conservative treatments to mitigate pain and to restore function. Growing evidence has indicated that some, but not all, conservative treatments can benefit older people with LBP [255, 256]. While the efficacy of various physiotherapy modalities in treating older people with LBP remains controversial [256], a recent meta-analysis has highlighted that Tai Chi, a mind-body exercise therapy, is an effective intervention for older patients with chronic pain (including LBP, osteoarthritis, fibromyalgia, and osteoporotic pain) as compared to education or stretching [255]. Importantly, in addition to pain relief, various systematic reviews on Tai Chi have revealed promising outcomes in improving balance [257], fear of falling [258], lower limb strength [259], physical function [260], hypertension [261], cognitive performance [262], and depression [263] in seniors as compared to no treatment or usual care. Given the high frequency of physical and psychological comorbidity among older adults (e.g., depression, hypertension, and osteoarthritis), Tai Chi appears to be a viable LBP treatment option for older adults with LBP. Future studies should determine the dose response of Tai Chi in treating older people with LBP in community and institutional settings.

### Lumbar surgery

Surgical intervention is indicated for older people only if there is a definite diagnosis of lumbar pathology (e.g., degenerative LSS, cauda equine syndrome, or spinal tumor) that needs to be treated by surgery or that is unresponsive to conservative intervention. While there are many different lumbar surgical interventions, the objective of these approaches is to minimize compression of neural tissues and/or enhance spinal stability. Decompression surgery (i.e., laminectomy, laminotomy, and discectomy) is used to partially or completely remove lumbar structures that are impinging neural tissues [264, 265]. Recent evidence suggests that minimally invasive spine surgery techniques have higher success rate than open lumbar decompression surgery [266]. Unlike decompression surgery, spinal fusion surgery utilizes bone grafts (autograft or allograft) or surgical devices to fuse adjacent vertebrae anteriorly, posteriorly, or circumferentially. Such surgery immobilizes the spinal motion segment, in theory removes key pain generating sources and eliminates intersegmental movement of vertebrae that may compress neural structures in order to alleviate symptoms [267]. In general, both simple and complex spinal fusion surgeries are associated with a higher risk of major complications and postoperative mortality as compared to decompression surgery [264]. While decompressive laminectomy/laminotomy with or without spinal fusion is a common surgical intervention for older patients with degenerative LSS [268], isolated decompression without spinal fusion is a preferred choice for older patients with lumbar degenerative spondylolisthesis without severe LBP/instability [269]. However, two recent randomized controlled trials have reported conflicting results regarding the effectiveness of decompression surgery plus spinal fusion versus decompression surgery alone in treating patients with LSS and degenerative spondylolisthesis [270, 271]. Decompression and spinal fusion are also indicated for patients with symptomatic degenerative lumbar scoliosis [272, 273] although these procedures may increase the risk of complications in older adults (especially those with comorbidities) [268, 272, 274–276]. Recently, disc arthroplasty has been adopted to restore the mobility of an intervertebral joint by replacing a degenerative disc with an artificial disc and minimizing the risk of adjacent segment degeneration/disease [277]. Although current evidence notes the safety and efficacy of such intervention for indication for cervical spine pathology in comparison to conventional interbody fusion procedures, outcomes for lumbar disc disorders remain under further evaluation.

Percutaneous transpedicular vertebroplasty and balloon kyphoplasty are two minimally invasive techniques for treating patients with painful osteoporotic vertebral compression fracture [278]. These procedures involve the injection of a small amount of bone cement into the collapsed vertebral body to alleviate excruciating pain and stabilize the fractured vertebral body [279]. However, individual studies have found that these procedures may heighten the risk of new vertebral fractures at the treated or adjacent vertebrae, and other complications (e.g., cement leakage into the lungs, veins, and the vertebral body) [280–283]. However, a recent meta-analysis reveals that these vertebral augmentation procedures may attenuate pain and correct deformity of patients with osteoporotic vertebral compression fractures without increasing the risk of complications or new vertebral fractures along the spine [278].

In addition, the past decade alone has seen a significant interest in the concept of sagittal alignment and balance with respect to the preoperative planning and predictive outcome analyses of patients with various lumbar spinal disorders and spinal deformities [284, 285]. Novel imaging software has been developed to quantify such parameters, such as pelvic incidence and tilt, and sacral slope, in a semi-automatic fashion [286, 287]. Numerous studies have noted the clinical utility assessing spinal alignment/balance [288–292] a field that

continues to gain widespread momentum and motivate future research.

Like conservative LBP treatments, some patients may experience persistent LBP (with or without sciatica) even after spinal surgery. The reasons for the failed back surgery syndrome (FBSS) may be ascribed to technical failure, incorrect selection of surgical patients, surgical complications, or related sequelae [267]. Additionally, since spinal surgery may alter the load distribution at vertebral structures adjacent to the operated segments (e.g., sacroiliac joint), this may result in the adjacent segment disease and pain. Because patients with FBSS are unlikely to benefit from revision surgery, spinal cord stimulation has been suggested to manage pain in these patients. Specifically, spinal cord stimulation involves the placement of electrodes into the epidural space and the generation of electrical current by a pulse generator placed subcutaneously. Studies have noted that there is fair evidence to support moderate effectiveness of spinal cord stimulation in attenuating persistent radicular pain of appropriately selected patients with FBSS although device-related complications are also common [267].

It is noteworthy that while surgical intervention may benefit some patients with LBP, clinicians should weigh the risks and benefits of surgery for each individual patient. A recent Cochrane review summarized the evidence regarding the effectiveness of surgical and conservative treatments for patients with LSS [293]. Two of the five included randomized controlled trials reported that patients undergoing spinal decompression with or without fusion had no significant difference in pain-related disability (measured by Oswestry Disability Index) from those receiving multi-modal conservative care at 6 and 12 months although the decompression group demonstrated improved disability at 24 months [294, 295]. Similarly, a small-scale included study found no significant difference in pain outcomes between decompression and usual non-surgical care (bracing and exercise) at 3 months, and 4- and 10-year follow-ups [296]. Another included study revealed that minimally invasive mild decompression was no better than epidural steroid injections in improving Oswestry Disability Index scores at 6 weeks although decompression had significantly better pain reduction but less improvement in Zurich Claudication Questionnaire scores [297]. Conversely, an included trial found that an interspinous spacer was significantly better than usual non-operative care in reducing symptoms and restoring physical function at 6 weeks, and 6 and 12 months [298]. Regardless of the treatment effects, approximately 10 to 24% of participants experienced peri or postoperative complications (e.g., lesion to the dural sac, hematoma, infection, spinous process fracture, respiratory distress, coronary ischemia, stroke, and even death secondary to pulmonary edema) while no side effect was documented for any conservative treatments [293]. Given above, back surgery should be considered carefully for high-risk patients (e.g., older adults with medical comorbidity). High-quality randomized controlled trials are warranted to compare the effectiveness of surgical versus nonsurgical interventions for older patients with LSS.

**Future research**

While anecdotal evidence and clinical experience suggest that older people appear to have higher rates of LBP with definite pathology (e.g., vertebral osteomyelitis, degenerative spondylolisthesis, and DNDLS), only a few studies have properly evaluated this issue. Given this knowledge gap, future research should quantify the prevalence of various LBP diagnoses so that health care resources can be better allocated to effectively manage the epidemic of LBP in the older population.

Although self-report of LBP is the gold standard for evaluating subjective pain experience, some patients with cognitive impairment may be unable to effectively verbalize their pain. Clinicians (especially those working in the geriatric field) should improve their competence in assessing nonverbal pain expression in patients with cognitive impairment. While multiple observational pain assessment scales have been developed, there is no consensus on the use of a particular assessment tool. Different clinical guidelines have recommended different scales [223, 225]. Given the rapid development and validation of different observational scales in the last decade, it is necessary to update existing guidelines on this issue.

While the scores of several observational pain behavior assessment tools (e.g., the Abbey Pain Scale and Pain Assessment in Advanced Dementia) have been found to be closely related to self-report of pain [299, 300], there is a paucity of research on the interpretation of scale/subscale scores in relation to pain or other psychological comorbidity (e.g., depression). Future studies should establish this relation. Further, most of the existing behavioral observational pain scales have only been validated in the nursing home setting. Future studies are warranted to compare various existing scales and evaluate their responsiveness and sensitivity to changes in pain following treatments in different settings, which can identify best assessment tools for different settings.

Since recent findings suggest that facial expression can provide many useful indirect information of pain, training health-care providers on the recognition and interpretation of facial expression of pain may improve the accuracy and reliability of pain assessment among patients with dementia. Importantly, future studies should adopt computer vision technology to develop automatic, real-time assessment of pain-related facial expression so as to facilitate the evaluation of pain condition in noncommunicable patients with LBP [301].

Currently, clinical assessments of LBP among older adults rely heavily on self-report or surrogate report of LBP or manual physical assessments. With recent advances in technology, clinicians can use reliable novel objective measurements (e.g., mechanical spinal stiffness assessments [302–304], ultrasonic measurements of paraspinal muscles [305], advanced medical imaging [306, 307], or genetic analysis [308]) to examine patients at affordable costs. Given that age-related physical changes (e.g., sarcopenia or fatty infiltration of paraspinal muscles) in older adults may worsen LBP-related physical changes, the adoption of validated objective measurements may enhance the reliability and sensitivity in detecting physical deficits or monitoring posttreatment improvements of LBP in older adults. For example, ultrasonography may be used to quantify atrophy of lumbar multifidus that can guide clinical treatments (e.g., spinal stabilization exercises). Likewise, computerized spinal stiffness tests can be used to identify patients with LBP who are likely to benefit from spinal manipulation [309]. Novel yet more sensitive imaging, such as chemical exchange saturation transfer, T2 mapping, T1-rho, ultra-short time-to-echo and sodium MRI, may identify the pain-generating source allowing for more targeted therapies [50, 310]. Furthermore, a refinement of some of the imaging phenotypes (e.g., disc degeneration, endplate changes, facet joint changes, paraspinal muscle integrity, and sagittal alignment/balance) or the utility of "phenomics" may further aid in proper diagnosis, management options, and the potential development of novel therapeutics. Knowledge gained from such approaches may enhance the exploration of new pathways of pain and potential treatment options in appropriate animal models. Moreover, the role of pain genetics and its actual utility toward the management of LBP in older individuals needs to be further explored. Taken together, while novel technology may gather new information from patients with LBP, clinicians should integrate these objective outcomes with other clinical findings in order to make proper diagnosis and clinical decision.

Given the multifactorial causes of LBP in older adults, it is necessary to consider the entire spectrum of "omic" approaches (e.g., genomics, metabolomics, phenomics, etc), ethnic variations, and all aforementioned risk factors in order to derive appropriate predictive models for future LBP development or severity of pain. These models can then be used to develop cost-effective and personalized LBP intervention for older adults.

## Conclusions

Although LBP is ubiquitous among older adults, the dearth of literature on the trajectories of LBP, determinants of chronic LBP, and effective LBP managements in older adults highlights the research gaps in this area. Given that multiple factors (e.g., dementia, psychiatric and physical comorbidities, maladaptive coping, and age-related physical and psychosocial changes) can modify the LBP experience in older adults, clinicians should incorporate comprehensive subjective, observational, and physical examinations, as well as proxy reports to make accurate diagnosis. For patients with persistent LBP, medical imaging may be ordered to rule out malignant causes of pain. To minimize undertreatment of older adults with LBP, it is necessary to recognize the presence of LBP and to titrate pain medications in accordance with individual needs. Through understanding various factors contributing to severe/chronic LBP in older adults, timely and proper treatment strategies can be formulated. In addition, with the expansive understanding of "omic" technologies, study designs, and findings, new pathways of pain may be identified and novel therapeutics may be developed. As such, it is with a hope that with the understanding of pain being broadened and deepened, the management of older patients with LBP may eventually become more personalized or precise and outcomes optimized, leading to a healthier and productive society.

## Abbreviations

APS: Abbey Pain Scale; BMI: Body mass index; CNPI: Checklist of Nonverbal Pain Indicators; DNDLS: De novo degenerative lumbar scoliosis; FAB: Fear avoidance beliefs; FPS: Faces Pain Scale; IPT: Iowa Pain Thermometer; LBP: Low back pain; LSS: Lumbar spinal stenosis; MRI: Magnetic resonance imaging; NOPPAIN: Noncommunicative Patient's Pain Assessment Instrument; NRS: Numeric Rating Scale; NSAID: Non-steroidal anti-inflammatory drug; PACSLAC: Pain Assessment Checklist for Seniors with Limited Ability to Communicate; PAINAD: Pain Assessment in Advanced Dementia Scale; SNP: Single-nucleotide polymorphism; VAS: Visual Analogue Scale; VDS: Verbal Descriptor Scale; VO: Vertebral osteomyelitis

## Acknowledgements

Not applicable.

## Funding

This work was supported by grants from the Hong Kong Theme-Based Research Scheme (T12-708/12N), the Hong Kong Research Grants Council (17117814), The Hong Kong Polytechnic University Start-up fund (1-ZE4G), and PolyU Central Research Grant-Fund for GRF Project Rated 3.5 (G-YBP9).

## Authors' contributions

AW, JK, and DS all actively contributed to the conception and content of the review. AW conducted the literature searches, abstract, and full-text screening, as well as data extraction. AW prepared the initial draft of the manuscript. All authors critically revised it for main intellectual content. All authors approved the final manuscript.

## Competing interests

The authors declare that they have no competing interests.

## Author details

[1]Department of Rehabilitation Sciences, Faculty of Health and Social Sciences, The Hong Kong Polytechnic University, Hung Hom, Hong Kong, SAR, China. [2]Medical Research Center Oulu, Department of Physical and Rehabilitation Medicine, University of Oulu and Oulu University Hospital, Oulu, Finland. [3]Finnish Institute of Occupational Health, Oulu, Finland. [4]Department of Orthopaedics and Traumatology, The University of Hong Kong, Pokfulam, Hong Kong, SAR, China.

## References

1. Tse MMY, Pun SPY, Benzie IFF. Pain relief strategies used by older people with chronic pain: an exploratory survey for planning patient-centred intervention. J Clin Nurs. 2005;14:315–20.
2. DoEaSA UN. World population ageing 2009. New York: United Nations Publication; 2010.
3. Greengross S, Murphy E, Quam L, Rochon P, Smith R. Aging: a subject that must be at the top of world agendas. BMJ. 1997;315:1029.
4. Bressler HB, Keyes WJ, Rochon PA, Badley E. The prevalence of low back pain in the elderly: a systematic review of the literature. Spine. 1999;24: 1813–9.
5. Podichetty VK, Mazanec DJ, Biscup RS. Chronic non-malignant musculoskeletal pain in older adults: clinical issues and opioid intervention. Postgrad Med J. 2003;79:627–33.
6. Edmond SL, Felson DT. Prevalence of back symptoms in elders. J Rheumatol. 2000;27:220–5.
7. Prince MJ, Wu F, Guo Y, Gutierrez Robledo LM, O'Donnell M, Sullivan R, et al. The burden of disease in older people and implications for health policy and practice. Lancet. 2015;385:549–62.
8. Leveille SG, Guralnik JM, Hochberg M, Hirsch R, Ferrucci L, Langlois J, et al. Low back pain and disability in older women: independent association with difficulty but not inability to perform daily activities. J Gerontol A Biol Sci Med Sci. 1999;54:M487–93.
9. Reid MC, Williams CS, Gill TM. Back pain and decline in lower extremity physical function among community-dwelling older persons. J Gerontol A Biol Sci Med Sci. 2005;60:793–7.
10. Hoy D, Bain C, Williams G, March L, Brooks P, Blyth F, et al. A systematic review of the global prevalence of low back pain. Arthritis Rheum. 2012;64: 2028–37.
11. Cypress BK. Characteristics of physician visits for back symptoms: a national perspective. Am J Public Health. 1983;73:389–95.
12. Balagué F, Pellisé F. Adolescent idiopathic scoliosis and back pain. Scoliosis Spinal Disord. 2016;11:27.
13. Thomas E, Peat G, Harris L, Wilkie R, Croft PR. The prevalence of pain and pain interference in a general population of older adults: cross-sectional findings from the North Staffordshire Osteoarthritis Project (NorStOP). Pain. 2004;110:361–8.
14. Papageorgiou AC, Croft PR, Ferry S, Jayson MIV, Silman AJ. Estimating the prevalence of low back pain in the general population: evidence from the south Manchester back pain survey. Spine. 1995;20:1889–994.
15. Walsh K, Cruddas M, Coggon D. Low back pain in eight areas of Britain. J Epidemiol Community Health. 1992;46:227–30.
16. Dijken CB-V, Fjellman-Wiklund A, Hildingsson C. Low back pain, lifestyle factors and physical activity: a population-based study. J Rehabil Med. 2008; 40:864–9.

17. Docking RE, Fleming J, Brayne C, Zhao J, Macfarlane GJ, Jones GT, et al. Epidemiology of back pain in older adults: prevalence and risk factors for back pain onset. Rheumatology (Oxford). 2011;50:1645–53.

18. Bernabei R, Gambassi G, Lapane K, Landi F, Gatsonis C, Dunlop R, et al. Management of pain in elderly patients with cancer. JAMA. 1998;279:1877–82.

19. Gibson SJ, Helme RD. Age-related differences in pain perception and report. Clin Geriatr Med. 2001;17:433–56.

20. Palacios-Ceña D, Alonso-Blanco C, Hernández-Barrera V, Carrasco-Garrido P, Jiménez-García R, Fernández-de-las-Peñas C. Prevalence of neck and low back pain in community-dwelling adults in Spain: an updated population-based national study. Eur Spine J. 2015;24:482–92.

21. Fernández-de-las-Peñas C, Alonso-Blanco C, Hernández-Barrera V, Palacios-Ceña D, Jiménez-García R, Carrasco-Garrido P. Has the prevalence of neck pain and low back pain changed over the last 5 years? A population-based national study in Spain. Spine J. 2013;13:1069–76.

22. Leopoldino AAO, Diz JBM, Martins VT, Henschke N, Pereira LSM, Dias RC, et al. Prevalence of low back pain in older Brazilians: a systematic review with meta-analysis. Rev Bras Reumatol Engl Ed. 2016;56:258–69.

23. Woo J, Leung J, Lau E. Prevalence and correlates of musculoskeletal pain in Chinese elderly and the impact on 4-year physical function and quality of life. Public Health. 2009;123:549–56.

24. Patel KV, Guralnik JM, Dansie EJ, Turk DC. Prevalence and impact of pain among older adults in the United States: Findings from the 2011 National Health and Aging Trends Study. Pain. 2013;154:2649–57.

25. Ferrell BA. Pain evaluation and management in the nursing home. Ann Intern Med. 1995;123:681–7.

26. Sengstaken EA, King SA. The problems of pain and its detection among geriatric nursing home residents. J Am Geriatr Soc. 1993;41:541–4.

27. Tarzian AJ, Hoffmann DE. Barriers to managing pain in the nursing home: findings from a statewide survey. J Am Med Dir Assoc. 2005;6:S13–9.

28. D'Astolfo CJ, Humphreys BK. A record review of reported musculoskeletal pain in an Ontario long term care facility. BMC Geriatr. 2006;6:5.

29. Cassidy JD, Carroll LJ, Côté P. The Saskatchewan health and back pain survey. The prevalence of low back pain and related disability in Saskatchewan adults. Spine. 1998;23:1860–6. discussion 1867.

30. Dionne CE, Dunn KM, Croft PR. Does back pain prevalence really decrease with increasing age? A systematic review. Age Ageing. 2006;35:229–34.

31. Williams JS, Ng N, Peltzer K, Yawson A, Biritwum R, Maximova T, et al. Risk factors and disability associated with low back pain in older adults in low- and middle-income countries. Results from the WHO Study on Global AGEing and Adult Health (SAGE). PLoS ONE. 2015;10:e0127880.

32. Cayea D, Perera S, Weiner DK. Chronic low back pain in older adults: what physicians know, what they think they know, and what they should be taught. J Am Geriatr Soc. 2006;54:1772–7.

33. Hartvigsen J, Frederiksen H, Christensen K. Back and neck pain in seniors—prevalence and impact. Eur Spine J. 2005;15:802–6.

34. Jiménez-Sánchez S, Fernández-de-las-Peñas C, Carrasco-Garrido P, Hernández-Barrera V, Alonso-Blanco C, Palacios-Ceña D, et al. Prevalence of chronic head, neck and low back pain and associated factors in women residing in the autonomous region of Madrid (Spain). Gac Sanit. 2012;26:534–40.

35. Jacobs JM, Hammerman-Rozenberg R, Cohen A, Stessman J. Chronic back pain among the elderly: prevalence, associations, and predictors. Spine. 2006;31:E203–7.

36. Won AB, Lapane KL, Vallow S, Schein J, Morris JN, Lipsitz LA. Persistent nonmalignant pain and analgesic prescribing patterns in elderly nursing home residents. J Am Geriatr Soc. 2004;52:867–74.

37. American Geriatrics Society Panel on the pharmacological management of persistent pain in older persons, (null). Pharmacological management of persistent pain in older persons. Pain Med. 2009;10:1062–83.

38. Cramer GW, Galer BS, Mendelson MA, Thompson GD. A drug use evaluation of selected opioid and nonopioid analgesics in the nursing facility setting. J Am Geriatr Soc. 2000;48:398–404.

39. Molton IR1, Terrill AL1. Overview of persistent pain in older adults. Am Psychol. 2014;69:197–207.

40. Robinson CL. Relieving pain in the elderly. Health Prog. 2007;88:48–53.

41. Gouke C, Scherer S, Katz B, Gibson S, Farrel M. Pain in residential aged care facilities: management strategies. Australian Pain Society; 2005.

42. Chou R, Fanciullo GJ, Fine PG, Adler JA, Ballantyne JC, Davies P, et al. Clinical guidelines for the use of chronic opioid therapy in chronic noncancer pain. J Pain. 2009;10:113–22.

43. Middleton K, Fish DE. Lumbar spondylosis: clinical presentation and treatment approaches. Curr Rev Musculoskelet Med. 2009;2:94–104.

44. Panta OB, Songmen S, Maharjan S, Subedi K, Ansari MA, Ghimire RK. Morphological changes in degenerative disc diseaseon magnetic resonance imaging: comparison between young and elderly. J Nepal Health Res Counc. 2016;13:209–13.

45. Magee DJ, Sueki D. Orthopedic physical assessment atlas and video. Selected special tests and movements. St. Louis: Elsevier Saunders; 2011.

46. Weinstein JN, Lurie JD, Tosteson TD, Zhao W, Blood EA, Tosteson ANA, et al. Surgical compared with nonoperative treatment for lumbar degenerative spondylolisthesis. J Bone Joint Surg Am. 2009;91:1295–304.

47. Kalichman L, Hunter DJ. Diagnosis and conservative management of degenerative lumbar spondylolisthesis. Eur Spine J Springer-Verlag. 2008;17:327–35.

48. Boden SD, Davis DO, Dina TS, Patronas NJ, Wiesel SW. Abnormal magnetic-resonance scans of the lumbar spine in asymptomatic subjects. A prospective investigation. J Bone Joint Surg Am. 1990;72:403–8.

49. Borenstein DG, O'Mara JW, Boden SD, Lauerman WC, Jacobson A, Platenberg C, et al. The value of magnetic resonance imaging of the lumbar spine to predict low-back pain in asymptomatic subjects: a seven-year follow-up study. J Bone Joint Surg Am. 2001;83-A:1306–11.

50. Samartzis D, Borthakur A, Belfer I, Bow C, Fong DY, Wang H-Q, et al. Novel diagnostic and prognostic methods for disc degeneration and low back pain. Spine J. 2015;15:1919–32.

51. Weiner DK, Sakamoto S, Perera S, Breuer P. Chronic low back pain in older adults: prevalence, reliability, and validity of physical examination findings. J Am Geriatr Soc. 2006;54:11–20.

52. Yoshihara H. Sacroiliac joint pain after lumbar/lumbosacral fusion: current knowledge. Eur Spine J. 2012;21:1788–96.

53. Travell JG, Simons DG. Myofascial pain and dysfunction: the trigger point manual. Baltimore: Williams and Wilkins; 1993.

54. Jirathanathornnukul N, Limthongkul W, Yingsakmongkol W, Singhatanadgige W, Parkpian V, Honsawek S. Increased expression of vascular endothelial growth factor is associated with hypertrophic ligamentum flavum in lumbar spinal canal stenosis. J Investig Med. 2016;64:882–7.

55. Singh K, Samartzis D, Biyani A, An HS. Lumbar spinal stenosis. J Am Acad Orthop Surg. 2008;16:171.

56. Singh K, Samartzis D, Vaccaro AR, Nassr A, Andersson GB, Yoon ST, et al. Congenital lumbar spinal stenosis: a prospective, control-matched, cohort radiographic analysis. Spine J. 2005;5:615–22.

57. Tomkins-Lane C, Melloh M, Lurie J, Smuck M, Battié MC, Freeman B, et al. ISSLS prize winner: consensus on the clinical diagnosis of lumbar spinal stenosis: results of an international delphi study. Spine. 2016;41:1239–46.

58. Fritz JM, Delitto A, Welch WC, Erhard RE. Lumbar spinal stenosis: a review of current concepts in evaluation, management, and outcome measurements. Arch Phys Med Rehabil. 1998;79:700–8.

59. Verbiest H. A radicular syndrome from developmental narrowing of the lumbar vertebral canal. J Bone Joint Surg (Br). 1954;36-B(2):230–7.

60. Verbiest H. Results of surgical treatment of idiopathic developmental stenosis of the lumbar vertebral canal. A review of twenty-seven years' experience. J Bone Joint Surg (Br). 1977;59:181–8.

61. Miller MD, Thompson SR, Hart J. Review of orthopaedics. 6th ed. Philadelphia: Elsevier; 2012.

62. Fanuele JC, Birkmeyer NJ, Abdu WA, Tosteson TD, Weinstein JN. The impact of spinal problems on the health status of patients: have we underestimated the effect? Spine. 2000;25:1509–14.

63. De Villiers PD, Booysen EL. Fibrous spinal stenosis. A report on 850 myelograms with a water-soluble contrast medium. Clin Orthop Relat Res. 1976;115:140–4.

64. Kamihara M, Nakano S, Fukunaga T, Ikeda K, Tsunetoh T, Tanada D, et al. Spinal cord stimulation for treatment of leg pain associated with lumbar spinal stenosis. Neuromodulation. 2014;17:340–4. discussion 345.

65. Old JL, Calvert M. Vertebral compression fractures in the elderly. Am Fam Physician. 2004;69:111–6.

66. Wong AYL. Musculoskeletal pain in postmenopausal women—implications for future research. Hong Kong Physiotherapy Journal. 2016;34:A1–2.

67. O'Neill TW, Cockerill W, Matthis C, Raspe HH, Lunt M, Cooper C, et al. Back pain, disability, and radiographic vertebral fracture in European women: a prospective study. Osteoporos Int. 2004;15:760–5.

68. Appelt CJ, Burant CJ, Siminoff LA, Kwoh CK, Ibrahim SA. Arthritis-specific health beliefs related to aging among older male patients with knee and/or hip osteoarthritis. J Gerontol A Biol Sci Med Sci. 2007;62:184–90.

69.  Downie A, Williams CM, Henschke N, Hancock MJ, Ostelo RWJG, de Vet HCW, et al. Red flags to screen for malignancy and fracture in patients with low back pain: systematic review. BMJ. 2013;347:f7095-5.

70.  Alexandru D, So W. Evaluation and management of vertebral compression fractures. Perm J. 2012;16:46-51.

71.  Kanis JA, Pitt FA. Epidemiology of osteoporosis. Bone. 1992;13:S7-15.

72.  Melton III LJ, Kan SH, Frye MA, Wahner HW, O'Fallon WM, Riggs BL. Epidemiology of vertebral fractures in women. Am J Epidemiol. 1989;129: 1000-11.

73.  Dewar C. Diagnosis and treatment of vertebral compression fractures. Radiol Technol. 2015;86:321-3.

74.  Schwab FJ, Smith VA, Biserni M, Gamez L, Farcy J-PC, Pagala M. Adult scoliosis: a quantitative radiographic and clinical analysis. Spine. 2002;27: 387-92.

75.  Bradford DS, Tay BK, Hu SS. Adult scoliosis: surgical indications, operative management, complications, and outcomes. Spine. 1999;24:2617-29.

76.  Bradford DS, Tribus CB. Current concepts and management of patients with fixed decompensated spinal deformity. Clin Orthop Relat Res. 1994;306:64-72.

77.  Faraj SSA, Holewijn RM, van Hooff ML, de Kleuver M, Pellisé F, Haanstra TM. De novo degenerative lumbar scoliosis: a systematic review of prognostic factors for curve progression. Eur Spine J. 2016;25:2347-58.

78.  Carter OD, Haynes SG. Prevalence rates for scoliosis in US adults: results from the first national health and nutrition examination survey. Int J Epidemiol. 1987;16:537-44.

79.  Kebaish KM, Neubauer PR, Voros GD, Khoshnevisan MA, Skolasky RL. Scoliosis in adults aged forty years and older: prevalence and relationship to age, race, and gender. Spine. 2011;36:731-6.

80.  Xu L, Sun X, Huang S, Zhu Z, Qiao J, Zhu F, et al. Degenerative lumbar scoliosis in Chinese Han population: prevalence and relationship to age, gender, bone mineral density, and body mass index. Eur Spine J. 2013;22:1326-31.

81.  Schwab F, Dubey A, Gamez L, El Fegoun AB, Hwang K, Pagala M, et al. Adult scoliosis: prevalence, SF-36, and nutritional parameters in an elderly volunteer population. Spine. 2005;30:1082-5.

82.  Shin J-H, Ha K-Y, Jung S-H, Chung Y-J. Genetic predisposition in degenerative lumbar scoliosis due to the copy number variation. Spine. 2011;36:1782-93.

83.  Youssef JA, Orndorff DO, Patty CA, Scott MA, Price HL, Hamlin LF, et al. Current status of adult spinal deformity. Glob Spine J. 2012;3:51-62.

84.  Kobayashi T, Atsuta Y, Takemitsu M, Matsuno T, Takeda N. A prospective study of de novo scoliosis in a community based cohort. Spine. 2006;31:178-82.

85.  Stokes IAF. Analysis and simulation of progressive adolescent scoliosis by biomechanical growth modulation. Eur Spine J. 2007;16:1621-8.

86.  Wu H-L, Ding W-Y, Shen Y, Zhang Y-Z, Guo J-K, Sun Y-P, et al. Prevalence of vertebral endplate modic changes in degenerative lumbar scoliosis and its associated factors analysis. Spine. 2012;37:1958-64.

87.  Nakamae T, Yamada K, Shimbo T, Kanazawa T, Okuda T, Takata H, et al. Bone marrow edema and low back pain in elderly degenerative lumbar scoliosis: a cross-sectional study. Spine. 2016;41:885-92.

88.  Pompei F, Wilson R. Age distribution of cancer: the incidence turnover at old age. Hum Ecol Risk Assess. 2010;7:1619-50.

89.  Henschke N, Maher CG, Ostelo R. Red flags to screen for malignancy in patients with low-back pain. Cochrane Database Syst Rev. 2013;2, CD008686.

90.  Jones LD, Pandit H, Lavy C. Back pain in the elderly: a review. Maturitas. 2014;78:258-62.

91.  Dekutoski MB, Clarke MJ, Rose P, Luzzati A, Rhines LD, Varga PP, et al. Osteosarcoma of the spine: prognostic variables for local recurrence and overall survival, a multicenter ambispective study. J Neurosurg Spine. 2016; 25:59-68.

92.  Bettegowda C, Yip S, Lo S-FL, Fisher CG, Boriani S, Rhines LD, et al. Spinal column chordoma: prognostic significance of clinical variables and T (brachyury) gene SNP rs2305089 for local recurrence and overall survival. Neuro Oncol. 2016 [Epub ahead of print].

93.  Dahlin DC. Pathology of osteosarcoma. Clin Orthop Relat Res. 1975;111:23-32.

94.  Chou D, Bilsky MH, Luzzati A, Fisher CG, Gokaslan ZL, Rhines LD, et al. Malignant peripheral nerve sheath tumors of the spine: results of surgical management from a multicenter study. J Neurosurg Spine. 2016 [Epub ahead of print].

95.  Ropper AE, Cahill KS, Hanna JW, McCarthy EF, Gokaslan ZL, Chi JH. Primary vertebral tumors: a review of epidemiologic, histological and imaging findings, part II: locally aggressive and malignant tumors. Neurosurgery. 2012;70:211-9.

96.  Weinstein JN, McLain RF. Primary tumors of the spine. Spine. 1987;12:843-51.

97.  Cunha BA. Osteomyelitis in elderly patients. Clin Infect Dis. 2002;35:287-93.

98.  Kehrer M, Pedersen C, Jensen TG, Lassen AT. Increasing incidence of pyogenic spondylodiscitis: a 14-year population-based study. J Infect. 2014; 68:313-20.

99.  Akiyama T, Chikuda H, Yasunaga H, Horiguchi H, Fushimi K, Saita K. Incidence and risk factors for mortality of vertebral osteomyelitis: a retrospective analysis using the Japanese diagnosis procedure combination database. BMJ. 2013;3:e002412.

100. Nagashima H, Nanjo Y, Tanida A, Dokai T, Teshima R. Clinical features of spinal infection in individuals older than eighty years. Int Orthop. 2012;36:1229-34.

101. Grammatico L, Baron S, Rusch E, Lepage B, Surer N, Desenclos JC, et al. Epidemiology of vertebral osteomyelitis (VO) in France: analysis of hospital-discharge data 2002-2003. Epidemiol Infect. 2008;136:653-60.

102. Colmenero JD, Jimenez-Mejias ME, Sánchez-Lora FJ, Reguera JM, Palomino-Nicás J, Martos F, et al. Pyogenic, tuberculous, and brucellar vertebral osteomyelitis: a descriptive and comparative study of 219 cases. Ann Rheum Dis. 1997;56:709-15.

103. Norman DC, Yoshikawa TT. Infections of the bone, joint, and bursa. Clin Geriatr Med. 1994;10:703-18.

104. Butler JS, Shelly MJ, Timlin M, Powderly WG, O'Byrne JM. Nontuberculous pyogenic spinal infection in adults: a 12-year experience from a tertiary referral center. Spine. 2006;31:2695-700.

105. Thompson D, Bannister P, Murphy P. Vertebral osteomyelitis in the elderly. Br Med J (Clin Res Ed). 1988;296:1309-11.

106. Beronius M, Bergman B, Andersson R. Vertebral osteomyelitis in Göteborg, Sweden: a retrospective study of patients during 1990-95. Scand J Infect Dis. 2001;33:527-32.

107. Hutchinson C, Hanger C, Wilkinson T, Sainsbury R, Pithie A. Spontaneous spinal infections in older people. Intern Med J. 2009;39:845-8.

108. Yee DKH, Samartzis D, Wong Y-W, Luk KDK, Cheung KMC. Infective spondylitis in Southern Chinese: a descriptive and comparative study of ninety-one cases. Spine. 2010;35:635-41.

109. Modic MT, Feiglin DH, Piraino DW, Boumphrey F, Weinstein MA, Duchesneau PM, et al. Vertebral osteomyelitis: assessment using MR. Radiology. 1985;157:157-66.

110. Klineberg E, Mazanec D, Orr D, Demicco R. Masquerade: medical causes of back pain. Cleve Clin J Med. 2007;74:905-13.

111. Lavy C, James A, Wilson-MacDonald J, Fairbank J. Cauda equina syndrome. BMJ. 2009;338:b936.

112. Kim W, Jin YS, Lee CS, Hwang CJ, Lee SY, Chung SG, et al. Relationship between the type and amount of physical activity and low back pain in Koreans aged 50 years and older. PM R. 2014;6:893-9.

113. Gibson SJ, Farrell M. A review of age differences in the neurophysiology of nociception and the perceptual experience of pain. Clin J Pain. 2004;20:227-39.

114. Cole LJ, Farrell MJ, Gibson SJ, Egan GF. Age-related differences in pain sensitivity and regional brain activity evoked by noxious pressure. Neurobiol Aging. 2010;31:494-503.

115. Zheng Z, Gibson SJ, Khalil Z, Helme RD, McMeeken JM. Age-related differences in the time course of capsaicin-induced hyperalgesia. Pain. 2000;85:51-8.

116. Lautenbacher S, Kunz M, Strate P, Nielsen J, Arendt-Nielsen L. Age effects on pain thresholds, temporal summation and spatial summation of heat and pressure pain. Pain. 2005;115:410-8.

117. Tseng M-T, Chiang M-C, Yazhuo K, Chao C-C, Tseng W-YI, Hsieh S-T. Effect of aging on the cerebral processing of thermal pain in the human brain. Pain. 2013;154:2120-9.

118. Lautenbacher S. Experimental approaches in the study of pain in the elderly. Pain Med. 2012;13 Suppl 2:S44-50.

119. Edwards RR, Fillingim RB. Age-associated differences in responses to noxious stimuli. J Gerontol A Biol Sci Med Sci. 2001;56:M180-5.

120. Harkins SW, Price DD, Martelli M. Effects of age on pain perception: thermonociception. J Gerontol. 1986;41:58-63.

121. Allen JS, Bruss J, Brown CK, Damasio H. Normal neuroanatomical variation due to age: the major lobes and a parcellation of the temporal region. Neurobiol Aging. 2005;26:1245-60.

122. Benedetti B, Charil A, Rovaris M, Judica E, Valsasina P, Sormani MP, et al. Influence of aging on brain gray and white matter changes assessed by conventional, MT, and DT MRI. Neurology. 2006;66:535-9.

123. Good CD, Johnsrude IS, Ashburner J, Henson RN, Friston KJ, Frackowiak RS. A voxel-based morphometric study of ageing in 465 normal adult human brains. Neuroimage. 2001;14:21-36.

124. Greenberg DL, Messer DF, Payne ME, Macfall JR, Provenzale JM, Steffens DC, et al. Aging, gender, and the elderly adult brain: an examination of analytical strategies. Neurobiol Aging. 2008;29:290–302.

125. Raz N, Rodrigue KM, Kennedy KM, Head D, Gunning-Dixon F, Acker JD. Differential aging of the human striatum: longitudinal evidence. AJNR Am J Neuroradiol. 2003;24:1849–56.

126. Walhovd KB, Fjell AM, Reinvang I, Lundervold A, Dale AM, Eilertsen DE, et al. Effects of age on volumes of cortex, white matter and subcortical structures. Neurobiol Aging. 2005;26:1261–70. discussion1275–8.

127. Washington LL, Gibson SJ, Helme RD. Age-related differences in the endogenous analgesic response to repeated cold water immersion in human volunteers. Pain. 2000;89:89–96.

128. Riley JL, King CD, Wong F, Fillingim RB, Mauderli AP. Lack of endogenous modulation and reduced decay of prolonged heat pain in older adults. Pain. 2010;150:153–60.

129. Edwards RR, Fillingim RB, Ness TJ. Age-related differences in endogenous pain modulation: a comparison of diffuse noxious inhibitory controls in healthy older and younger adults. Pain. 2003;101:155–65.

130. Naugle KM, Cruz-Almeida Y, Fillingim RB, Riley JL. Offset analgesia is reduced in older adults. Pain. 2013;154:2381–7.

131. Wood PB, Schweinhardt P, Jaeger E, Dagher A, Hakyemez H, Rabiner EA, et al. Fibromyalgia patients show an abnormal dopamine response to pain. Eur J Neurosci. 2007;25:3576–82.

132. Baliki MN, Petre B, Torbey S, Herrmann KM, Huang L, Schnitzer TJ, et al. Corticostriatal functional connectivity predicts transition to chronic back pain. Nat Neurosci. 2012;15:1117–9.

133. Riley JL, Cruz-Almeida Y, Glover TL, King CD, Goodin BR, Sibille KT, et al. Age and race effects on pain sensitivity and modulation among middle-aged and older adults. J Pain. 2014;15:272–82.

134. Farrell M, Gibson S. Age interacts with stimulus frequency in the temporal summation of pain. Pain Med. 2007;8:514–20.

135. Edwards RR, Fillingim RB. Effects of age on temporal summation and habituation of thermal pain: clinical relevance in healthy older and younger adults. J Pain. 2001;2:307–17.

136. Scherder EJA, Sergeant JA, Swaab DF. Pain processing in dementia and its relation to neuropathology. Lancet Neurol. 2003;2:677–86.

137. Carlino E, Benedetti F, Rainero I, Asteggiano G, Cappa G, Tarenzi L, et al. Pain perception and tolerance in patients with frontotemporal dementia. Pain. 2010;151:783–9.

138. Benedetti F, Vighetti S, Ricco C, Lagna E, Bergamasco B, Pinessi L, et al. Pain threshold and tolerance in Alzheimer's disease. Pain. 1999;80:377–82.

139. Gibson SJ, Voukelatos X, Ames D, Flicker L, Helme RD. An examination of pain perception and cerebral event-related potentials following carbon dioxide laser stimulation in patients with Alzheimer's disease and age-matched control volunteers. Pain Res Manag. 2001;6:126–32.

140. Jensen-Dahm C, Werner MU, Dahl JB, Jensen TS, Ballegaard M, Hejl A-M, et al. Quantitative sensory testing and pain tolerance in patients with mild to moderate Alzheimer disease compared to healthy control subjects. Pain. 2014;155:1439–45.

141. Mansour A, Baria AT, Tetreault P, Vachon-Presseau E, Chang P-C, Huang L, et al. Global disruption of degree rank order: a hallmark of chronic pain. Sci Rep. 2016;6:34853.

142. Mutso AA, Radzicki D, Baliki MN, Huang L, Banisadr G, Centeno MV, et al. Abnormalities in hippocampal functioning with persistent pain. J Neurosci. 2012;32:5747–56.

143. Mutso AA, Petre B, Huang L, Baliki MN, Torbey S, Herrmann KM, et al. Reorganization of hippocampal functional connectivity with transition to chronic back pain. J Neurophysiol. 2014;111:1065–76.

144. Apkarian VA, Hashmi JA, Baliki MN. Pain and the brain: specificity and plasticity of the brain in clinical chronic pain. Pain. 2011;152:S49–64.

145. Baliki MN, Chialvo DR, Geha PY, Levy RM, Harden RN, Parrish TB, et al. Chronic pain and the emotional brain: specific brain activity associated with spontaneous fluctuations of intensity of chronic back pain. J Neurosci. 2006; 26:12165–73.

146. Isnard J, Magnin M, Jung J, Mauguière F, Garcia-Larrea L. Does the insula tell our brain that we are in pain? Pain. 2011;152:946–51.

147. Staud R, Robinson ME, Vierck CJ, Price DD. Diffuse noxious inhibitory controls (DNIC) attenuate temporal summation of second pain in normal males but not in normal females or fibromyalgia patients. Pain. 2003;101:167–74.

148. Bartley EJ, Fillingim RB. Sex differences in pain: a brief review of clinical and experimental findings. Br J Anaesth. 2013;111:52–8.

149. Ge HY, Madeleine P, Arendt-Nielsen L. Sex differences in temporal characteristics of descending inhibitory control: an evaluation using repeated bilateral experimental induction of muscle pain. Pain. 2004; 110:72–8.

150. Sarlani E, Greenspan JD. Gender differences in temporal summation of mechanically evoked pain. Pain. 2002;97:163–9.

151. Ward K, Ogilvie JW, Singleton MV, Chettier R, Engler G, Nelson LM. Validation of DNA-based prognostic testing to predict spinal curve progression in adolescent idiopathic scoliosis. Spine. 2010;35:E1455–64.

152. Cheung KMC, Samartzis D, Karppinen J, Mok FPS, Ho DWH, Fong DYT, et al. Intervertebral disc degeneration: new insights based on "skipped" level disc pathology. Arthritis Rheum. 2010;62:2392–400.

153. Mok FPS, Samartzis D, Karppinen J, Luk KDK, Fong DYT, Cheung KMC. ISSLS prize winner: prevalence, determinants, and association of Schmorl nodes of the lumbar spine with disc degeneration: a population-based study of 2449 individuals. Spine. 2010;35:1944–52.

154. Joshi AA, Leporé N, Joshi SH, Lee AD, Barysheva M, Stein JL, et al. The contribution of genes to cortical thickness and volume. NeuroReport. 2011;22:101–5.

155. Dick DM. Gene-environment interaction in psychological traits and disorders. Annual review of clinical psychology. Ann Rev Clin Psychol. 2011; 7:383–409.

156. Diatchenko L, Slade GD, Nackley AG, Bhalang K, Sigurdsson A, Belfer I, et al. Genetic basis for individual variations in pain perception and the development of a chronic pain condition. Hum Mol Genet. 2005;14:135–43.

157. Diatchenko L, Nackley AG, Slade GD, Bhalang K, Belfer I, Max MB, et al. Catechol-O-methyltransferase gene polymorphisms are associated with multiple pain-evoking stimuli. Pain. 2006;125:216–24.

158. Skouen JS, Smith AJ, Warrington NM, O' Sullivan PB, McKenzie L, Pennell CE, et al. Genetic variation in the beta-2 adrenergic receptor is associated with chronic musculoskeletal complaints in adolescents. Eur J Pain. 2012;16: 1232–42.

159. Karppinen J, Daavittila I, Noponen N, Haapea M, Taimela S, Vanharanta H, et al. Is the interleukin-6 haplotype a prognostic factor for sciatica? Eur J Pain. 2008;12:1018–25.

160. Oertel B, Lötsch J. Genetic mutations that prevent pain: implications for future pain medication. Pharmacogenomics. 2008;9:179–94.

161. Yang Y, Wang Y, Li S, Xu Z, Li H, Ma L, et al. Mutations in SCN9A, encoding a sodium channel alpha subunit, in patients with primary erythermalgia. J Med Genet. 2004;41:171–4.

162. Reimann F, Cox JJ, Belfer I, Diatchenko L, Zaykin DV, McHale DP, et al. Pain perception is altered by a nucleotide polymorphism in SCN9A. Proc Natl Acad Sci. 2010;107:5148–53.

163. Tegeder I, Costigan M, Griffin RS, Abele A, Belfer I, Schmidt H, et al. GTP cyclohydrolase and tetrahydrobiopterin regulate pain sensitivity and persistence. Nat Med. 2006;12:1269–77.

164. Belfer I, Young EE, Diatchenko L. Letting the gene out of the bottleOPRM1 interactions. Anesthesiology. 2014;121:678–80.

165. Hwang IC, Park J-Y, Myung S-K, Ahn HY, Fukuda K-I, Liao Q. OPRM1 A118G gene variant and postoperative opioid requirement: a systematic review and meta-analysis. Anesthesiology. 2014;121:825–34.

166. Bond C, LaForge KS, Tian M, Melia D, Zhang S, Borg L, et al. Single-nucleotide polymorphism in the human mu opioid receptor gene alters beta-endorphin binding and activity: possible implications for opiate addiction. Proc Natl Acad Sci U S A. 1998;95:9608–13.

167. Landau R, Liu S-K, Blouin J-L, Carvalho B. The effect of OPRM1 and COMT genotypes on the analgesic response to intravenous fentanyl labor analgesia. Anesth Analg. 2013;116:386–91.

168. Kolesnikov Y, Gabovits B, Levin A, Veske A, Qin L, Dai F, et al. Chronic pain after lower abdominal surgery: do catechol-O-methyl transferase/opioid receptor μ-1 polymorphisms contribute? Mol Pain. 2013;9:19.

169. Shabalina SA, Zaykin DV, Gris P, Ogurtsov AY, Gauthier J, Shibata K, et al. Expansion of the human μ-opioid receptor gene architecture: novel functional variants. Hum Mol Genet. 2009;18:1037–51.

170. Olsen MB, Jacobsen LM, Schistad EI, Pedersen LM, Rygh LJ, Gjerstad J. Pain intensity the first year after lumbar disc herniation is associated with the A118G polymorphism in the opioid receptor mu 1 gene: evidence of a sex and genotype interaction. J Neurosci. 2012;32:678–80.

171. Heneweer H, Picavet HSJ, Staes F, Kiers H, Vanhees L. Physical fitness, rather than self-reported physical activities, is more strongly associated with low back pain: evidence from a working population. Eur Spine J. 2012;21:1265–72.

172. Plouvier S, Chastang J-F, Cyr D, Bonenfant S, Descatha A, Goldberg M, et al. Occupational biomechanical exposure predicts low back pain in older age among men in the Gazel Cohort. Int Arch Occup Environ Health. 2015;88:501–10.

173. Sobti A, Cooper C, Inskip H, Searle S, Coggon D. Occupational physical activity and long-term risk of musculoskeletal symptoms: a national survey of post office pensioners. Am J Ind Med. 1997;32:76–83.

174. Traeger AC, Moseley GL, Hübscher M, Lee H, Skinner IW, Nicholas MK, et al. Pain education to prevent chronic low back pain: a study protocol for a randomised controlled trial. BMJ Open. 2014;4:e005505–5.

175. Martin BI, Deyo RA, Mirza SK, Turner JA, Comstock BA, Hollingworth W, et al. Expenditures and health status among adults with back and neck problems. JAMA. 2008;299:656–64.

176. Dunn KM, Hestbaek L, Cassidy JD. Low back pain across the life course. Best Pract Res Clin Rheumatol. 2013;27:591–600.

177. Reid MC, Williams CS, Concato J, Tinetti ME, Gill TM. Depressive symptoms as a risk factor for disabling back pain in community-dwelling older persons. J Am Geriatr Soc. 2003;51:1710–7.

178. Demyttenaere K, Bruffaerts R, Lee S, Posada-Villa J, Kovess V, Angermeyer MC, et al. Mental disorders among persons with chronic back or neck pain: results from the world mental health surveys. Pain. 2007;129:332–42.

179. Basler H-D, Luckmann J, Wolf U, Quint S. Fear-avoidance beliefs, physical activity, and disability in elderly individuals with chronic low back pain and healthy controls. Clin J Pain. 2008;24:604–10.

180. Camacho-Soto A, Sowa GA, Perera S, Weiner DK. Fear avoidance beliefs predict disability in older adults with chronic low back pain. PM R. 2012;4:493–7.

181. Sions JM, Hicks GE. Fear-avoidance beliefs are associated with disability in older American adults with low back pain. Phys Ther. 2011;91:525–34.

182. Vincent HK, Seay AN, Montero C, Conrad BP, Hurley RW, Vincent KR. Kinesiophobia and fear-avoidance beliefs in overweight older adults with chronic low-back pain: relationship to walking endurance—part II. Am J Phys Med Rehabil. 2013;92:439–45.

183. Kovacs F, Noguera J, Abraira V, Royuela A, Cano A, Gil del Real MT, et al. The influence of psychological factors on low back pain-related disability in community dwelling older persons. Pain Med. 2008;9:871–80.

184. Vincent HK, George SZ, Seay AN, Vincent KR, Hurley RW. Resistance exercise, disability, and pain catastrophizing in obese adults with back pain. Med Sci Sports Exerc. 2014;46:1693–701.

185. Ledoux E, Dubois J-D, Descarreaux M. Physical and psychosocial predictors of functional trunk capacity in older adults with and without low back pain. J Manipulative Physiol Ther. 2012;35:338–45.

186. Monie AP, Fazey PJ, Singer KP. Low back pain misdiagnosis or missed diagnosis: core principles. Man Ther. 2016;22:68–71.

187. Shi Y, Weingarten TN, Mantilla CB, Hooten WM, Warner DO. Smoking and pain pathophysiology and clinical implications. Anesthesiology. 2010;113:977–92.

188. Wang D, Nasto LA, Roughley P, Leme AS, Houghton AM, Usas A, et al. Spine degeneration in a murine model of chronic human tobacco smokers. Osteoarthritis Cartilage. 2012;20:896–905.

189. Líndal E, Stefánsson JG. Connection between smoking and back pain—findings from an Icelandic general population study. Scand J Rehabil Med. 1996;28:33–8.

190. Glassman SD, Anagnost SC, Parker A, Burke D, Johnson JR, Dimar JR. The effect of cigarette smoking and smoking cessation on spinal fusion. Spine. 2000;25:2608–15.

191. Battié MC, Videman T, Gill K, Moneta GB, Nyman R, Kaprio J, et al. 1991 Volvo Award in clinical sciences. Smoking and lumbar intervertebral disc degeneration: an MRI study of identical twins. Spine. 1991;16:1015–21.

192. Jordan KP, Thomas E, Peat G, Wilkie R, Croft P. Social risks for disabling pain in older people: a prospective study of individual and area characteristics. Pain. 2008;137:652–61.

193. Ben-Shlomo Y, Kuh D. A life course approach to chronic disease epidemiology: conceptual models, empirical challenges and interdisciplinary perspectives. Int J Epidemiol. 2002;31:285–93.

194. Rognerud MA, Krüger O, Gjertsen F, Thelle DS. Strong regional links between socio-economic background factors and disability and mortality in Oslo, Norway. Eur J Epidemiol. 1998;14:457–63.

195. Ebrahim S, Papacosta O, Wannamethee G, Adamson J. British Regional Heart Study. Social inequalities and disability in older men: prospective findings from the British regional heart study. Soc Sci Med. 2004;59:2109–20.

196. Matthews RJ, Smith LK, Hancock RM, Jagger C, Spiers NA. Socioeconomic factors associated with the onset of disability in older age: a longitudinal study of people aged 75 years and over. Soc Sci Med. 2005;61:1567–75.

197. Hartvigsen J, Christensen K, Frederiksen H. Back and neck pain exhibit many common features in old age: a population-based study of 4,486 Danish twins 70–102 years of age. Spine. 2004;29:576–80.

198. Drake DF, Harkins S, Qutubuddin A. Pain in Parkinson's disease: pathology to treatment, medication to deep brain stimulation. Neuro Rehabilitation. 2005;20:335–41.

199. Mott S, Kenrick M, Dixon M, Bird G. Pain as a sequela of Parkinson disease. Aust Fam Physician. 2004;33:663–4.

200. Witjas T, Kaphan E, Azulay JP, Blin O, Ceccaldi M, Pouget J, et al. Nonmotor fluctuations in Parkinson's disease: frequent and disabling. Neurology. 2002;59:408–13.

201. Wong AY, Samartzis D. Low back pain in older adults—the need for specific outcome and psychometric tools. J Pain Research. 2016;9:989–91.

202. Weiner DK, Peterson BL, Logue P, Keefe FJ. Predictors of pain self-report in nursing home residents. Aging Clin Exp Res. 1998;10:411–20.

203. Scherder EJ, Bouma A. Visual analogue scales for pain assessment in Alzheimer's disease. Gerontology. 2000;46:47–53.

204. Herr K, Spratt KF, Garand L, Li L. Evaluation of the Iowa Pain Thermometer and other selected pain intensity scales in younger and older adult cohorts using controlled clinical pain: a preliminary study. Pain Med. 2007;8:585–600.

205. Bieri D, Reeve RA, Champion DG, Addicoat L, Ziegler JB. The faces pain scale for the self-assessment of the severity of pain experienced by children: development, initial validation, and preliminary investigation for ratio scale properties. Pain. 1990;41:139–50.

206. Herr KA, Mobily PR, Kohout FJ, Wagenaar D. Evaluation of the faces pain scale for use with the elderly. Clin J Pain. 1998;14:29–38.

207. Miró J, Huguet A, Nieto R, Paredes S, Baos J. Evaluation of reliability, validity, and preference for a pain intensity scale for use with the elderly. J Pain. 2005;6:727–35.

208. Stuppy DJ. The faces pain scale: reliability and validity with mature adults. Appl Nurs Res. 1998;11:84–9.

209. Li L, Liu X, Herr K. Postoperative pain intensity assessment: a comparison of four scales in Chinese adults. Pain Med. 2007;8:223–34.

210. Ware LJ, Epps CD, Herr K, Packard A. Evaluation of the revised faces pain scale, verbal descriptor scale, numeric rating scale, and Iowa pain thermometer in older minority adults. Pain Manag Nurs. 2006;7:117–25.

211. Porter FL, Malhotra KM, Wolf CM, Morris JC, Miller JP, Smith MC. Dementia and response to pain in the elderly. Pain. 1996;68:413–21.

212. Kunz M, Scharmann S, Hemmeter U, Schepelmann K, Lautenbacher S. The facial expression of pain in patients with dementia. Pain. 2007;133:221–8.

213. Cole LJ, Farrell MJ, Duff EP, Barber JB, Egan GF, Gibson SJ. Pain sensitivity and fMRI pain-related brain activity in Alzheimer's disease. Brain. 2006;129:2957–65.

214. Shega JW, Rudy T, Keefe FJ, Perri LC, Mengin OT, Weiner DK. Validity of pain behaviors in persons with mild to moderate cognitive impairment. J Am Geriatr Soc. 2008;56:1631–7.

215. Parmelee PA, Smithy B, Katz IR. Pain complaints and cognitive status among elderly institution residents. J Am Geriatr Soc. 2015;41:517–22.

216. Won A, Lapane K, Gambassi G, Bernabei R, Mor V, Lipsitz LA. Correlates and management of nonmalignant pain in the nursing home. J Am Geriatr Soc. 1999;47:936–42.

217. Herr K. Pain in the older adult: an imperative across all health care settings. Pain Manag Nurs. 2010;11:S1–10.

218. Hugo J, Ganguli M. Dementia and cognitive impairment: epidemiology, diagnosis, and treatment. Clin Geriatr Med. 2014;30:421–42.

219. Nasreddine ZS, Phillips NA, Bédirian V, Charbonneau S, Whitehead V, Collin I, et al. The Montreal Cognitive Assessment, MoCA: a brief screening tool for mild cognitive impairment. J Am Geriatr Soc. 2005;53:695–9.

220. Borson S, Scanlan JM, Chen P, Ganguli M. The Mini-Cog as a screen for dementia: validation in a population-based sample. J Am Geriatr Soc. 2003;51:1451–4.

221. Borson S, Scanlan J, Brush M, Vitaliano P, Dokmak A. The Mini-Cog: a cognitive "vital signs" measure for dementia screening in multi-lingual elderly. Int J Geriatr Psychiatry. 2000;15:1021–7.

222. Tariq SH, Tumosa N, Chibnall JT, Perry III MH, Morley JE. Comparison of the Saint Louis University Mental Status Examination and the Mini-Mental State Examination for detecting dementia and mild neurocognitive disorder—a pilot study. Am J Geriatr Psychiatry. 2006;14:900–10.

223. Wright R, Malec M, Shega JW, Rodriguez E, Kulas J, Morrow L, et al. Deconstructing chronic low back pain in the older adult-step by step evidence and expert-based recommendations for evaluation and treatment: part XI: dementia. Pain Med. 2016;17:1993–2002.

224. Husebo BS, Ballard C, Sandvik R, Nilsen OB, Aarsland D. Efficacy of treating pain to reduce behavioural disturbances in residents of nursing homes with dementia: cluster randomised clinical trial. BMJ. 2011;343:d4065–5.

225. Herr K, Bursch H, Ersek M, Miller LL, Swafford K. Use of pain-behavioral assessment tools in the nursing home: expert consensus recommendations for practice. J Gerontol Nurs. 2012;36:18–29.

226. Aubin M, Giguère A, Hadjistavropoulos T, Verreault R. The systematic evaluation of instruments designed to assess pain in persons with limited ability to communicate. Pain Res Manag. 2007;12:195–203.

227. Zwakhalen SMG, Hamers JPH, Abu-Saad HH, Berger MPF. Pain in elderly people with severe dementia: a systematic review of behavioural pain assessment tools. BMC Geriatr. 2006;6:3.

228. Warden V, Hurley AC, Volicer L. Development and psychometric evaluation of the Pain Assessment in Advanced Dementia (PAINAD) scale. J Am Med Dir Asso. 2003;4:9–15.

229. Kunz M, Mylius V, Schepelmann K, Lautenbacher S. Effects of age and mild cognitive impairment on the pain response system. Gerontology. 2009;55:674–82.

230. Kunz M, Mylius V, Scharmann S, Schepelman K, Lautenbacher S. Influence of dementia on multiple components of pain. Eur J Pain. 2009;13:317–25.

231. Kenny GP, Yardley JE, Martineau L, Jay O. Physical work capacity in older adults: implications for the aging worker. Am J Ind Med. 2008;51:610–25.

232. Fitzgerald MD, Tanaka H, Tran ZV, Seals DR. Age-related declines in maximal aerobic capacity in regularly exercising vs. sedentary women: a meta-analysis. J Appl Physiol (1985). 1997;83:160–5.

233. Morley JE. Sarcopenia in the elderly. Fam Pract. 2012;29:i44–8.

234. Patel KV, Phelan EA, Leveille SG, Lamb SE, Missikpode C, Wallace RB, et al. High prevalence of falls, fear of falling, and impaired balance in older adults with pain in the United States: findings from the 2011 National Health and Aging Trends Study. J Am Geriatr Soc. 2014;62:1844–52.

235. Muraki S, Akune T, Oka H, En-Yo Y, Yoshida M, Nakamura K, et al. Prevalence of falls and the association with knee osteoarthritis and lumbar spondylosis as well as knee and lower back pain in Japanese men and women. Arthritis Care Res. 2011;63:1425–31.

236. Kitayuguchi J, Kamada M, Inoue S, Kamioka H, Abe T, Okada S, et al. Association of low back and knee pain with falls in Japanese community-dwelling older adults: a 3-year prospective cohort study. Geriatr Gerontol Int. 2016. doi:10.1111/ggi.12799 [Epub ahead of print].

237. Stevens JA, Hasbrouck LM, Durant TM, Dellinger AM, Batabyal PK, Crosby AE, et al. Surveillance for injuries and violence among older adults. MMWR CDC Surveill Summ. 1999;48:27–50.

238. Tomita Y, Arima K, Kanagae M, Okabe T, Mizukami S, Nishimura T, et al. Association of physical performance and pain with fear of falling among community-dwelling Japanese women aged 65 years and older. Medicine (Baltimore). 2015;94:e1449.

239. AGS Panel on Persistent Pain in Older Persons. The management of persistent pain in older persons. J Am Geriatr Soc. 2002;50:S205–24.

240. Marquardt KA, Alsop JA, Albertson TE. Tramadol exposures reported to statewide poison control system. Ann Pharmacother. 2005;39:1039–44.

241. Huang AR, Mallet L, Rochefort CM, Eguale T, Buckeridge DL, Tamblyn R. Medication-related falls in the elderly: causative factors and preventive strategies. Drugs Aging. 2012;29:359–76.

242. Field TS, Gurwitz JH, Avorn J, McCormick D, Jain S, Eckler M, et al. Risk factors for adverse drug events among nursing home residents. Arch Intern Med. 2001;161:1629–34.

243. Shorr RI, Griffin MR, Daugherty JR, Ray WA. Opioid analgesics and the risk of hip fracture in the elderly—codeine and propoxyphene. J Gerontol. 1992;47:M111–5.

244. Allain H, Bentue-Ferrer D, Polard E, Akwa Y, Patat A. Postural instability and consequent falls and hip fractures associated with use of hypnotics in the elderly—a comparative review. Drugs Aging. 2005;22:749–65.

245. Coupland C, Dhiman P, Morriss R, Arthur A, Barton G, Hippisley-Cox J. Antidepressant use and risk of adverse outcomes in older people: population based cohort study. BMJ. 2011;343:d4551.

246. Khong TP, de Vries F, Goldenberg JSB, Klungel OH, Robinson NJ, Ibáñez L, et al. Potential impact of benzodiazepine use on the rate of hip fractures in five large European countries and the United States. Calcif Tissue Int. 2012; 91:24–31.

247. Beakley BD, Kaye AM, Kaye AD. Tramadol, pharmacology, side effects, and serotonin syndrome: a review. Pain Physician. 2015;18:395–400.

248. Tashakori A, Afshari R. Tramadol overdose as a cause of serotonin syndrome: a case series. Clin Toxicol. 2010;48:337–41.

249. Hall AJ, Logan JE, Toblin RL, Kaplan JA, Kraner JC, Bixler D, et al. Patterns of abuse among unintentional pharmaceutical overdose fatalities. JAMA. 2008; 300:2613–20.

250. Hasegawa K, Brown DFM, Tsugawa Y, Camargo Jr CA. Epidemiology of emergency department visits for opioid overdose: a population-based study. Mayo Clin Proc. 2014;89:462–71.

251. Calcaterra S, Glanz J, Binswanger IA. National trends in pharmaceutical opioid related overdose deaths compared to other substance related overdose deaths: 1999–2009. Drug Alcohol Depend. 2013;131:263–70.

252. Cheatle MD. Depression, chronic pain, and suicide by overdose: on the edge. Pain Med. 2011;12:S43–8.

253. Volkow ND, McLellan AT. Opioid abuse in chronic pain—misconceptions and mitigation strategies. N Engl J Med. 2016;374:1253–63.

254. Wheeler E, Jones TS, Gilbert MK, Davidson PJ, Centers for Disease Control and Prevention (CDC). Opioid overdose prevention programs providing naloxone to laypersons—United States, 2014. MMWR Morb Mortal Wkly Rep. 2015;64:631–5.

255. Kong LJ, Lauche R, Klose P, Bu JH, Yang XC, Guo CQ, et al. Tai chi for chronic pain conditions: a systematic review and meta-analysis of randomized controlled trials. Sci Rep. 2016;6:25325.

256. Kuss K, Becker A, Quint S, Leonhardt C. Activating therapy modalities in older individuals with chronic non-specific low back pain: a systematic review. Physiotherapy. 2015;101:310–8.

257. Leung DP, Chan CK, Tsang HW, Tsang WW, Jones AY. Tai chi as an intervention to improve balance and reduce falls in older adults: a systematic and meta-analytical review. Altern Ther Health Med. 2011;17:40–8.

258. Rand D, Miller WC, Yiu J, Eng JJ. Interventions for addressing low balance confidence in older adults: a systematic review and meta-analysis. Age Ageing. 2011;40:297–306.

259. Liu B, Liu Z-H, Zhu H-E, Mo J-C, Cheng D-H. Effects of tai chi on lower-limb myodynamia in the elderly people: a meta-analysis. J Tradit Chin Med. 2011; 31:141–6.

260. Yan J-H, Gu W-J, Sun J, Zhang W-X, Li B-W, Pan L. Efficacy of Tai Chi on pain, stiffness and function in patients with osteoarthritis: a meta-analysis. PLoS One. 2013;8, e61672.

261. Wang J, Feng B, Yang X, Liu W, Teng F, Li S, et al. Tai chi for essential hypertension. Evid Based Complement Alternat Med. 2013;2013:215254–10.

262. Wayne PM, Walsh JN, Taylor-Piliae RE, Wells RE, Papp KV, Donovan NJ, et al. Effect of tai chi on cognitive performance in older adults: systematic review and meta-analysis. J Am Geriatr Soc. 2014;62:25–39.

263. Chi I, Jordan-Marsh M, Guo M, Xie B, Bai Z. Tai chi and reduction of depressive symptoms for older adults: a meta-analysis of randomized trials. Geriatr Gerontol Int. 2013;13:3–12.

264. Gibson JNA, Waddell G. Surgical interventions for lumbar disc prolapse: updated Cochrane Review. Spine. 2007;32:1735–47.

265. Gibson JNA, Waddell G. Surgery for degenerative lumbar spondylosis: updated Cochrane Review. Spine. 2005;30:2312–20.

266. Smith ZA, Fessler RG. Paradigm changes in spine surgery: evolution of minimally invasive techniques. Nat Rev Neurol. 2012;8:443–50.

267. Morlion B. Chronic low back pain: pharmacological, interventional and surgical strategies. Nat Rev Neurol. 2013;9:462–73.

268. Deyo RA, Mirza SK, Martin BI, Kreuter W, Goodman DC, Jarvik JG. Trends, major medical complications, and charges associated with surgery for lumbar spinal stenosis in older adults. JAMA. 2010;303:1259–65.

269. Schroeder GD, Kepler CK, Kurd MF, Vaccaro AR, Hsu WK, Patel AA, et al. Rationale for the surgical treatment of lumbar degenerative spondylolisthesis. Spine. 2015;40:E1161–6.

270. Försth P, Ólafsson G, Carlsson T, Frost A, Borgström F, Fritzell P, et al. A randomized, controlled trial of fusion surgery for lumbar spinal stenosis. N Engl J Med. 2016;374:1413–23.

271. Ghogawala Z, Dziura J, Butler WE, Dai F, Terrin N, Magge SN, et al. Laminectomy plus fusion versus laminectomy alone for lumbar spondylolisthesis. N Engl J Med. 2016;374:1424–34.

272. Shapiro GS, Taira G, Boachie-Adjei O. Results of surgical treatment of adult idiopathic scoliosis with low back pain and spinal stenosis: a study of long-term clinical radiographic outcomes. Spine. 2003;28:358–63.

273. Simmons ED, Simmons EH. Spinal stenosis with scoliosis. Spine. 1992;17: S117–20.

274. Eck KR, Bridwell KH, Ungacta FF, Riew KD, Lapp MA, Lenke LG, et al. Complications and results of long adult deformity fusions down to l4, l5, and the sacrum. Spine. 2001;26:E182–92.

275. Glassman SD, Hamill CL, Bridwell KH, Schwab FJ, Dimar JR, Lowe TG. The impact of perioperative complications on clinical outcome in adult deformity surgery. Spine. 2007;32:2764–70.

276. Takahashi S, Delécrin J, Passuti N. Surgical treatment of idiopathic scoliosis in adults: an age-related analysis of outcome. Spine. 2002;27:1742–8.

277. van Tulder MW, Koes B, Seitsalo S, Malmivaara A. Outcome of invasive treatment modalities on back pain and sciatica: an evidence-based review. Eur Spine J Springer-Verlag. 2006;15 Suppl 1:S82–92.

278. Zhang H, Xu C, Zhang T, Gao Z, Zhang T. Does percutaneous vertebroplasty or balloon kyphoplasty for osteoporotic vertebral compression fractures increase the incidence of new vertebral fracture? A meta-analysis. Pain Physician. 2017;20:E13–28.

279. Evans AJ, Jensen ME, Kip KE, DeNardo AJ, Lawler GJ, Negin GA, et al. Vertebral compression fractures: pain reduction and improvement in functional mobility after percutaneous polymethylmethacrylate vertebroplasty retrospective report of 245 cases. Radiology. 2003;226:366–72.

280. Hulme PA, Krebs J, Ferguson SJ, Berlemann U. Vertebroplasty and kyphoplasty: a systematic review of 69 clinical studies. Spine. 2006;31:1983–2001.

281. Civelek E, Cansever T, Yilmaz C, Kabatas S, Gülşen S, Aydemir F, et al. The retrospective analysis of the effect of balloon kyphoplasty to the adjacent-segment fracture in 171 patients. J Spinal Disord Tech. 2014;27:98–104.

282. Rothermich MA, Buchowski JM, Bumpass DB, Patterson GA. Pulmonary cement embolization after vertebroplasty requiring pulmonary wedge resection. Clin Orthop Relat. 2014;472:1652–7.

283. Lindsay R, Silverman SL, Cooper C, Hanley DA, Barton I, Broy SB, et al. Risk of new vertebral fracture in the year following a fracture. JAMA. 2001;285:320–3.

284. Fakurnejad S, Scheer JK, Lafage V, Smith JS, Deviren V, Hostin R, et al. The likelihood of reaching minimum clinically important difference and substantial clinical benefit at 2 years following a 3-column osteotomy: analysis of 140 patients. J Neurosurg Spine. 2015;23:340–8.

285. Ailon T, Scheer JK, Lafage V, Schwab FJ, Klineberg E, Sciubba DM, et al. Adult spinal deformity surgeons are unable to accurately predict postoperative spinal alignment using clinical judgment alone. Spine Deform. 2016;4:323–9.

286. Champain S, Benchikh K, Nogier A, Mazel C, De Guise J, Skalli W. Validation of new clinical quantitative analysis software applicable in spine orthopaedic studies. Eur Spine J. 2006;15:982–91.

287. Berthonnaud E, Labelle H, Roussouly P, Grimard G, Vaz G, Dimnet J. A variability study of computerized sagittal spinopelvic radiologic measurements of trunk balance. J Spinal Disord Tech. 2005;18:66–71.

288. Schwab F, Lafage V, Boyce R, Skalli W, Farcy J-P. Gravity line analysis in adult volunteers: age-related correlation with spinal parameters, pelvic parameters, and foot position. Spine. 2006;31:E959–67.

289. Schwab F, Farcy J-P, Bridwell K, Berven S, Glassman S, Harrast J, et al. A clinical impact classification of scoliosis in the adult. Spine. 2006;31:2109–14.

290. Lafage V, Schwab F, Patel A, Hawkinson N, Farcy J-P. Pelvic tilt and truncal inclination: two key radiographic parameters in the setting of adults with spinal deformity. Spine. 2009;34:E599–606.

291. Lazennec JY, Ramaré S, Arafati N, Laudet CG, Gorin M, Roger B, et al. Sagittal alignment in lumbosacral fusion: relations between radiological parameters and pain. Eur Spine J. 2000;9:47–55.

292. Roussouly P, Pinheiro-Franco JL. Biomechanical analysis of the spino-pelvic organization and adaptation in pathology. Eur Spine J. 2011;20:S609–18.

293. Zaina F, Tomkins-Lane C, Carragee E, Negrini S. Surgical versus non-surgical treatment for lumbar spinal stenosis. (null), editor. Cochrane Database Syst Rev. 2016;1:CD010264.

294. Malmivaara A, Slätis P, Heliövaara M, Sainio P, Kinnunen H, Kankare J, et al. Surgical or nonoperative treatment for lumbar spinal stenosis? Spine. 2007;32:1–8.

295. Weinstein JN, Tosteson TD, Lurie JD, Tosteson ANA, Blood E, Hanscom B, et al. Surgical versus nonsurgical therapy for lumbar spinal stenosis. N Engl J Med. 2008;358:794–810.

296. Amundsen T, Weber H, Nordal HJ, Magnaes B, Abdelnoor M, Lilleas F. Lumbar spinal stenosis: conservative or surgical management? A prospective 10-year study. Spine. 2000;25:1424–35.

297. Brown LL. A double-blind, randomized, prospective study of epidural steroid injection vs. the mild® procedure in patients with symptomatic lumbar spinal stenosis. Pain Practice. 2012;12:333–41.

298. Zucherman JF, Hsu KY, Hartjen CA, Mehalic TF, Implicito DA, Martin MJ, et al. A prospective randomized multi-center study for the treatment of lumbar spinal stenosis with the X STOP interspinous implant: 1-year results. Eur Spine J. 2004;13:22–31.

299. Kaasalainen S, Akhtar-Danesh N, Hadjistavropoulos T, Zwakhalen S, Verreault R. A comparison between behavioral and verbal report pain assessment tools for use with residents in long term care. Pain Management Nursing. 2013;14:e106–14.

300. Lukas A, Barber JB, Johnson P, Gibson SJ. Observer-rated pain assessment instruments improve both the detection of pain and the evaluation of pain intensity in people with dementia. Eur J Pain. 2013;17:1558–68.

301. Hadjistavropoulos T, Hunter P, Dever Fitzgerald T. Pain assessment and management in older adults: conceptual issues and clinical challenges. Can Psychol. 2009;50:241–54.

302. Wong AYL, Kawchuk G, Parent E, Prasad N. Within- and between-day reliability of spinal stiffness measurements obtained using a computer controlled mechanical indenter in individuals with and without low back pain. Man Ther. 2013;18:395–402.

303. Wong AYL, Kawchuk GN. The clinical value of assessing lumbar posteroanterior segmental stiffness: a narrative review of manual and instrumented methods. PM R. 2016 [Epub ahead of print].

304. Kawchuk GN, Edgecombe TL, Wong AYL, Cojocaru A, Prasad N. A non-randomized clinical trial to assess the impact of nonrigid, inelastic corsets on spine function in low back pain participants and asymptomatic controls. Spine J. 2015;15:2222–7.

305. Wong AYL, Parent E, Kawchuk G. Reliability of 2 ultrasonic imaging analysis methods in quantifying lumbar multifidus thickness. J Orthop Sports Phys Ther. 2013;43:251–62.

306. Samartzis D, Cheung JPY, Rajasekaran S, Kawaguchi Y, Acharya S, Kawakami M, et al. Is lumbar facet joint tropism developmental or secondary to degeneration? An international, large-scale multicenter study by the AOSpine Asia Pacific Research Collaboration Consortium. Scoliosis Spinal Disord. 2016;11:9.

307. Samartzis D, Karppinen J, Cheung JPY, Lotz J. Disk degeneration and low back pain: are they fat-related conditions? Glob Spine J. 2013;03:133–44.

308. Sadhasivam S, Chidambaran V. Pharmacogenomics of opioids and perioperative pain management. Pharmacogenomics. 2012;13:1719–40.

309. Wong AYL, Parent EC, Dhillon SS, Prasad N, Kawchuk GN. Do participants with low back pain who respond to spinal manipulative therapy differ biomechanically from nonresponders, untreated controls or asymptomatic controls? Spine. 2015;40:1329–37.

310. Karppinen J, Shen FH, Luk KDK, Andersson GBJ, Cheung KMC, Samartzis D. Management of degenerative disk disease and chronic low back pain. Orthop Clin North Am. 2011;42:513–28.

311. van Dijk JFM, Kappen TH, van Wijck AJM, Kalkman CJ, Schuurmans MJ. The diagnostic value of the numeric pain rating scale in older postoperative patients. J Clin Nurs. 2012;21:3018–24.

312. Wood BM, Nicholas MK, Blyth F, Asghari A, Gibson S. Assessing pain in older people with persistent pain: the NRS is valid but only provides part of the picture. J Pain. 2010;11:1259–66.

313. Lukas A, Niederecker T, Günther I, Mayer B, Nikolaus T. Self- and proxy report for the assessment of pain in patients with and without cognitive impairment. Experiences gained in a geriatric hospital. Z Gerontol Geriatr. 2013;46:214–21.

314. Li L, Herr K, Chen P. Postoperative pain assessment with three intensity scales in Chinese elders. J Nurs Scholarsh. 2009;41:241–9.

315. Zhou Y, Petpichetchian W, Kitrungrote L. Psychometric properties of pain intensity scales comparing among postoperative adult patients, elderly patients without and with mild cognitive impairment in China. Int J Nurs Stud. 2011;48:449–57.

316. Robert G, Le Jeune F, Dondaine T, Drapier S, Péron J, Lozachmeur C, et al. Apathy and impaired emotional facial recognition networks overlap in Parkinson's disease: a PET study with conjunction analyses. J Neurol Neurosurg Psychiatr. 2014;85:1153–8.

317. Jones KR, Vojir CP, Hutt E, Fink R. Determining mild, moderate, and severe pain equivalency across pain-intensity tools in nursing home residents. J Rehabil Res Dev. 2007;44:305–14.

318. Pesonen A, Kauppila T, Tarkkila P, Sutela A, Ninisto L, Rosenberg PH. Evaluation of easily applicable pain measurement tools for the assessment of pain in demented patients. Acta Anaesthesiol Scand. 2009;53:657–64.

319. Herr KA, Mobily PR. Comparison of selected pain assessment tools for use with the elderly. Appl Nurs Res. 1993;6:39–46.

320. Horgas AL, Elliott AF, Marsiske M. Pain assessment in persons with dementia: relationship between self-report and behavioral observation. J Am Geriatr Soc. 2009;57:126–32.

321. Pautex S, Michon A, Guedira M, Emond H, Le Lous P, Samaras D, et al. Pain in severe dementia: self-assessment or observational scales? J Am Geriatr Soc. 2006;54:1040–5.

322. Feldt KS. The checklist of nonverbal pain indicators (CNPI). Pain Manag Nurs. 2000;1:13–21.

323. Ersek M, Herr K, Neradilek MB, Buck HG, Black B. Comparing the psychometric properties of the Checklist of Nonverbal Pain Behaviors (CNPI) and the Pain Assessment in Advanced Dementia (PAIN-AD) instruments. Pain Med. 2010;11:395–404.

324. Lints-Martindale AC, Hadjistavropoulos T, Lix LM, Thorpe L. A comparative investigation of observational pain assessment tools for older adults with dementia. Clin J Pain. 2012;28:226–37.

325. Neville C, Ostini R. A psychometric evaluation of three pain rating scales for people with moderate to severe dementia. Pain Manag Nurs. 2014;15:798–806.

326. Abbey J, Piller N, De Bellis A, Esterman A. The Abbey pain scale: a 1-minute numerical indicator for people with end-stage dementia. Int J Palliat Nurs. 2004;10:6–13.

327. Liu JYW, Briggs M, Closs SJ. The psychometric qualities of four observational pain tools (OPTs) for the assessment of pain in elderly people with osteoarthritic pain. J Pain Symptom Manage. 2010;40:582–98.

328. Gregersen M, Melin AS, Nygaard IS, Nielsen CH, Beedholm-Ebsen M. Reliability of the Danish Abbey Pain Scale in severely demented and non-communicative older patients. Int J Palliat Nurs. 2016;22:482–8.

329. Hølen JC, Saltvedt I, Fayers PM, Bjørnnes M, Stenseth G, Hval B, et al. The Norwegian Doloplus-2, a tool for behavioural pain assessment: translation and pilot-validation in nursing home patients with cognitive impairment. Palliat Med. 2005;19:411–7.

330. Hølen JC, Saltvedt I, Fayers PM, Hjermstad MJ, Loge JH, Kaasa S. Doloplus-2, a valid tool for behavioural pain assessment? BMC Geriatr. 2007;7:29.

331. Snow AL, Weber JB, O'Malley KJ, Cody M, Beck C, Bruera E, et al. NOPPAIN: a nursing assistant-administered pain assessment instrument for use in dementia. Dement Geriatr Cogn Disord. 2004;17:240–6.

332. Horgas AL, Nichols AL, Schapson CA, Vietes K. Assessing pain in persons with dementia: relationships among the non-communicative patient's pain assessment instrument, self-report, and behavioral observations. Pain Manag Nurs. 2007;8:77–85.

333. Fuchs-Lacelle S, Hadjistavropoulos T, Lix L. Pain assessment as intervention: a study of older adults with severe dementia. Clin J Pain. 2008;24:697–707.

334. Chan S, Hadjistavropoulos T, Williams J, Lints-Martindale A. Evidence-based development and initial validation of the pain assessment checklist for seniors with limited ability to communicate-II (PACSLAC-II). Clin J Pain. 2014;30:816–24.

335. Persons APOPPIO. The management of persistent pain in older persons. J Am Geriatr Soc. 2002;50:205–24.

336. Zwakhalen SMG, Hamers JPH, Berger MPF. The psychometric quality and clinical usefulness of three pain assessment tools for elderly people with dementia. Pain. 2006;126:210–20.

337. Fuchs-Lacelle S, Hadjistavropoulos T. Development and preliminary validation of the pain assessment checklist for seniors with limited ability to communicate (PACSLAC). Pain Manag Nurs. 2004;5:37–49.

338. Horgas A, Miller L. Pain assessment in people with dementia. AJN. 2008;108:62–70.

339. DeWaters T, Faut-Callahan M, McCann JJ, Paice JA, Fogg L, Hollinger-Smith L, et al. Comparison of self-reported pain and the PAINAD scale in hospitalized cognitively impaired and intact older adults after hip fracture surgery. Orthop Nurs. 2008;27:21–8.

340. Zwakhalen SMG, van der Steen JT, Najim MD. Which score most likely represents pain on the observational PAINAD pain scale for patients with dementia? J Am Med Dir Asso. 2012;13:384–9.

341. Leong IY-O, Chong MS, Gibson SJ. The use of a self-reported pain measure, a nurse-reported pain measure and the PAINAD in nursing home residents with moderate and severe dementia: a validation study. Age Ageing. 2006;35:252–6.

342. Schuler MS, Becker S, Kaspar R, Nikolaus T, Kruse A, Basler H-D. Psychometric properties of the German "Pain Assessment in Advanced Dementia Scale" (PAINAD-G) in nursing home residents. J Am Med Dir Asso. 2007;8:388–95.

343. Mosele M, Inelmen EM, Toffanello ED, Girardi A, Coin A, Sergi G, et al. Psychometric properties of the pain assessment in advanced dementia scale compared to self assessment of pain in elderly patients. Dement Geriatr Cogn Disord. 2012;34:38–43.

# 9

# An immediate effect of PNF specific mobilization on the angle of trunk rotation and the Trunk-Pelvis-Hip Angle range of motion in adolescent girls with double idiopathic scoliosis

A. Stępień[1*], K. Fabian[2], K. Graff[1], M. Podgurniak[3^] and A. Wit[1]

## Abstract

**Background:** Impairment of spine rotation is a key concept in several theories explaining the pathogenesis and progression of scoliosis. In previous studies, a more limited range of motion in scoliotic girls compared to their non-scoliotic peers was noted. The Trunk-Pelvis-Hip Angle measurement is a test used to assess the range of motion in the trunk-pelvis-hip complex in the transverse plane. The aim of this study was to assess an immediate effect of Proprioceptive Neuromuscular Facilitation specific mobilization (mPNF) on the angle of trunk rotation and Trunk-Pelvis-Hip Angle range of motion in adolescent girls with double scoliosis.

**Methods:** The study was conducted on 83 girls aged 10 to 17 years (mean $13.7 \pm 1.9$) with double idiopathic scoliosis consisting of a right-sided thoracic curve (mean $25.1° \pm 13.9°$) and a left-sided thoracolumbar or lumbar curve (mean $20.8° \pm 11.4°$). The angle of trunk rotation and Trunk-Pelvis-Hip Angle were measured at baseline and after PNF mobilization. Bilateral lower limb patterns of Proprioceptive Neuromuscular Facilitation were used in combination with the "contract–relax" technique and stimulation of asymmetrical breathing. In the statistical analysis, the SAS rel. 13.2 software was used. Preliminary statistical analysis was performed using descriptive statistics. According to Shapiro-Wilk criterion of normality, the Wilcoxon test was used to compare paired samples. Next, the data was analyzed using multivariate GLM models.

**Results:** In adolescent girls with double scoliosis, significant differences between the left and right side of the body concerning the Trunk-Pelvis-Hip Angle ranges were noted. A single, unilateral PNF mobilization significantly decreased the angle of trunk rotation in the thoracic ($p < 0.001$) and lumbar spine ($p < 0.001$). Unilateral PNF mobilization also increased the Trunk-Pelvis-Hip Angle ranges on the left ($p < 0.001$) and right ($p < 0.001$) side significantly.

**Conclusions:** Unilateral PNF mobilization led to a decrease in the angle of trunk rotation, improvement in the range of motion, and the symmetry of mobility in the transverse plane in the trunk-pelvis-hip complex in adolescent girls with double idiopathic scoliosis. The effects should be treated only as immediate. Further studies are required to determine long-term effects of PNF mobilization on the spinal alignment.

**Keywords:** Idiopathic scoliosis, PNF, Angle of trunk rotation, Rotation, Physiotherapy

* Correspondence: orthosas@wp.pl
^Deceased
[1]Department of Rehabilitation, Józef Piłsudski University of Physical Education, Warsaw, Poland
Full list of author information is available at the end of the article

## Background

Idiopathic scoliosis is one of the most common spinal deformities in children and adolescents. It is defined as three-dimensional torsional deformity characterized by lateral deviation of the spine equal to or greater than 10°, vertebral rotation and reduced normal thoracic kyphosis [1, 2]. According to the literature, adolescent idiopathic scoliosis (AIS) affects 0.93 to 12% of adolescents aged 10–18 years and is more common in girls [2, 3].

Vertebral rotation with the associated rib hump and/ or lumbar hump is a major sign of scoliosis. That is why measurement of the angle of trunk rotation (ATR) with a scoliometer is an important element of scoliosis examination. To date, however, a standard physical examination has not included an assessment of the spine rotation range. It may stem from the fact that scoliotic individuals demonstrate generalized joint hypermobility significantly more often [4, 5]. On the other hand, previous studies showed a more limited range of motion (ROM) in the transverse plane in scoliotic girls compared to their non-scoliotic peers [6–8]. It was noted that the limitation in the range of rotation increased with the Cobb angle [6]. The greatest differences in ROM between the left and right side of the body were observed in girls with double scoliosis [7]. The Trunk-Pelvis-Hip Angle (TPHA) measurement is a test used to assess the range of motion in the trunk-pelvis-hip complex in the transverse plane. The TPHA test showed rotational asymmetry in girls with double scoliosis [8]. According to some theories, an impairment of spine rotation is considered a factor predisposing to the development and progression of scoliosis [9, 10].

Proprioceptive Neuromuscular Facilitation (PNF) method is used in patients with various motor problems and offers a large number of movement patterns, procedures, and techniques, including effective techniques to improve ROM [11–13]. Precisely described movement patterns allow the therapist to act selectively on particular parts of the musculoskeletal system, including the spine [12]. To date, the effectiveness of PNF in the conservative treatment of individuals with idiopathic scoliosis has not been confirmed.

The aim of this study was to assess an immediate effect of PNF specific mobilization on the ATR and the TPHA range of motion in adolescent girls with double scoliosis.

## Methods

The study was approved by the Senate Research Ethics Committee at Jozef Pilsudski University of Physical Education in Warsaw, Poland, SKE 01-04/2015.

### Study subjects

Scoliotic girls who visited one of the three centers specializing in the conservative treatment of scoliosis were consecutively enrolled in the study which lasted 6 months. The inclusion criteria were as follows: female, double idiopathic scoliosis consisting of a right-sided thoracic curve and a left-sided lumbar/thoracolumbar curve diagnosed on antero-posterior radiogram, absence of systemic diseases, age 10–17 years, and participation consent. Girls with other types of scoliosis, a spinal curvature with a Cobb angle of less than 10°, with pain or a history of traumatic injury were excluded from the study.

The girls and their parents or legal guardians were informed about the aims of the study and signed the consent to participate in the study and publish anonymous data form.

### Measurement methods

The study was performed by three physiotherapists who were experienced in treating scoliosis and were trained and certified in PNF. The physiotherapists were also trained regarding the application of the TPHA test.

At one session, the girls underwent a physiotherapy examination twice, at the beginning and at the end of the session. The examination, carried out by a physiotherapist, included test 1, i.e., a standard measurement of the ATR, and test 2, i.e., an assessment of the active ROM in the trunk-pelvis-hip complex using the TPHA test (Fig. 1a, b). After the first examination, the girls

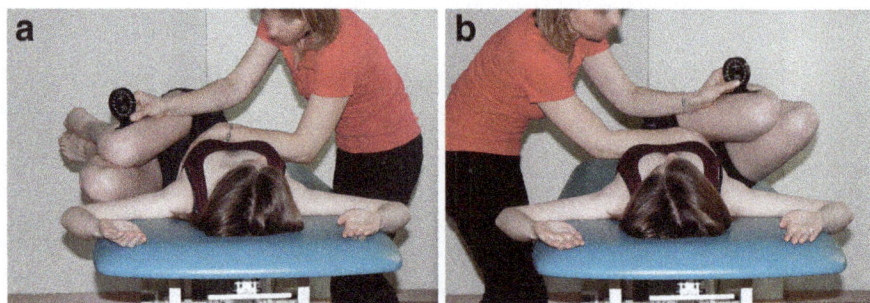

**Fig. 1 a** The Trunk-Pelvis-Hip Angle on the *left* (TPHAleft). **b** The Trunk-Pelvis-Hip Angle on the *right* (TPHAright)

underwent mobilization using the bilateral lower limb PNF patterns (mPNF) and were again assessed (test 1 and test 2) to find out whether the mobilization had any effect on the ATR and TPHA.

The ATR (test 1) was measured with a scoliometer (Orthopedic Systems Inc. OSI 1995), which showed excellent reliability in the previous studies [14–16]. One measurement was performed on the thoracic and lumbar segments of the spine with the subject standing. The range of motion in the TPHA (test 2) was assessed with a Rippstein plurimeter (Rippstein, Switzerland). The assessment of the TPHA test reliability demonstrated excellent agreement of measurements—the inter-rater reliability for three investigators was 0.97 (THPAleft) and 0.98 (TPHAright) and the intraobserver reliability was 0.87 (TPHAleft) and 0.81 (TPHAright) [8].

The TPHA measurements were performed on an adjustable-height table with the subject in a supine position, arms perpendicular to the trunk, and elbows flexed at a 90° angle. Next, lower limbs were flexed at the hips and knees until the sacral bone was involved in the motion and the lumbar segment remained on the surface of the table. Standing at the subject's side, the examiner stabilized her chest with his or her own forearm kept across the chest at the level of the costal arches and measured the ROM with the other hand. The plurimeter base was held along the long axis of the femur on the lateral aspect of the thigh, at the knee fissure. The subject was asked to move the flexed lower limbs towards the elbow opposite to the examiner. The motion of the lower limbs was stopped when the examiner felt the ribs move under his or her forearm or the subject experienced pain. The actual measurement was performed at the upper ROM limit, 5 s after it had been reached. Before the measurement, the plurimeter was reset to zero in relation to the surface. The angle of the hip position below the surface level was marked as "–"and that above the surface level as "+". The measurements were performed in triplicate, alternately on the left and right side. The highest ROM values were used in the statistical analysis.

### Mobilization techniques

The therapeutic session consisted of unilateral PNF specific muscle mobilization (mPNF), which was safe and painless. The direction of mPNF was determined on the basis of the results of previous research which revealed limitations of the range of motion in the TPHAright compared to the TPHAleft both in girls with double scoliosis and healthy girls [8]. Bilateral lower limb patterns (flexion to the right and extension to the left) were used in subjects in a supine position with a stable chest in combination with the "contract–relax" technique and stimulation of asymmetrical breathing. The subject had

to maintain muscle tension for 5 s three times in succession and then actively increase ROM. This cycle was repeated three times at 10-s intervals. The last phase of mobilization consisted of 10 active movements of lower limbs towards mobilization and asymmetrical breathing—5 slow inspirations and expirations (Table 1). The total duration of mobilization was approximately 3 min.

After mPNF, the measurement of the ATR and TPHA was repeated and compared with the measurements obtained at baseline.

In the statistical analysis, the SAS rel. 13.2 software was used. Preliminary statistical analysis was performed using descriptive statistics. According to Shapiro-Wilk criterion of normality, the Wilcoxon test was used to compare paired samples. Next, the data was analyzed using multivariate GLM models. The analysis of power and sample size was performed in the SAS System. As shown in the sample size analysis based on a pilot data and confirmed by the results of the main study, the power of the tests used in this manuscript should exceed 0.80.

### Results

In the period of 6 months, 87 girls with double scoliosis were qualified for participation in the study. Four girls did not come to the meeting with a physiotherapist. Ultimately, the study was performed on 83 girls with double idiopathic scoliosis with different levels of deformity diagnosed according to the recommended classification [2]. The basic characteristics of the group are presented in Table 2.

When the classification by a degree of spinal curvature was used in compliance with the guidelines [2], 24 girls (28.9%) were found to have low scoliosis (10°–15°); 16 girls (19.3%), low to moderate scoliosis (16°–24°); 19 girls (22.9%), moderate scoliosis (25°–34°); 16 girls (19.3%), moderate to severe scoliosis (35°–44°); and 8 girls (9.6%) had severe and very severe scoliosis. The Risser grade was as follows: 0 in 8 girls (9.6%), 1 in 13 girls (15.7%), 2 in 10 girls (12.0%), 3 in 16 girls (19.3%), 4 in 27 girls (32.5%), and 5 in 9 girls (10.8%). Twenty-five subjects (30.1%) wore a brace. Most study participants ($n = 62$, 74.7%) underwent some physiotherapy, while 21 girls did not receive any physiotherapeutic treatment. In this group, 11 girls had low scoliosis.

Mean values of the ATR and TPHA obtained before and after mPNF are presented in Table 3. The comparison of the initial values of the TPHA on both sides of the body in the entire study group revealed that the TPHAleft was significantly greater than the TPHAright ($p < 0.001$).

The mPNF significantly reduced the ATR in the thoracic (ATRT, $p < 0.001$) and lumbar spine (ARTL, $p < 0.001$).

**Table 1** PNF mobilization method

| Step | Description | Photograph |
|---|---|---|
| 1. | Starting position: the patient in a supine position with the arms perpendicular to the trunk and elbows flexed at a 90° angle. | |
| 2. | The physiotherapist (PT) standing by the patient at the side with limited ROM. The patient's lower limbs are flexed and pulled towards the chest until the sacral bone is lifted up. | |
| 3. | The patient's chest stabilized by the PT's forearm; the lower limbs moved towards the elbow until the rib movement is felt by the PT. | |
| 4. | Lower limbs stabilized by the PT with the other forearm and the chest. The patient's chest remains stable: "Contract–relax" against-resistance—an attempt to move the lower limbs (isometric contraction) towards the bilateral extension pattern for the lower limbs (3 × 5 s). | |
| 5. | Active movement of the lower limbs towards the bilateral flexion pattern at the end of ROM without manual resistance, movement repeated 10 times, the patient's chest remains stable. | |
| 6. | The lower limbs kept stable, inhalation and exhalation repeated five times with the rib movement on the opposite side towards the table surface | |
| 7. | Back to the starting position (1). | |

*mPNF* PNF mobilization, *PT* physiotherapist, *ROM* range of motion

**Table 2** Characteristics of the study group (age, weight, height, BMI, Th Cobb, L Cobb)

| | Mean (N = 83) | SD | Min. | Max. |
|---|---|---|---|---|
| Age (years) | 13.7 | 1.9 | 10 | 17 |
| Weight (kg) | 51.8 | 10.9 | 23 | 75 |
| Height (m) | 1.62 | 9.5 | 1.29 | 1.77 |
| BMI (kg/m²) | 19.5 | 2.7 | 13.8 | 24.7 |
| Th Cobb (°) | 25.1 | 13.9 | 10 | 82 |
| L Cobb (°) | 20.8 | 11.4 | 10 | 53 |

*BMI* body mass index, *N* number, *Th Cobb* Cobb measurements in the thoracic spine, *L Cobb* Cobb measurements in the lumbar spine, *SD* standard deviation, *SE* standard error, *Min* minimum, *Max* maximum

In the majority of the subjects, the decrease in the ATR in the thoracic (ATRT) and lumbar (ATRL) segment was obtained. In 35 girls, ATR values decreased by at least 2° both in the thoracic and in the lumbar segment. A simultaneous analysis of both curve angles revealed that in 55% of the subjects, one of the ATR values changed by at least 3°. An improvement in the ATR in the thoracic or lumbar spine from 0 to 2 was noted in 37 subjects. The biggest changes in the ATR were noted in the thoracic segment of the spine in girls with scoliosis deeper than 35°. Changes in the ATRT (Fig. 2) and ATRL (Fig. 3) occurring after mPNF in particular girls are presented below.

**Table 3** Values of the ATR in the thoracic/lumbar part of the spine and the TPHA before and after mPNF in girls with double scoliosis

|  | ATRT ± SEM | ATRL ± SEM | TPHAleft ± SEM | TPHAright ± SEM | TPHAleft vs TPHAright |
|---|---|---|---|---|---|
| Before mPNF | 7.96° ± 0.75° | 4.90° ± 0.39° | − 7.65° ± 0.94 | + 1.82° ± 1.18° | p < 0.001 |
| After mPNF | 5.71° ± 0.61° | 3.23° ± 0.33° | − 12.48° ± 0.47 | − 9.78° ± 0.85° | p < 0.001 |
| Significance | p < 0.001 | p < 0.001 | p < 0.001 | p < 0.001 |  |

Significant difference p < 0.05

*ATR* angle of trunk rotation, *ATRT/ATRL* angle of trunk rotation in the thoracic/lumbar part of the spine; *TPHA* Trunk-Pelvis-Hip Angle; *TPHAleft/TPHAright* TPHA to the left/right; *mPNF* PNF mobilization; SEM standard error of measurement

The mPNF significantly increased the ROM in both the mTPHAleft (TPHAleft measured after mobilization) and mTPHAright (TPHAright measured after mobilization). After mobilization, the difference between the values of the mTPHAleft and mTPHAright decreased although it remained significant ($p < 0.001$). Figures 4 and 5 present the TPHAleft and TPHAright values before and after mobilization in particular girls.

In 12 out of 83 girls, no lower values of the TPHAright compared to the TPHAleft before the mobilization were revealed. Despite the lack of movement limitation, unilateral mobilization decreased the ATR and changed the ranges of motion in all the girls from this subgroup.

In order to reflect the changes in the TPHA test and to determine symmetries of the movements, a conventional line was set—the bisector deviation (BD) of the angle between the two extreme ranges of motion, i.e., the TPHAleft and TPHAright (Fig. 6). BD, initially transposed to the left in 86% of the subjects, was shifted to the sagittal axis of the body following mobilization (mBD). Before the mPNF, the bisector deviation between the TPHAleft and TPHAright was transposed to the left from the sagittal axis of the body by 4.73° (± SEM 0.50), and after mPNF, the shift to the left was by 1.35° (± SEM 0.37). This change was statistically significant ($p < 0.001$). The biggest shift of BD was noted in girls with scoliosis deeper that 35°.

Taking into account Akaike information criterion (AIC), the model with the normal distribution of identity link function was the most appropriate multivariate GLM model. In this model, repeated measurements were represented by a factor affecting the analyzed parameters (ATR, TPHA, BD). This factor was significant in models both with and without other factors such as Th Cobb, L Cobb, a brace, physiotherapy, and Risser test. That means that the mPNF influenced significant changes in the ATR, TPHA, and BD.

## Discussion

In the present research, it was revealed that a single use of unilateral mPNF significantly decreased the ATR, increased the TPHA range of motion, and improved motion symmetry reflected in the shift of BD to the sagittal axis of the body in girls with double idiopathic scoliosis. A multivariate analysis confirmed a considerable influence of mPNF on the changes of the ATR, TPHA, and BD. Additionally, the influence of mPNF was also considered significant when other parameters such as curve size in the thoracic and lumbar segment, Risser test, a brace, and physiotherapy were taken into account.

A significant improvement in the ATR values in the thoracic and lumbar spine after mobilization was observed in the study group. However, caution in the interpretation of the results is advised since we do not know whether these differences are not only statistically but also clinically significant. In 37 subjects, a difference of 0°–2° was found in the thoracic or lumbar spine after mPNF and such a change may be seen as clinically insignificant. Nevertheless, a greater improvement was noted in the majority of the subjects. It is also worth

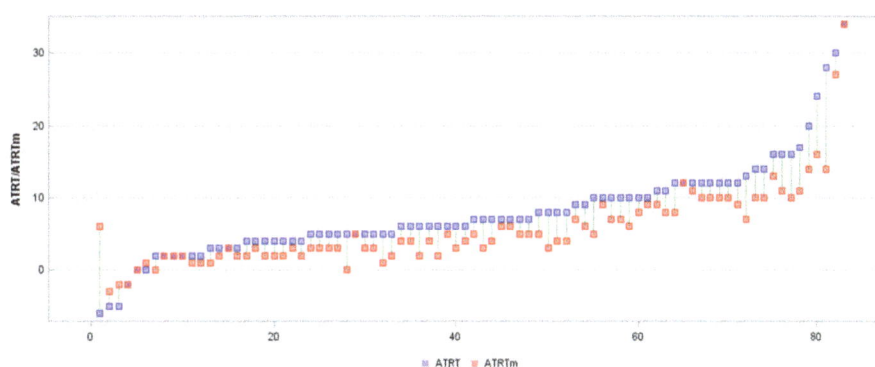

**Fig. 2** Measurements (°) of the ATRT and ATRTm in individual participants (*ATRT* angle of trunk rotation in the thoracic spine before mPNF, *ATRTm* angle of trunk rotation in the thoracic spine after mPNF, *mPNF* PNF mobilization)

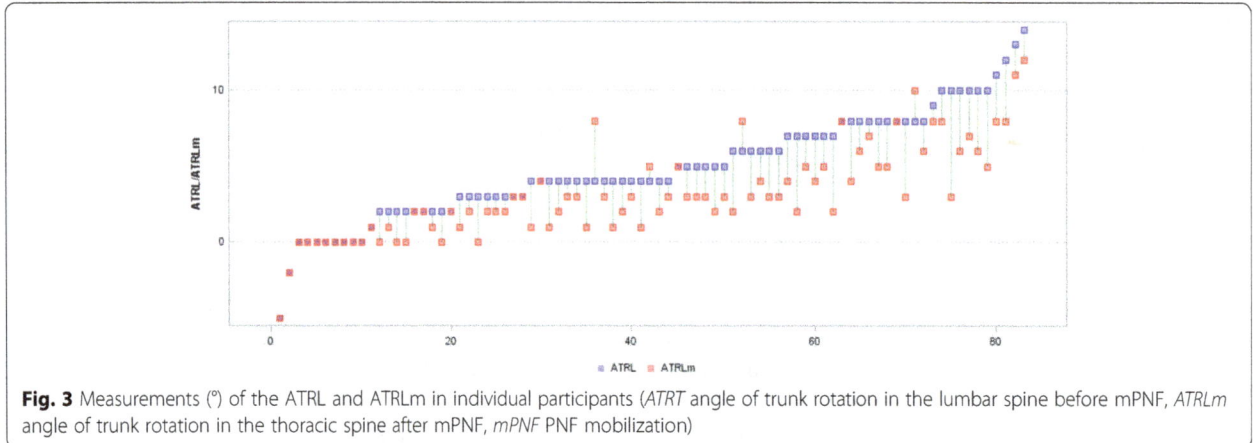

**Fig. 3** Measurements (°) of the ATRL and ATRLm in individual participants (*ATRT* angle of trunk rotation in the lumbar spine before mPNF, *ATRLm* angle of trunk rotation in the thoracic spine after mPNF, *mPNF* PNF mobilization)

noting that in a number of girls, the ATR values decreased both in the thoracic and in the lumbar segment, which may affect the way clinical significance of these changes is seen. The biggest changes were noted in girls with scoliosis deeper than 35°.

In the literature of the subject, the issue of an immediate effect of particular techniques on the ATR values in scoliosis has not been frequently discussed. No publication has been found which would describe the application of muscle mobilization similar to the one used in our research. Wnuk et al. revealed an immediate positive effect of derotation manual therapy on a decrease in the ATR in two groups of girls with single and double scoliosis. The greatest effect reflected by the decreased ATR was achieved in girls with single scoliosis [17]. These results cannot be directly compared to our research results due to a different type of mobilization technique applied in the studies.

Derotation techniques are frequently used by manual therapists, chiropractors, and osteopaths. Certain studies indicate the effectiveness of treating scoliosis with manual therapy techniques, including derotation techniques [18, 19], but the authors of other studies are not certain about the long-term effects of manual therapy or chiropractic [20, 21]. Morningstar et al. revealed an improvement in radiological image in the group of 22 subjects aged 15–65 with scoliosis after a 4- to 6-week-long manipulative and rehabilitation therapy [18]. Lewis et al. applied Active Therapeutic Movement Version 2 device and home exercises using the Mulligan's mobilization for 4 weeks and revealed an improvement in body position in 43 individuals with scoliosis from various age groups [19]. On the other hand, following a literature review, Romano and Negrini revealed that the level of the previous studies does not make it possible to draw conclusions regarding the effectiveness of manual therapy in treating scoliosis [21].

A change in the TPHA ranges was another effect of the applied mPNF. The value of the TPHAright in the study group before mobilization was significantly lower than the value of the TPHAleft. After the application of mPNF, the ranges of motion of the TPHA changed but the difference between the TPHAleft and TPHAright remained significant although it was smaller.

The noted limitation of the TPHAright in relation to the TPHAleft in the study group is in line with earlier findings reported by Stępień et al. [7]. This earlier study, conducted with the use of computer-assisted motion

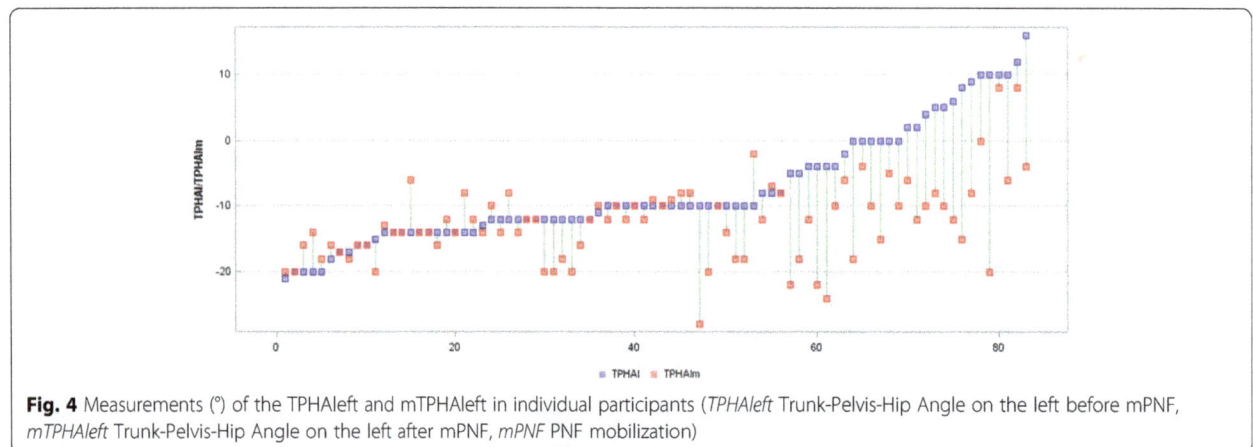

**Fig. 4** Measurements (°) of the TPHAleft and mTPHAleft in individual participants (*TPHAleft* Trunk-Pelvis-Hip Angle on the left before mPNF, *mTPHAleft* Trunk-Pelvis-Hip Angle on the left after mPNF, *mPNF* PNF mobilization)

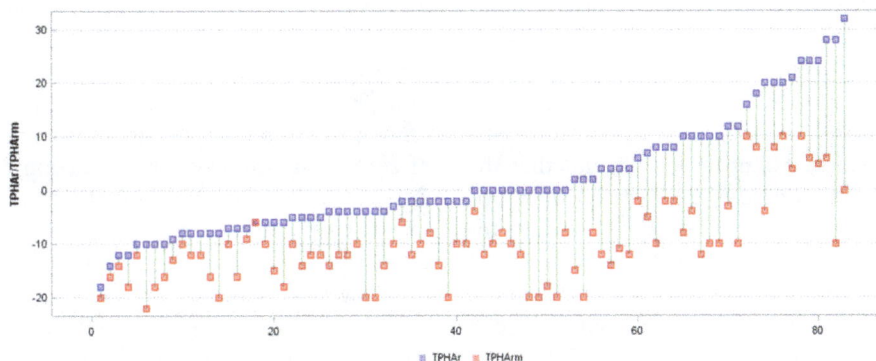

**Fig. 5** Measurements (°) of the TPHAright and mTPHAright in individual participants (*TPHAright* Trunk-Pelvis-Hip Angle on the right before mPNF, *mTPHAleft* Trunk-Pelvis-Hip Angle on the *right* after mPNF, *mPNF* PNF mobilization)

analysis on a group of adolescent girls with double scoliosis, found significant differences between ranges of motion in the transverse plane. The trunk rotation to the right was greater than the trunk rotation to the left, and the measured rotation of the pelvis to the left was significantly greater than the rotation to the right. The ranges of trunk rotation to the left and pelvis rotation to the right were significantly smaller in scoliotic girls than in their healthy peers [7].

Asymmetry of spinal rotation in the girls with scoliosis was also demonstrated in the latest studies using the TPHA test. In the research including 49 adolescent girls with double scoliosis and 49 healthy girls, a significant limitation in the TPHAright was noted in the group of girls with spinal deformity. The range of motion of the TPHAright was significantly lower not only than the

range of motion of the TPHAleft in this group but also than the range of motion of the TPHAright noted in the group of healthy girls. A significant limitation of the range of motion of the TPHAright compared to the TPHAleft was also noted within the group of girls without scoliosis [8], which indicates the existence of a certain physiological asymmetry of rotational movements that increases in individuals with double scoliosis. The bilateral lower limb patterns used in unilateral mPNF were selected due to the determined direction of the limitation of the TPHAright.

An impairment of rotation in adolescent girls with progressive idiopathic scoliosis was also observed in much earlier studies conducted by other authors. Poussa and Mellin, who studied spinal mobility in 71 girls with idiopathic thoracic scoliosis, noted lower ranges of

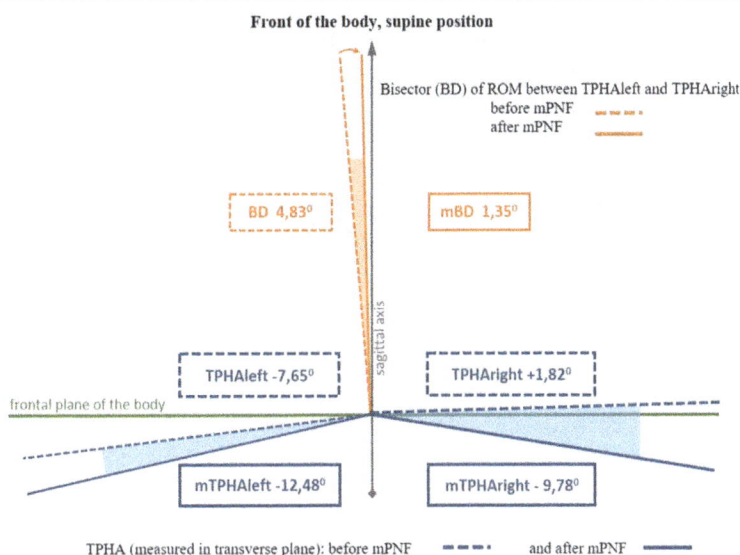

**Fig. 6** The bisector BD of the angle between the TPHAleft and TPHAright before and after mPNF (*ROM* range of motion, *mPNF* PNF mobilization, *TPHAleft* Trunk-Pelvis-Hip Angle on the left before mPNF, *mTPHAleft* Trunk-Pelvis-Hip Angle on the *left* after mPNF, *TPHAright* Trunk-Pelvis-Hip Angle on the *right* before mPNF, *mTPHAright* Trunk-Pelvis-Hip Angle on the right after mPNF, *BD* bisector deviation angle from the sagittal axis of the body, *mBD* BD after mPNF)

rotation in girls with a greater curvature of the spine. The authors concluded that decreased thoracic rotation and the straightening of the spine may serve as factors affecting the progression of scoliosis in the thoracic segment of the spine [6]. In another research on the girls with idiopathic scoliosis, McIntire et al. found that the strength of rotation towards the concavity of their primary curve was lower than the strength of rotation towards the convex side. The authors concluded that factors which might potentially lead to differences in the strength of muscles participating in rotation included soft tissue tension and limited rotation range [22].

To date, few authors have analyzed an influence of the therapy on an increase in the spinal range of motion. In their research, Lewis et al. noted an improvement in spinal ranges of motion in all directions except for flexion and extension. However, the research included subjects from a broad range of age groups, which made it difficult to analyze and compare the results [19].

An improvement in ROM in patients with scoliosis should be carefully analyzed. Usually, increased mobility of the spine is thought to be dangerous in scoliosis [4, 5, 23]. Czaprowski et al. found that generalized joint hypermobility occurred significantly more often in girls and boys with scoliosis compared to their healthy peers [5]. In their study, they used the Beighton scale which assesses mobility of the spine in the sagittal plane and does not take into consideration motion in the transverse plane. Generalized joint laxity and a higher incidence of scoliosis were found in rhythmic gymnastics trainees [4] and ballet dancers [23], but rotation was not assessed in these groups, either. To sum up, it should be concluded that the process of increasing spine mobility in scoliotic patients should be conducted carefully and further research in this field is necessary. In our opinion, it should be established every time in which plane a limited or increased range of motion of the spine occurs.

It is difficult to say what mechanism was responsible for an immediate effect in our research. There is a lot of evidence leading to the conclusion that the decreased ATR and the increased TPHA result from muscle relaxation, but muscle tension was not assessed in our study. A number of earlier studies revealed differences in the activity of paravertebral muscles between the concave and the convex sides of the curve in the subjects with scoliosis [24, 25]. A correlation was found between muscle function asymmetry and axial rotation of the spine [24]. In the present study, the muscle contract–relax technique was used, which in addition to the "hold–relax" technique, is utilized by PNF to relax tense muscles [12, 13]. Several authors have demonstrated the effectiveness of PNF muscle relaxation techniques [11, 26–29], but in none of the studies, an attempt

was made at improving spinal rotation. It was observed that maximal muscle contraction is not required to achieve muscle relaxation and increase the range of motion [30–32]. For this reason, in the present study, the physiotherapists used moderate resistance. The technique of contracting muscles for 5 s used in our study did not differ from that proposed by other authors [11, 30, 33], while the number of repetitions of muscle contractions chosen by the present authors was based on their earlier observations and clinical experience.

In the present study, the study group included all the girls with double scoliosis who were in the required age group, regardless of the results of the TPHA test conducted prior to the test. It results from the fact that at this stage of research, it is difficult to define what values of the TPHAleft and TPHAright should be seen as a norm and what values indicate movement limitation. Determining the norm requires further research on bigger samples including healthy individuals and subjects with various types of scoliosis. In the examined group of 83 girls with double scoliosis, there were 12 girls who did not reveal lower values of the TPHAright. This subgroup mainly included girls with non-progressive low scoliosis and low to moderate scoliosis. Two girls had scoliosis of over 30°. After the application of unilateral mPNF in this subgroup, an improvement in the ATR and a change of the TPHA values were noted in all the girls. The results indicate that there exists a certain mechanism, apart from a unilateral movement limitation, which affects the body position in scoliosis. The mechanism which underlies the improvement of the ATR and the increased mobility is not fully understood and needs further investigation.

In the past, rotation limitations were seen as one of the main factors affecting the development of idiopathic scoliosis [9, 10]. Burwell et al. stated that scoliosis results from a cyclical failure of mechanisms of rotation control in the trunk during gait [9]. Wong concluded that thoracic rotational instability leads to the development of scoliosis [10]. Asymmetries of rotational movements noted in the present research may serve as a completion of the aforementioned theories.

To sum up, it can be concluded that an improvement in the ATR, TPHA, and BD parameters in this research indicates an immediate effect in girls with double scoliosis. However, it does not prove the effectiveness of the undertaken actions. Therefore, further long-term observation and radiological confirmation are needed. According to the international guidelines, such long-term effectiveness is perceived as a higher satisfaction with appearance and a better quality of life in scoliotic adolescents, arrested progression of deformity, alleviation of pain and improved respiratory function and exercise efficiency [34].

## Limitations of the study

The study has certain limitations. It was revealed that an immediate effect of mPNF occurred only in the girls with double idiopathic scoliosis. An immediate effect seen as a decrease in the ATR and an increase in the TPHA with the reduction in the differences between the right and left sides does not prove the effectiveness of the method used since that would require long-term observation confirmed by radiographic evidence. It is recommended to assess the long-term efficiency of physiotherapy. In order to confirm the efficiency of the applied interventions, further studies are needed with a control group in which a different stretching method would be applied. Another obvious limitation is the fact that the ATR and TPHA measurements were performed by the physiotherapists applying mPNF.

The results of the study should be considered as a preliminary observation which allows better understanding of the spinal biomechanics in double idiopathic scoliosis. Although the effect achieved may be clinically insignificant, it may indicate a promising direction in the physiotherapy of scoliosis.

## Conclusions

Unilateral mPNF has an impact on the reduction in the angle of trunk rotation, improvement in the range of motion, and the symmetry of mobility in the transverse plane in the trunk-pelvis-hip complex in adolescent girls with double idiopathic scoliosis. The effects should be treated only as immediate. Further studies are required to determine long-term effects of mPNF on the spinal alignment.

## Abbreviations

AIS: Adolescent idiopathic scoliosis; ATR: Angle of trunk rotation; ATRL: Angle of trunk rotation in the lumbar spine; ATRT: Angle of trunk rotation in the thoracic spine; BD: Bisector deviation; L: Lumbar; mBD: BD after mPNF; mPNF: PNF mobilization; mTPHA: TPHA after mPNF; PNF: Proprioceptive Neuromuscular Facilitation; PT: Physiotherapist; ROM: Range of motion; SD: Standard deviation; SEM: Standard error of measurement; T: Thoracic; TPHA: Trunk-Pelvis-Hip Angle; TPHAleft/TPHAright: TPHA on the left/right

## Acknowledgements

The authors give many thanks to Professor Andrzej Seyfried for valuable teaching and initiating the study in the past. We are grateful to Anna Karwańska for her support in data analysis.

## Funding

There are no sources of funding for the research. The publication fee was contributed by the authors.

## Authors' contributions

AS conceptualized and designed the study; participated in the recruitment of participants, the examination of participants, and therapeutic session as PT; collected the data; analyzed and interpreted the data; and drafted the manuscript. KF participated in the recruitment of participants, the examination of participants, and therapeutic session as PT and collected the data. KG participated in the recruitment of participants, the examination of participants, and therapeutic session as PT and collected the data. MP performed a statistical analysis. AW revised the manuscript critically. All the authors read and approved the final manuscript.

## Competing interests

AS is a certificated teacher of PNF method. The authors declare that they have no competing interests.

## Author details

[1]Department of Rehabilitation, Józef Piłsudski University of Physical Education, Warsaw, Poland. [2]Regional Children's Hospital, Jastrzębie Zdrój, Poland. [3]Department of Physiological Sciences, University of Life Science, Warsaw, Poland.

## References

1. Grivas TB, Burwell GR, Vasiliadis ES, Webb JK. A segmental radiological study of the spine and rib-cage in children with progressive infantile idiopathic scoliosis. Scoliosis 2006;1:17.
2. Negrini S, Aulisa AG, Aulisa L, Circo AB, de Mauroy JC, Durmala JC, Grivas TB, Knott P, Kotwicki T, Maruyama T, Minozzi S, O'Brien JP, Papadopoulos D, Rigo M, Rivard CR, Romano M, Wynne JH, Villagrasa M, Weiss HR, Zaina F. 2011 SOSORT guidelines: Orthopaedic and rehabilitation treatment of idiopathic scoliosis during growth. Scoliosis. 2012;7:3.
3. Konieczny MR, Senyurt H, Krauspe R. Epidemiology of adolescent idiopathic scoliosis. J Child Orthop. 2013;7:3–9.
4. Tanchev PI, Dzherov AD, Parushev AD, Dikov DM, Todorov MB. Scoliosis in rhythmic gymnasts. Spine (Phila Pa 1976). 2000;25(11):1367–72.
5. Czaprowski D, Kotwicki T, Pawłowska P, Stoliński Ł. Joint hypermobility in children with idiopathic scoliosis: SOSORT award 2011 winner. Scoliosis. 2011;6:22.
6. Poussa M, Mellin G. Spinal mobility and posture in adolescent idiopathic scoliosis at three stages of curve magnitude. Spine. 1992;17:757–60.
7. Stępień A. A range of rotation of the trunk and pelvis in girls with idiopathic scoliosis. Advances in Rehabilitation. 2011;25(3):5–12.
8. Stępień A, Guzek K, Rekowski W, Radomska I, Stępowska J. Assessment of the lumbo-pelvic-hip complex mobility with the Trunk-Pelvis-Hip Angle test: intraobserver reliability and differences in ranges of motion between girls with idiopathic scoliosis and their healthy counterparts. Advances in Rehabilitation. 2016;30(3):27–39.
9. Burwell RG, Cole AA, Cook TA, Grivas TB, Kiel AW, Moulton A, Thirwall AS, Upadhay SS, Webb JK, Wemyss-Holden SA, Whitwell DJ, Wojcik AS, Wythers DJ. Pathogenesis of idiopathic scoliosis. The Nottingham concept Acta Orthop Belg. 1992;58:33–58.
10. Wong CH. Mechanism of right thoracic adolescent idiopathic scoliosis at risk for progression; a unifying pathway of development by normal growth and imbalance. Scoliosis. 2015;10:2.
11. Sharman MJ, Cresswell AG, Riek S. Proprioceptive neuromuscular facilitation stretching: mechanisms and clinical implications. Sports Med. 2006;36(11):929–39.
12. Adler SS, Becker D, Buck M. PNF in practice. 4th ed. Berlin Heidelberg: Springer – Verlag; 2014.
13. Smedes F, Heidmann M, Schäfer C, Fischer N, Stępień A. The proprioceptive neuromuscular facilitation concept; the state of the evidence, a narrative review. Phys Ther Rev. 2016;21(1):17–31. doi:10.1080/10833196.2016.1216764.
14. Amendt LE, Ause-Ellias KL, Eybers JL, Wadsworth CT, Nielsen DH, Weinstein SL. Validity and reliability testing of the Scoliometer. Phys Ther. 1990;70(2):108–17.
15. Korovessis PG. Scoliometer is useful instrument with high reliability and repeatability. Spine (Phila Pa 1976). 1999;24(3):307–8.
16. Bonagamba GH, Coelho DM, Oliveira A. Inter and intra-rater reliability of the scoliometer. Rev Bras Fisioter. 2010;14(5):432–8.
17. Wnuk B, Blicharska I, Błaszczak B, Durmała J. The impact of the derotational mobilization of manual therapy according to Kaltenborn-Evjenth on the angle of trunk rotation in patients with adolescent idiopathic scoliosis—pilot study, direct observation. Ortop Trumatol Rehabil. 2015;4(6):343–50.
18. Morningstar MW, Woggon D, Lawrence G. Scoliosis treatment using a combination of manipulative and rehabilitative therapy: a retrospective case series. BMC Musculoskelet Disord. 2004;5:32.
19. Lewis C, Diaz R, Lopez G, Marki N, Olivio B. A preliminary study evaluate postural improvement in subject with scoliosis: active therapeutic movement

version 2 device and home exercises using Mulliga's mobilization –with movement concept. JMPT. 2014;20:1–8.

20.  Lantz CA, Chen J. Effect of chiropractic intervention on small scoliotic curves in younger subjects: a time-series cohort design. J Manip Physiol Ther. 2001;24:385–93.

21.  Romano M, Negrini S. Manual therapy as a conservative treatment for adolescent idiopathic scoliosis. Scoliosis. 2008;3:2.

22.  McIntire KL, Asher MA, Burton DC, Liu W. Trunk rotational strength asymmetry in adolescents with idiopathic scoliosis: an observational study. Scoliosis. 2007;2:9.

23.  Warren MP, Brooks-Gunn J, Hamilton LH, Warren LF, Hamilton WG. Scoliosis and fractures in young ballet dancers. Relation to delayed menarche and secondary amenorrhea. N Engl J Med. 1986;314(21):1348–53.

24.  Cheung J, Veldhuizen AG, Halberts JP, Sluiter WJ, Van Horn JR. Geometric and electromyographic assessments in the evaluation of curve progression in idiopathic scoliosis. Spine. 2006;31(3):322–9.

25.  Chwała W, Koziana A, Kasperczyk T, Walaszek R, Płaszewski M. Electromyographic assessment of functional symmetry of paraspinal muscles during static exercises in adolescents with idiopathic scoliosis. Biomed Res Int. 2014; doi:10.1155/573276.

26.  Godges JJ, Mattson-Bell M, Thorpe D, Shah D. The immediate effects of soft tissue mobilization with proprioceptive neuromuscular facilitation on glenohumeral external rotation and overhead reach. J Orthop Sports Phys Ther. 2003;33(12):713–8.

27.  Hindle KB, Whitcomb TJ, Briggs WO, Hong J. Proprioceptive Neuromuscular Facilitation (PNF): its mechanisms and effects on range of motion and muscular function. J Hum Kinet. 2012;31(1):105–13.

28.  Funk DC, Swank AM, Mikla BM, Fagan TA, Farr BK. Impact of prior exercise on hamstring flexibility: a comparison of proprioceptive neuromuscular facilitation and static stretching. J Strength Cond Res. 2003;17(3):489–92.

29.  Al Dajah SB. Soft tissue mobilization and PNF improve range of motion and minimize pain level in shoulder impingement. J Phys Ther Sci. 2014;26(11):1803–5.

30.  Feland JB, Marin HN. Effect of submaximal contraction intensity in contract-relax proprioceptive neuromuscular facilitation stretching. Br J Sports Med. 2004;38(4):E18.

31.  Sheard PW, Paine TJ. Optimal contraction intensity during proprioceptive neuromuscular facilitation for maximal increase of range of motion. J Strength Cond Res. 2010;24(2):416–21.

32.  Kwak DH, Ryu YU. Applying proprioceptive neuromuscular facilitation stretching: optimal contraction intensity to attain the maximum increase in range of motion in young males. J Phys Ther Sci. 2015;27(7):2129–32.

33.  Rowlands AV, Marginson VF, Lee J. Chronic flexibility gains: effect of isometric contraction duration during proprioceptive neuromuscular facilitation stretching techniques. Res Q Exerc Sport. 2003;74(1):47–51.

34.  Negrini S, Grivas TB, Kotwicki T, Maruyama T, Rigo M, Weiss HR. Why do we treat adolescent idiopathic scoliosis? What we want to obtain and to avoid for our patients. SOSORT 2005 consensus paper. Scoliosis. 2006;1:4.

# 10

# Associations between sarcopenia and degenerative lumbar scoliosis in older women

Yawara Eguchi[1*], Munetaka Suzuki[1], Hajime Yamanaka[1], Hiroshi Tamai[1], Tatsuya Kobayashi[1], Sumihisa Orita[2], Kazuyo Yamauchi[2], Miyako Suzuki[2], Kazuhide Inage[2], Kazuki Fujimoto[2], Hirohito Kanamoto[2], Koki Abe[2], Yasuchika Aoki[3], Tomoaki Toyone[4], Tomoyuki Ozawa[4], Kazuhisa Takahashi[2] and Seiji Ohtori[2]

## Abstract

**Background:** Age-related sarcopenia can cause various forms of physical disabilities. We investigated how sarcopenia affects degenerative lumbar scoliosis (DLS) and lumbar spinal canal stenosis (LSCS).

**Methods:** Subjects comprised 40 elderly women (mean age 74 years) with spinal disease whose chief complaints were low back pain and lower limb pain. They included 15 cases of DLS (mean 74.8 years) and 25 cases of LSCS (mean age 72.9 years).
We performed whole-body dual-energy X-ray absorptiometry (DXA) to analyze body composition, including appendicular and trunk skeletal muscle mass index (SMI; lean mass (kg)/height (m)$^2$) and bone mineral density (BMD). A diagnostic criterion for sarcopenia was an appendicular SMI <5.46. To check spinal alignment, lumbar scoliosis (LS), sagittal vertical axis (SVA), thoracic kyphosis (TK), lumbar lordosis (LL), pelvic tilt (PT), pelvic incidence (PI), sacral slope (SS), and vertebral rotational angle (VRA) were measured. Clinical symptoms were determined from the Japanese Orthopedic Association scores, low back pain visual analog scale, and Roland-Morris Disability Questionnaire (RDQ). Criteria for DLS were lumbar scoliosis >10° and a sagittal vertical axis (SVA) >50 mm. Sarcopenia prevalence, correlations between spinal alignment, BMD, and clinical symptoms with appendicular and trunk SMIs, and correlation between spinal alignment and clinical symptoms were investigated.

**Results:** DLS cases had significantly lower body weight, BMI, lean mass arm, and total lean mass than LSCS cases. Sarcopenia prevalence rates were 4/25 cases (16%) in LSCS and 7/15 cases (46.6%) in DLS, revealing a high prevalence in DLS. Appendicular SMIs were DLS 5.61 and LSCS 6.13 ($p < 0.05$), and trunk SMIs were DLS 6.91 and LSCS 7.61 ($p < 0.01$) showing DLS to have significantly lower values than LSCS. Spinal alignment correlations revealed the appendicular SMI was negatively correlated with PT ($p < 0.05$) and the trunk SMI was found to have a significant negative correlation with SVA, PT, LS, and VRA ($p < 0.05$). The trunk SMI was found to have a significant positive correlation with BMD ($p < 0.05$). As for clinical symptoms, RDQ was negatively correlated with appendicular SMI and positively correlated with PT ($P < 0.05$).

(Continued on next page)

* Correspondence: yawara_eguchi@yahoo.co.jp
[1]Department of Orthopaedic Surgery, Shimoshizu National Hospital, 934-5, Shikawatashi, Yotsukaido, Chiba 284-0003, Japan
Full list of author information is available at the end of the article

(Continued from previous page)

**Conclusions:** Sarcopenia complications were noted in 16% of LSCS patients and a much higher percentage, or 46. 6%, of DLS patients. Appendicular and trunk SMIs were both lower in DLS, suggesting that sarcopenia may be involved in scoliosis. The appendicular skeletal muscle was related to posterior pelvic tilt, while the trunk muscle affected stooped posture, posterior pelvic tilt, lumbar scoliosis, and vertebral rotation. Decreases in trunk muscle mass were also associated with osteoporosis. Moreover, RDQ had a negative correlation with appendicular skeletal muscle mass and a positive correlation with PT, suggesting that sarcopenia may be associated with low back pain as a result of posterior pelvic tilt. Our research reveals for the first time how sarcopenia is involved in spinal deformations, suggesting decreases in pelvic/lumbar support structures such as trunk and appendicular muscle mass may be involved in the progression of spinal deformities and increased low back pain.

**Keywords:** Adult spinal deformity, Sarcopenia, Skeletal muscle, Low back pain, Sagittal alignment

## Background

As our society continues to age, more patients develop kyphotic deformities that affect their daily activities. Takemitsu et al. [1] reported that patients suffer disruption of their ADL and low back pain as a result of posterior lumbar tilt. A broad range of associated issues can impact ADL including low back pain due to spinal deformation, back pain, and gait disorders accompanying trunk imbalance, gastroesophageal reflux disease, and esthetic and psychological complaints [1–6]. Various causes of degenerative lumbar scoliosis (DLS) have been reported, including sex, age, osteoprotic vertebral fractures, kyphosis due to deformity, and factors due to spinal surgery, but the disease mechanism is yet to be elucidated [1–6]. Trunk muscles play an important role in the spinal support structure, and paraspinal muscle degeneration has been reported to be related to spinal deformity. However, there are no reports on the relationship between trunk and appendicular skeletal muscle mass and spinal deformation.

Sarcopenia is a syndrome characterized by progressive and systemic loss of skeletal muscle mass and muscle strength. It is an at-risk state where a fall could easily lead to the patient becoming bedridden, and it can lead to major physical and economic losses in an aging society [7–9]. It is believed to be caused by inactivity, but this mechanism has not yet been completely elucidated. Sarcopenia causes decreases in back strength, and this is believed to be a factor in aggravating kyphosis, but there are no clear research results on how sarcopenia affects DLS.

In this study, we looked at how sarcopenia is associated with degenerative lumbar scoliosis (DLS) and lumbar spinal canal stenosis (LSCS) and at the relationship between spinal alignment and skeletal musculature.

## Methods

Subjects included 40 women with spinal disease and a chief complaint of low back pain or lower limb pain (mean 74.0 ±

1.0 years). There were 15 cases (mean 74.8 ± 1.3 years) of DLS and 25 cases (mean 72.9 ± 1.4 years) of LSCS. There were 3 patients with L5 foraminal stenosis but without central canal stenosis in the DLS group. There were no patients with lumbar scoliosis in the LSCS group. Five cases in the DLS group recieved corrective surgery, while all cases in the LSCS group underwent laminectomies Exclusion criteria included a history of multiple fractures of the thoracolumbar spine, spinal surgery or hip joint surgery, and neuromuscular disorders such as Parkinson's disease. Criteria for DLS were lumbar scoliosis >10°, and a sagittal vertical axis (SVA) of >50 mm$^2$.

Body composition was measured using whole-body dual-energy X-ray absorptiometry (DXA) (Hologic, QDR-DELPHIW scanner DPX-NT; Hologic, Waltham, MA, USA). This system provided the mass of lean soft tissue, fat, and bone mineral for both the whole body and specific regions such as the arms, legs, and trunk.

Appendicular skeletal muscle mass was calculated as the sum of skeletal muscle mass in the arms and legs, assuming that the mass of lean soft tissue is a skeletal muscle. Appendicular skeletal mass index (SMI) was determined as the sum of the arm and leg lean mass (kg)/height$^2$ (m$^2$). Sarcopenia among the women was defined as an appendicular SMI value of <5.46 kg/m$^2$ based on normative data for sarcopenia in Japanese men and women [10]. Although the lean mass of the trunk contains the internal organs, relative trunk SMI was defined as the trunk lean mass (kg)/height$^2$ (m$^2$). Age, height, weight, body mass index (BMI), bone mineral density (BMD), lean mass arm, lean mass leg, lean mass trunk, appendicular lean mass, and total lean mass were recorded for all patients (Table 1).

The frontal view of the entire spine and the lateral view including the hip joints were photographed in a standing position. Radiographic measurements were made of lumbar scoliosis (LS), sagittal vertical axis (SVA), thoracic kyphosis (TK), lumbar lordosis (LL), pelvic tilt (PT), pelvic incidence (PI), and sacral slope (SS). Vertebral rotational angle (VRA) was measured in the axial computed tomography (CT) plane. The LS was measured as the angle between the lower end plate of

**Table 1** Patient characteristics

|  | DLS | LSCS | p value |
| --- | --- | --- | --- |
| Age (years) | 74.8 ± 1.3 | 72.9 ± 1.4 | 0.326 |
| Body weight (kg) | 46.6 ± 1.1 | 53.1 ± 1.9 | 0.008 |
| Height (m) | 1.51 ± 0.01 | 1.49 ± 0.01 | 0.391 |
| BMI (kg/m²) | 20.3 ± 0.5 | 23.8 ± 0.6 | 0.0004 |
| BMD | 0.962 ± 0.033 | 0.949 ± 0.013 | 0.703 |
| Lean mass arm (kg) | 2.82 ± 0.11 | 3.34 ± 0.10 | 0.003 |
| Lean mass leg (kg) | 9.88 ± 0.20 | 10.58 ± 0.38 | 0.201 |
| Lean mass trunk (kg) | 1.58 ± 0.32 | 1.69 ± 0.45 | 0.053 |
| Appendicular lean mass (kg) | 12.71 ± 0.35 | 13.93 ± 0.47 | 0.079 |
| Total lean mass (kg) | 29.59 ± 1.98 | 34.27 ± 0.94 | 0.021 |

L1 and the lower end plate of L5 on frontal radiographs. The SVA was measured as the distance from the C7 plumb line to a perpendicular line drawn from the superior posterior end plate of the S1 vertebral body on lateral radiographs. The TK was measured from the upper end plate of T5 to the lower end plate of T12. The LL was measured from the lower end plate of T12 to the upper end plate of S1. The PT was measured as the angle between the vertical line and the line joining the hip axis to the center of the superior end plate of S1. The PI was measured as the angle subtended by a perpendicular line from the upper end plate of S1 and a line connecting the center of the femoral head to the center of the cephalad end plate of S1. The SS was measured as the angle between the superior end plate of S1 and a horizontal line. Vertebral rotational angle (VRA) was defined as the angle between longitudinal axis of the apical vertebra and the midsagittal axis of the sacral vertebra.

Clinical symptoms were evaluated using the visual analog scale (VAS) score for low back pain from 100 (extreme amount of pain) to 0 (no pain), the Japanese Orthopedic Association (JOA; 0–29 points) scoring system and the Roland-Morris Disability Questionnaire (RDQ; 0–24 point). The normal JOA score is 29 points, based on 3 subjective symptoms (9 points), 3 clinical signs including straight-leg raising (6 points), and 7 activities of daily living (14 points). The normal RDQ is zero points with the total number of items checked from a minimum of 0 to a maximum of 24.

Study items were sarcopenia prevalence in each group, correlations between spinal alignment, BMD, and clinical symptoms with appendicular and trunk SMIs, and correlation between spinal alignment and clinical symptoms.

**Statistical analysis**

Statistical analyses were performed with Stat View software (version 5.0).

For each parameter, differences between both groups were evaluated by the unpaired $t$ test.

Pearson correlation coefficients were calculated to determine the correlation between appendicular SMI or trunk SMI and spinal parameters or clinical symptoms. A threshold of $p < 0.05$ was considered significant.

**Results**

Subject heights were DLS 1.51 ± 0.01 m and LSCS 1.49 ± 0.01 m ($p = 0.391$); body weight was DLS 46.6 ± 1.1 kg and LSCS 53.1 ± 1.9 kg ($p < 0.01$); BMI was DLS 20.3 ± 0.5 and LSCS 23.8 ± 0.6 ($p < 0.001$); BMD was DLS 0.962 ± 0.033 and LSCS 0.949 ± 0.013 ($p = 0.703$); lean mass arm was DLS 2.82 ± 0.11 kg and LSCS 3.34 ± 0.10 kg ($p < 0.01$); lean mass leg was DLS 9.88 ± 0.20 kg and LSCS 10.58 ± 0.38 kg ($p = 0.201$); lean mass trunk was DLS 1.58 ± 0.32 kg and LSCS 1.69 ± 0.45 kg ($p = 0.53$); appendicular lean mass was DLS 12.71 ± 0.35 kg and LSCS 13.93 ± 0.47 kg ($p = 0.079$); and total lean mass was DLS 29.59 ± 1.98 kg and LSCS 34.27 ± 0.94 kg ($p < 0.05$). DLS cases had significantly lower body weight, BMI, lean mass arm, and total lean mass than LSCS cases (Table 1).

Radiographical alignment in the DLS group revealed SVA 78.6 ± 7.3 mm, LS 29.9 ± 2.4°, TK 18.4 ± 3.8°, LL 26.2 ± 4.9°, PI 55.7 ± 3.5°, PT 32.3 ± 2.7°, and SS 25.6 ± 3.3°. In the LSCS group, SVA 32.2 ± 4.2 mm, LS 4.1 ± 0.8°, TK 24.5 ± 1.5°, LL 41.5 ± 2.5°, PI 49.0 ± 2.4°, PT 22.1 ± 1.2°, and SS 28.7 ± 2.0°.

Sarcopenia prevalence was DLS 7/15 cases (46.6%) and LSCS 4/25 cases (16%) with a high percentage of involvement in DLS cases. Appendicular SMIs were DLS 5.61 ± 0.16 and LSCS 6.13 ± 0.15 ($p < 0.05$); trunk SMI values were DLS 6.91 ± 0.17 and LSCS 7.61 ± 0.15 ($p < 0.01$) with DLS significantly lower than LSCS (Fig. 1). In this study, since there are more severe coronal deformity parameters (LS 29.9°) than sagittal balance parameter (SVA 78.6 mm) in DLS cases, we analyzed DLS cases into coronal scoliosis subgroups, high coronal scoliosis (HS) group (LS > 30°; average 36.8°), and low coronal scoliosis (LS) group (LS < 30°; average 23.0°). Appendicular SMI was 5.92 ± 0.30 in the HS group, versus 5.36 ± 0.07 in the LS group ($p = 0.10$); trunk SMI was 6.90 ± 0.30 in the HS group, versus 6.97 ± 0.21 in the LS group ($p = 0.85$). Differences were not found between appendicular or trunk SMI in the HS group and in LS group.

Correlations with spinal alignment revealed a significant negative correlation between appendicular SMI and PT ($p < 0.05$) (Fig. 2). Negative correlations between trunk SMI and SVA, PT, LS, and VRA were also statistically significant ($p < 0.05$) (Fig. 3a–d). Trunk SMI was found to have a significant positive correlation with BMD ($p < 0.05$) (Fig. 3e). As for clinical symptoms, there was a negative correlation ($p < 0.05$) between appendicular SMI and RDQ (Fig. 4a) and a positive correlation ($p < 0.05$) between PT and RDQ (Fig. 4b).

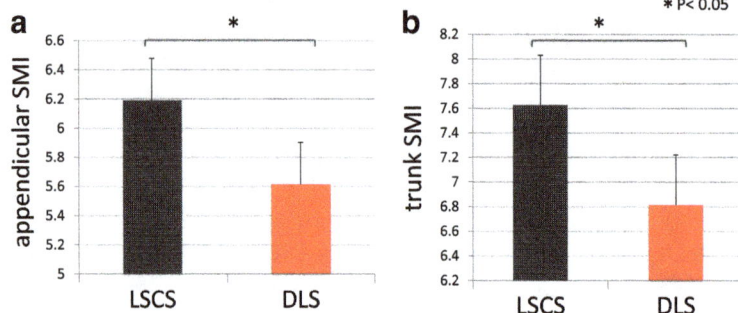

**Fig. 1** Appendicular and trunk SIMs in both groups. **a** Appendicular SIMs were ASD 5.61 ± 0.16 and LSCS 6.13 ± 0.15 (*p* < 0.05), and **b** trunk SIMs were DLS 6.91 ± 0.17 and LSCS 7.61 ± 0.15 (*p* < 0.01). DLS values were significantly lower than those of LSCS

## Discussion

Reports have been published on research using MRI to assess paraspinal muscle in spinal deformities. Yagi et al. [11] reported that multifidus and iliopsoas muscle cross sections were smaller in spinal deformation, and that this correlated with sagittal alignment. A report found fatty degeneration of multifidus muscle on the concave side of degenerative scoliosis [12], while hyperplasia of the multifidus muscle and iliopsoas muscle has been reported regarding the convex side of degenerative scoliosis [13]. On the other hand, when Enomoto et al. [14] took surface electromyograms of paravertebral muscle activity, they found that compared to lumbar spinal canal stenosis (LSCS), patients with degenerative lumbar scoliosis (DLS) had high paravertebral muscle activity. Yagi et al. [11] measured appendicular skeletal muscle mass in patients with DLS and LSCS by DXA and reported that there was no significant difference between the two groups. However, postoperative measurements were only taken for appendicular weight, and height-corrected SMI values were not considered. Muscle assessment in adult spinal deformity had previously been limited to localized evaluation of appendicular and trunk muscle mass. How these might relate to sarcopenia has never been investigated until this time.

Sarcopenia is defined as the age-associated loss of skeletal muscle mass and function with a risk of adverse outcomes such as physical disability and poor quality of life [7, 8]. Sarcopenia is very common in older individuals, with a reported prevalence in 60- to 70-year-olds of 5–13% [9].

In a report on sarcopenia and spinal diseases, Miyakoshi et al. [15] reported 20% of Japanese patients with osteoporosis suffer sarcopenia complications while only 10% of healthy individuals have sarcopenia. In our study, trunk SMI was found to have a significant positive correlation with BMD, suggesting that decreases in trunk muscle mass were associated with osteoporosis. Another study found that patients with low back pain have a statistically significant decrease in lower appendicular muscle mass [16]. However, no studies have clearly defined the relationship between sarcopenia and spinal deformity.

With regard to spinal alignment which adversely affects QOL, Takemitsu et al. [1] reported that 95% of patients with lumbar degenerative kyphosis suffer low back pain with severe disruption of their ADL and raised these issues regarding kyphosis. Glassmann et al. [3] found that those cases with large SVAs, where the C7 plumb line shows anterior displacement, suffer the greatest disruption of QOL and stressed the importance of sagittal alignment. Lafage et al. [4] have associated posterior pelvic tilt and stooping posture to poor QOL and so consider PT and SVA to be vital factors. Schwab et al. [5] chose radiographical parameters PI-LL <10°, PT < 20°, and SVA < 50 mm as the thresholds for correction and mentioned the importance of a good sagittal plane balance.

In our research, sarcopenia complications were found in 16% of LSCS, and nearly half, or 46.6% of DLS. Appendicular SMI and trunk SMI were both reduced in DLS, suggesting that sarcopenia may be involved in scoliosis. In particular, lean mass arm and total lean mass were markedly reduced in DLS compared with

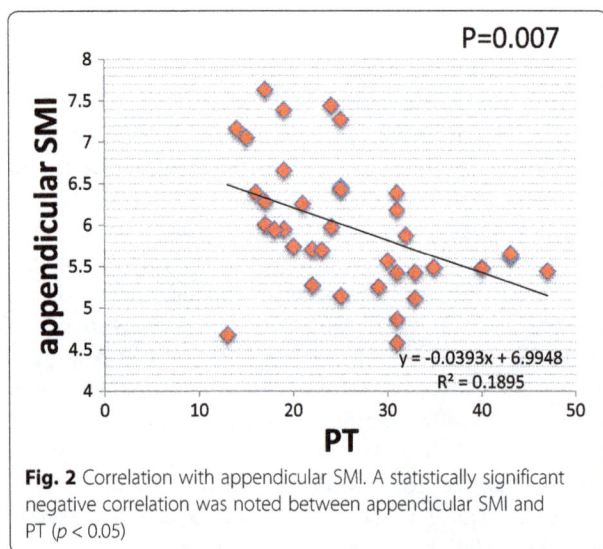

**Fig. 2** Correlation with appendicular SMI. A statistically significant negative correlation was noted between appendicular SMI and PT (*p* < 0.05)

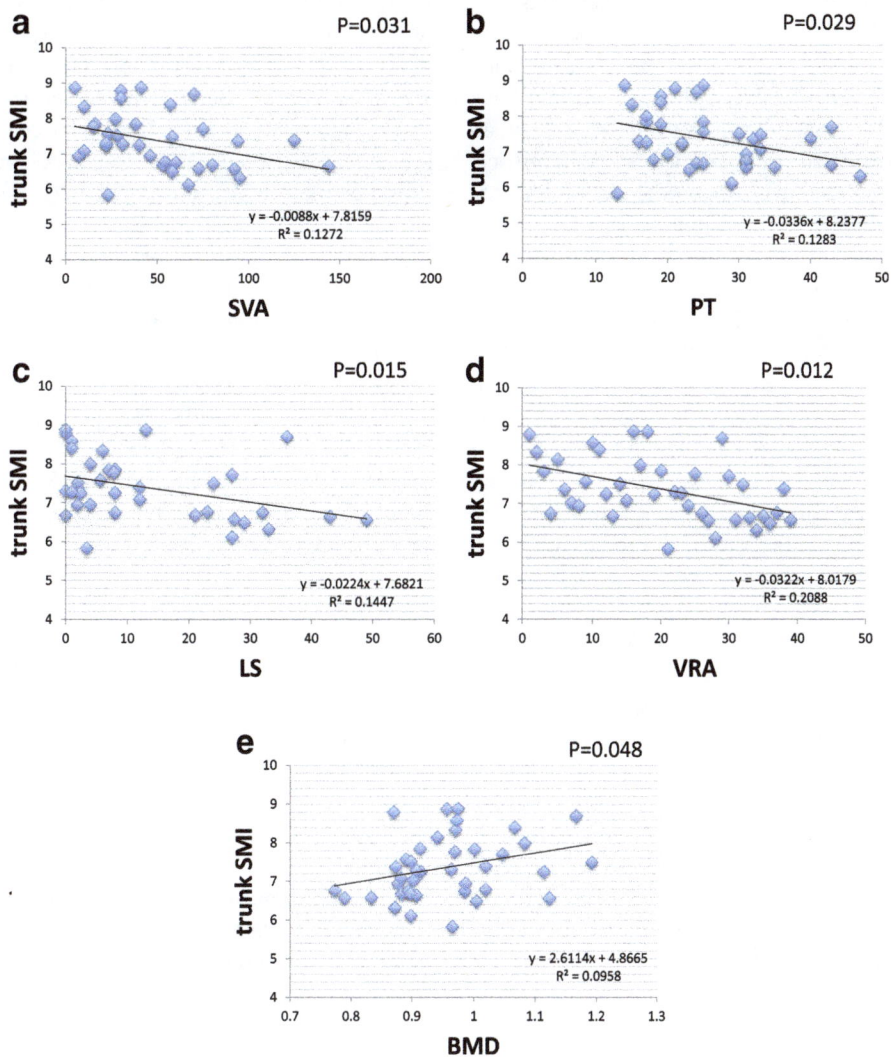

**Fig. 3** Correlation with trunk SMI. A statistically significant negative correlation was observed between trunk SMI and SVA (**a**), PT (**b**), LS (**c**), and VRA (**d**) ($p < 0.05$). A statistically significant positive correlation was observed between trunk SMI and BMD (**e**) ($p < 0.05$)

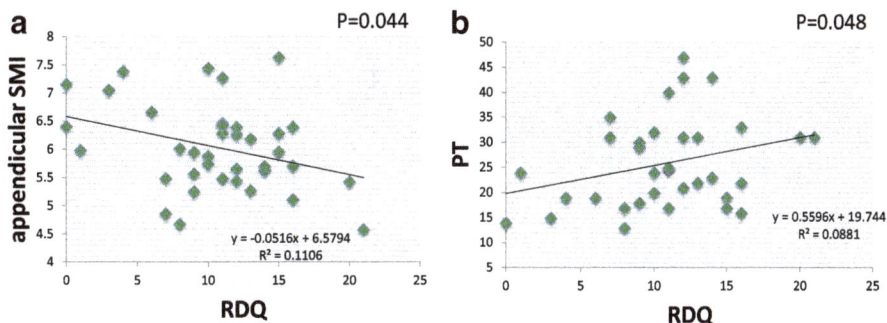

**Fig. 4** Correlation with a scale of clinical symptoms, RDQ. A statistically significant negative correlation was noted between appendicular SMI and RDQ (**a**) ($p < 0.05$). A statistically significant positive correlation was noted between PT and RDQ (**b**) ($p < 0.05$)

LSCS. Differences might be not found in lean mass leg between DLS and LSCS due to disuse atrophy from intermittent claudication in LSCS. In the future, results should be compared to a healthy volunteer without back problems. Moreover, appendicular skeletal muscle mass was negatively correlated with PT, while trunk muscle mass showed negative correlations with SVA, PT, LS, and VRA. Appendicular skeletal muscle was associated with posterior pelvic tilt, while trunk muscle mass was associated with stooped posture, posterior pelvic tilt, lumbar scoliosis, and vertebral rotation. In addition, RDQ had a negative correlation with appendicular skeletal muscle mass and a positive correlation with PT, suggesting a relationship between sarcopenia and low back pain as a result of posterior pelvic tilt (Fig. 5). Our results do not differ from those of published reports and confirm that sagittal plane alignment PT and SVA are important factors that affect QOL. Decreases in trunk muscle and appendicular muscle mass which form the pelvic/lumbar stabilization structure may be one of the causes of spinal deformation and low back pain.

Our study has several limitations. (1) The first is that only a small number of subjects were investigated, requiring confirmation of our findings in a larger population.

(2) DXA cannot measure individual spinal muscles such as paravertebral muscle and psoas. The trunk SMI defined in this study includes the internal organs so it is not an accurate measure of actual trunk muscle volume but merely a relative evaluation. However, trunk muscle accounts for approximately 15% of the lumboabdominal region and is second only to the 30% representing the femoral muscles, and so it cannot be ignored in terms of assessing whole-body skeletal muscle mass [17]. A new device has recently been introduced to evaluate the total and regional body composition—bioelectrical impedance analyzer (BIA). BIA estimates body composition using the difference of conductivity of the various tissues due to the difference of their biological characteristics. High agreement between DXA and BIA was high for lean mass trunk (95%IC 0.82) [18]. In the future, results should be compared to measure the trunk muscle with BIA and MRI evaluations. (3) The study is a cross-sectional analysis, not a longitudinal one. (4) This study was only compared to patient with spinal stenosis but not compared to a normal population without back problems and not compared to younger populations.

(5) We did not study postoperative spinal alignment, but multifidus muscular atrophy has been implicated in proximal junctional kyphosis (PJK) [19] after orthomorphic surgery [11] and should be investigated further in the future.

## Conclusions

We investigated how sarcopenia affected degenerative lumbar scoliosis (DLS) and lumbar spinal canal stenosis (LSCS) in elderly women. Corrected appendicular muscle mass and corrected trunk muscle mass were determined using DXA. Sarcopenia was noted in 16% of LSCS and a much higher 46.6% of patients with DLS. Both appendicular and trunk skeletal muscle mass was lower in the DLS group, suggesting sarcopenia may be involved in causing spinal deformities. Decreases in appendicular skeletal muscle mass were associated with posterior pelvic tilt and low back pain, while decreases in trunk muscle mass were associated with stooping posture, posterior pelvic tilt, lumbar scoliosis, vertebral

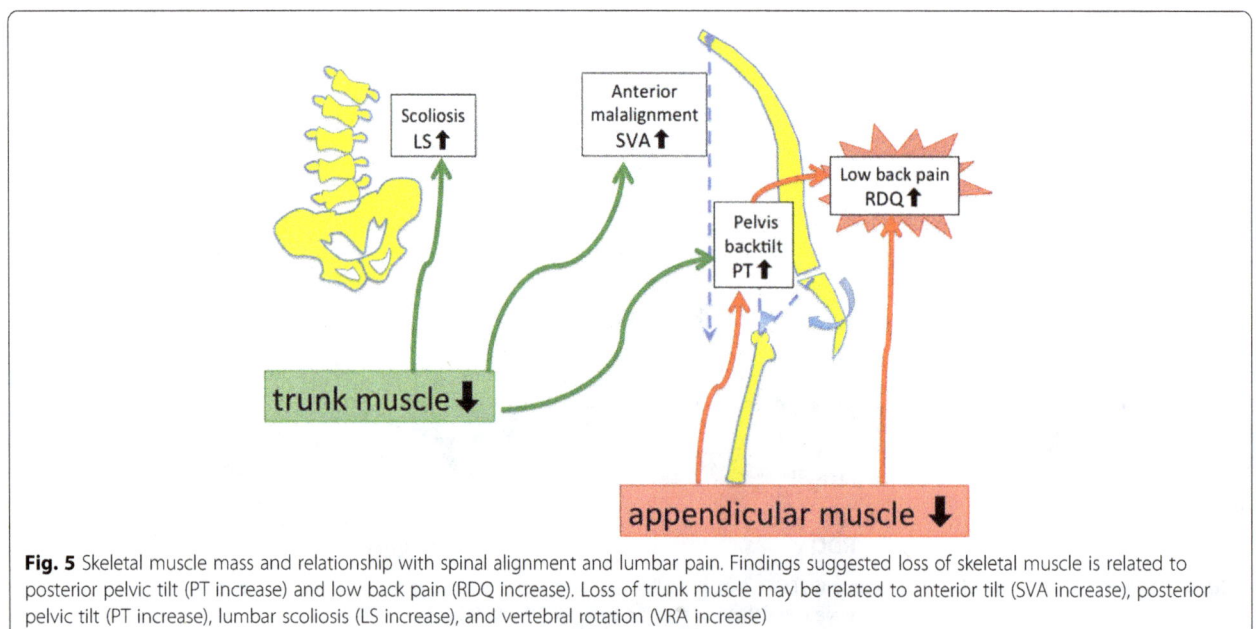

Fig. 5 Skeletal muscle mass and relationship with spinal alignment and lumbar pain. Findings suggested loss of skeletal muscle is related to posterior pelvic tilt (PT increase) and low back pain (RDQ increase). Loss of trunk muscle may be related to anterior tilt (SVA increase), posterior pelvic tilt (PT increase), lumbar scoliosis (LS increase), and vertebral rotation (VRA increase)

rotation, and osteoporosis. Low back pain was associated with decreased appendicular skeletal muscle mass and posterior pelvic tilt.

Loss of trunk and appendicular muscle, which form the truncal stabilization structure, is thought to be one of the causes of progressive deformation of the spine and low back pain.

## Abbreviations
BMD: Bone mineral density; DLS: Degenerative lumbar scoliosis; DXA: Dual-energy X-ray absorptiometry; LL: Lumbar lordosis; LS: Lumbar scoliosis; LSCS: Lumbar spinal canal stenosis; PI: Pelvic incidence; PT: Pelvic tilt; RDQ: Roland-Morris Disability Questionnaire; SMI: Skeletal muscle mass index; SS: Sacral slope; SVA: Sagittal vertical axis; TK: Thoracic kyphosis; VAS: Visual analog scale; VRA: Vertebral rotational angle

## Acknowledgements
The authors acknowledge all the staff at Shimoshizu National Hospital for providing the support in carrying out this study.

## Funding
We did not receive grants or external funding in support of our research or preparation of this manuscript. We did not receive payments or other benefits or a commitment or agreement to provide such benefits from any commercial entities.

## Authors' contributions
YE conducted data collection and data entry, and wrote the manuscript. All authors contributed to and have approved the final manuscript.

## Competing interests
The authors declare that they have no competing interests.

## Author details
[1]Department of Orthopaedic Surgery, Shimoshizu National Hospital, 934-5, Shikawatashi, Yotsukaido, Chiba 284-0003, Japan. [2]Department of Orthopaedic Surgery, Graduate School of Medicine, Chiba University, 1-8-1 Inohana, Chuo-ku, Chiba 260-8670, Japan. [3]Department of Orthopaedic Surgery, Eastern Chiba Medical Center, 3-6-2, Okayamadai, Togane, Chiba 283-8686, Japan. [4]Department of Orthopaedic Surgery, Showa University School of Medicine, 1-5-8 Hatanodai, Shinagawa-ku, Tokyo 142-8555, Japan.

## References
1. Takemitsu Y, Harada Y, Iwahara T, Miyamoto M, Miyatake Y. Lumbar degenerative kyphosis. Clinical, radiological and epidemiological studies. Spine (Phila Pa 1976). 1988;13(11):1317–26.
2. Aebi M. The adult scoliosis. Eur Spine J. 2005;14(10):925–48.
3. Glassman SD, Bridwell K, Dimar JR, Horton W, Berven S, Schwab F. The impact of positive sagittal balance in adult spinal deformity. Spine. 2005;30(18):2024–9.
4. Lafage V, Schwab F, Patel A, Hawkinson N, Farcy JP. Pelvic tilt and truncal inclination: two key radiographic parameters in the setting of adults with spinal deformity. Spine. 2009;34(17):E599–606.
5. Schwab F, Ungar B, Blondel B, Buchowski J, Coe J, Deinlein D, DeWald C, Mehdian H, Shaffrey C, Tribus C, Lafage V. Scoliosis Research Society-Schwab adult spinal deformity classification: a validation study. Spine. 2012;37(12):1077–82.
6. Ploumis A, Liu H, Mehbod AA, Transfeldt EE, Winter RB. A correlation of radiographic and functional measurements in adult degenerative scoliosis. Spine. 2009;34(15):1581–4.
7. Cruz-Jentoft AJ, Landi F, Schneider SM, Zúñiga C, Arai H, Boirie Y, Chen LK, Fielding RA, Martin FC, Michel JP, Sieber C, Stout JR, Studenski SA, Vellas B, Woo J, Zamboni M, Cederholm T. Prevalence of and interventions for sarcopenia in ageing adults: a systematic review. Report of the International Sarcopenia Initiative (EWGSOP and IWGS). Age Ageing. 2014;43(6):748–59.
8. Wu IC, Lin CC, Hsiung CA, Wang CY, Wu CH, Chan DC, Li TC, Lin WY, Huang KC, Chen CY, Hsu CC. Sarcopenia and Translational Aging Research in Taiwan Team. Epidemiology of sarcopenia among community-dwelling older adults in Taiwan: a pooled analysis for a broader adoption of sarcopenia assessments. Geriatr Gerontol Int. 2014;14 Suppl 1:52–60.
9. Morley JE. Sarcopenia: diagnosis and treatment. J Nutr Health Aging. 2008;12:452–6.
10. Sanada K, Miyachi M, Tanimoto M, Yamamoto K, Murakami H, Okumura S, Gando Y, Suzuki K, Tabata I, Higuchi M. A cross-sectional study of sarcopenia in Japanese men and women: reference values and association with cardiovascular risk factors. Eur J Appl Physiol. 2010;110:57–65.
11. Yagi M, Hosogane N, Watanabe K, Asazuma T, Matsumoto M; Keio Spine Research Group. The paravertebral muscle and psoas for the maintenance of global spinal alignment in patient with degenerative lumbar scoliosis. Spine J. 2015 in press.
12. Shafaq N, Suzuki A, Matsumura A, Terai H, Toyoda H, Yasuda H, Ibrahim M, Nakamura H. Asymmetric degeneration of paravertebral muscles in patients with degenerative lumbar scoliosis. Spine. 2012;37(16):1398–406.
13. Kim H, Lee CK, Yeom JS, Lee JH, Cho JH, Shin SI, Lee HJ, Chang BS. Asymmetry of the cross-sectional area of paravertebral and psoas muscle in patients with degenerative scoliosis. Eur Spine J. 2013;22(6):1332–8.
14. Enomoto M, Ukegawa D, Sakaki K, Tomizawa S, Arai Y, Kawabata S, Kato T, Yoshii T, Shinomiya K, Okawa A. Increase in paravertebral muscle activity in lumbar kyphosis patients by surface electromyography compared with lumbar spinal canal stenosis patients and healthy volunteers. J Spinal Disord Tech. 2012;25(6):E167–73.
15. Miyakoshi N, Hongo M, Mizutani Y, Shimada Y. Prevalence of sarcopenia in Japanese women with osteopenia and osteoporosis. J Bone Miner Metab. 2013;31(5):556–61.
16. Sakai Y. Sarcopenia and low back pain. Orthop Surg Traumatol. 2015;58:181–6.
17. Lee SJ, Janssen I, Heymsfield SB, Ross R. Relation between whole-body and regional measures of human skeletal muscle. Am J Clin Nutr. 2004;80(5):1215–21.
18. Buckinx F, Reginster JY, Dardenne N, Croisier JL, Kaux JF, Beaudart C, Slomian J, Bruyère O. Concordance between muscle mass assessed by bioelectrical impedance analysis and by dual energy X-ray absorptiometry: a cross-sectional study. BMC Musculoskelet Disord. 2015;16:60.
19. Watanabe K, Lenke LG, Bridwell KH, Kim YJ, Koester L, Hensley M. Proximal junctional vertebral fracture in adults after spinal deformity surgery using pedicle screw constructs: analysis of morphological features. Spine. 2010;35:138–45.

# 11

# The influence of sarcopenia in dropped head syndrome in older women

Yawara Eguchi[1*], Toru Toyoguchi[2], Masao Koda[3], Munetaka Suzuki[1], Hajime Yamanaka[1], Hiroshi Tamai[1], Tatsuya Kobayashi[1], Sumihisa Orita[3], Kazuyo Yamauchi[3], Miyako Suzuki[3], Kazuhide Inage[3], Kazuki Fujimoto[3], Hirohito Kanamoto[3], Koki Abe[3], Yasuchika Aoki[4], Kazuhisa Takahashi[3] and Seiji Ohtori[3]

## Abstract

**Background:** Age-related sarcopenia may cause physical dysfunction. We investigated the involvement of sarcopenia in dropped head syndrome (DHS).

**Methods:** Our study subjects were ten elderly women with idiopathic DHS (mean age 75.1 years, range 55–89). Twenty age- and sex-matched volunteers (mean age 73.0, range 58–83) served as controls. We used a bioelectrical impedance analyzer (BIA) to analyze body composition, including appendicular skeletal muscle mass index (SMI; appendicular lean mass (kg)/(height (m))$^2$). SMI <5.75 was considered diagnostic for sarcopenia. Cervical sagittal plane alignment: C2–7 sagittal vertical axis (SVA), C2–7 angle (C2–C7 A), and C2 slope (C2S) were also measured. We investigated sarcopenia prevalence in both groups, height, weight, BMI, lean mass arm, lean mass leg, lean mass trunk, appendicular lean mass, total lean mass, and SMI. In addition, we also examined the correlation between cervical spine alignment and SMI in DHS.

**Results:** Sarcopenia was observed at a high rate in DHS subjects: 70% compared to 25% of healthy controls. Height, weight, BMI, lean mass arm, lean mass leg, axial lean mass, appendicular lean mass, total lean mass, and SMI all had significantly lower values in the DHS group. In particular, total lean mass, lean mass arm, and lean mass trunk were considerably lower in the DHS group. There was no correlation noted between cervical spine alignment and SMI.

**Conclusions:** Sarcopenia prevalence was high in the DHS group—70 versus 25% in the control group, suggesting the involvement of sarcopenia in DHS. In particular, axial lean mass and lean mass arm were markedly reduced in the DHS group. DHS is due to significant weakness of the neck extensor group, and chin-on-chest deformity occurs. Until the present, evaluation of DHS has been done using only MRI; no studies have systematically examined skeletal muscle mass. In the present study, muscle mass decrease was noted not only in the neck muscles but also throughout the entire body. Involvement of trunk and upper limb muscles in particular suggests a disuse atrophy of the upper body and spinal muscles. BIA can easily and systemically evaluate skeletal muscle mass. We expect it to contribute to further elucidating the pathogenesis of DHS.

**Keywords:** Dropped head syndrome, Sarcopenia, Skeletal muscle, Bioelectrical impedance analyzer

* Correspondence: yawara_eguchi@yahoo.co.jp
[1]Department of Orthopeadic Surgery, Shimoshizu National Hospital, 934-5, Shikawatashi, Yotsukaido, Chiba 284-0003, Japan
Full list of author information is available at the end of the article

## Background

Dropped head syndrome (DHS) exhibits chin-on-chest deformity due to significant weakness of the neck extensor group [1–6]. DHS can impair quality of life, resulting in restrictions on forward gaze and ambulation, dysphagia, and neck pain. Neck extensor atrophy occurs in a variety of disease backgrounds, including neurological, neuromuscular, and muscular disorders [1, 2]. Among these, idiopathic DHS, due to neck extensor muscle failure of unknown cause, is a problem for many elderly patients. There is the possibility for further increase as society ages [5].

Sarcopenia is a syndrome characterized by progressive and systemic reduction in skeletal muscle mass. It carries a high risk of becoming bedridden from a fall, and there is great physical and economic loss in an aging society [7–10]. It is believed that sarcopenia results from inactivity, but the mechanism is not entirely clear. Decrease in back strength due to sarcopenia is believed to contribute to the development of DHS. Until the present, evaluation of DHS has consisted of only local neck MRI 5,6. There has been no report of the involvement of whole-body skeletal muscle mass in sarcopenia.

In the present study, we report the prevalence of sarcopenia in DHS and examine whole-body skeletal muscle mass.

## Methods

Our study subjects were ten elderly women with idiopathic DHS (mean age 75.1 years, range 55–89). Twenty age- and sex-matched volunteers (mean age 73.0, range 58–83) served as controls. DHS was clinically defined as a disabling condition in which severe weakness of the neck extensor muscles causes difficulty in lifting the head against gravity, which results in a correctable chin-on-chest deformity. Two patients with a single thoracolumbar compression fracture (case 1: L3, case 3: Th12) were included (Table 1). Subjects were excluded for multiple thoracolumbar compression fractures or a history of spinal surgery.

A multi-frequency bioelectrical impedance analyzer (BIA), the InBody 720 Biospace device (Biospace Co., Ltd., Korea), was used according to the manufacturer's guidelines. BIA estimates body composition using the difference of conductivity of the various tissues due to the difference of their biological characteristics. Conductivity is proportional to water content (more specifically to electrolytes), and conductivity decreases as the cell approaches a perfect spherical shape. Adipose tissue is composed of round cells and contains relatively little water compared to other tissues like muscle; therefore, conductivity decreases as body fat increases. In practice, electrodes are placed at eight precise tactile points of the body to achieve a multi-segmental frequency analysis. A total of 30 impedance measurements are obtained using six different frequencies (1, 5, 50, 250, 500, and 1000 kHz) for the following five segments of the body: right and left arms, trunk, and right and left legs.

Appendicular skeletal muscle mass was calculated as the sum of skeletal muscle mass in the arms and legs, assuming that mass of lean soft tissue is effectively equivalent to skeletal muscle mass. Appendicular skeletal mass index (SMI) was determined as the sum of arm and leg lean mass $(kg)/(height\ (m))^2$. The diagnosis of sarcopenia among women was defined as appendicular SMI value $<5.75\ kg/m^2$, determined using sarcopenia normative data [11].

**Table 1** Patient characteristics

| Case | Age | Sex | Height (m) | Weight (kg) | BMI (kg/m2) | Lean mass arm (kg) | Lean mass leg (kg) | Lean mass trunk (kg) | Appendicular lean mass (kg) | Total lean mass (kg) | SMI (kg/m2) | C2–7 SVA (m) | C2–7 A (°) | C2S (°) |
|---|---|---|---|---|---|---|---|---|---|---|---|---|---|---|
| | | | | | | Skeletal muscle | | | | | | Cervical sagittal alignment | | |
| 1 | 73 | F | 1.47 | 51.3 | 23.74 | 2.93 | 9.34 | 14.2 | 12.27 | 26.47 | 5.678 [a] | 30 | −22 | 36 |
| 2 | 69 | F | 1.47 | 35.3 | 16.33 | 1.6 | 7.16 | 10.6 | 8.76 | 19.36 | 4.053 [a] | 35 | 16 | 17 |
| 3 | 82 | F | 1.4 | 40.8 | 20.81 | 2.26 | 7.81 | 11.6 | 10.07 | 21.67 | 5.137 [a] | 63 | −13 | 55 |
| 4 | 77 | F | 1.44 | 33.4 | 16.10 | 1.74 | 8.1 | 10.6 | 9.84 | 20.44 | 4.745 [a] | 52 | −14 | 44 |
| 5 | 55 | F | 1.4 | 49.9 | 25.45 | 2.34 | 10.32 | 12.1 | 12.66 | 24.76 | 6.459 | 64 | −59 | 90 |
| 6 | 60 | F | 1.54 | 45.2 | 19.05 | 2.55 | 9.23 | 13.6 | 11.78 | 25.38 | 4.967 [a] | 61 | −56 | 50 |
| 7 | 89 | F | 1.47 | 48.3 | 22.35 | 2.58 | 12.29 | 12.7 | 14.87 | 27.57 | 6.881 | 60 | 20 | 30 |
| 8 | 88 | F | 1.43 | 43.5 | 21.27 | 2.29 | 10.1 | 11.9 | 12.39 | 24.29 | 6.058 | 47 | −14 | 35 |
| 9 | 74 | F | 1.4 | 39.7 | 20.25 | 2.83 | 8.01 | 13.1 | 10.84 | 23.94 | 5.530 [a] | 69 | −50 | 80 |
| 10 | 84 | F | 1.46 | 52.9 | 24.81 | 2.83 | 8.77 | 14 | 11.6 | 25.6 | 5.441 [a] | 30 | −1 | 28 |
| Mean | 75.1 | | 1.448 | 44.03 | 21.02 | 2.395 | 9.113 | 12.44 | 11.508 | 23.948 | 5.495 | 51.1 | −19.3 | 46.5 |

[a]Sarcopenia positive (SMI <5.75)

The radiographs were taken in the standing position. Cervical sagittal plane alignment was measured by C2–7 sagittal vertical axis (SVA), C2–7 angle (C2–C7 A), and C2 slope (C2 S) (Fig. 1).

We investigated sarcopenia prevalence in both groups, height, weight, BMI, lean mass arm, lean mass leg, lean mass trunk, appendicular lean mass, total lean mass, and SMI (Table 1). In addition, we also examined the correlation between cervical spine alignment and SMI in DHS.

### Statistical analysis

Statistical analyses were performed with StatView software (version 5.0).

For each parameter, differences between groups were evaluated using unpaired $t$ test.

Pearson correlation coefficients were calculated to determine the correlation between appendicular SMI and spinal parameters. A threshold of $p < 0.05$ was considered significant.

### Results

Height, weight, and BMI were significantly lower for the DHS group compared to controls (Fig. 2): height for the DHS group was $1.448 \pm 0.044$ m compared to $1.522 \pm 0.072$ m for controls ($p = 0.0072$); weight for the DHS group was $44.03 \pm 6.70$ kg compared to $54.33 \pm 6.65$ kg for controls ($p = 0.0005$); and BMI for the DHS group

was $21.02 \pm 3.23$ kg/m$^2$ compared to $23.48 \pm 2.65$ kg/m$^2$ for controls ($p = 0.036$).

Cervical spine parameters for the DHS group were C2–7SVA: $51.1 \pm 14.8$ mm, C2–7A: $-19.3 \pm 28.1°$, and C2S: $46.5 \pm 23.2°$, representing advanced anteversion and kyphosis. We detected no correlation of any of these parameters with SMI: C2–7SVA ($r = 0.300$, $p = 0.39$), C2–7A ($r = -0100$, $p = 0.78$), and C2S ($r = 0.301$, $p = 0.39$).

Sarcopenia prevalence was high in the DHS group, including 7 out of 10 cases (70%), versus 5 out of 20 controls (20%). Regarding skeletal muscle mass parameters: lean mass arm was $2.39 \pm 0.44$ kg in the DHS group versus $3.45 \pm 0.54$ kg in controls ($p = 0.000016$), lean mass leg was $9.11 \pm 1.50$ kg in DHS versus $10.86 \pm 1.67$ kg in controls ($p = 0.010$), lean mass trunk was $12.44 \pm 1.30$ kg in DHS versus $16.02 \pm 1.81$ kg in controls ($p = 0.0000081$), appendicular lean mass was $11.50 \pm 1.72$ kg in DHS versus $14.31 \pm 2.06$ kg in controls ($p = 0.0011$), total lean mass was $23.94 \pm 2.65$ kg in DHS versus $30.33 \pm 3.74$ kg in controls ($p = 0.000062$), and SMI was $5.49 \pm 0.83$ kg/m$^2$ in DHS versus $6.15 \pm 0.54$ kg/m$^2$ in controls ($p = 0.016$). The DHS group had significantly lower values for all items (Fig. 3).

### Discussion

Dropped head syndrome comprises a group of disorders associated with chin-on-chest deformity due to marked weakness of the neck extensor muscles. It has been reported in the setting of a wide variety of diseases, including neurological, neuromuscular, and muscular disorders [1–6], Parkinson disease [3], multiple system atrophy [4], amyotrophic lateral sclerosis, and isolated neck extensor myopathy (INEM). Katz et al. reported on DHS due to cervical extensor muscle weakness of unknown origin in INEM. They propose an isolated myopathy that occurs due to nonspecific inflammation in the extensor muscle due to continued abnormal posture. This is observed in those greater than 60 years of age and mainly confined to the neck extensor muscles. A subacute process is recognized that includes weakness of shoulder blade and upper arm muscles, myogenic changes in needle EMG, and muscle atrophy in MRI, but these features do not extend to the other parts of the body.

Until the present, evaluation of DHS has consisted of only local MRI examination of spinal muscles. There are no reports on the association between skeletal muscle mass and sarcopenia.

Sarcopenia is defined as age-associated loss of skeletal muscle mass and function, and it includes a risk of adverse outcomes such as physical disability and poor quality of life [7, 8]. Sarcopenia is very common in older individuals, with a reported prevalence in 60- to 70-year-olds of 5–13% [9].

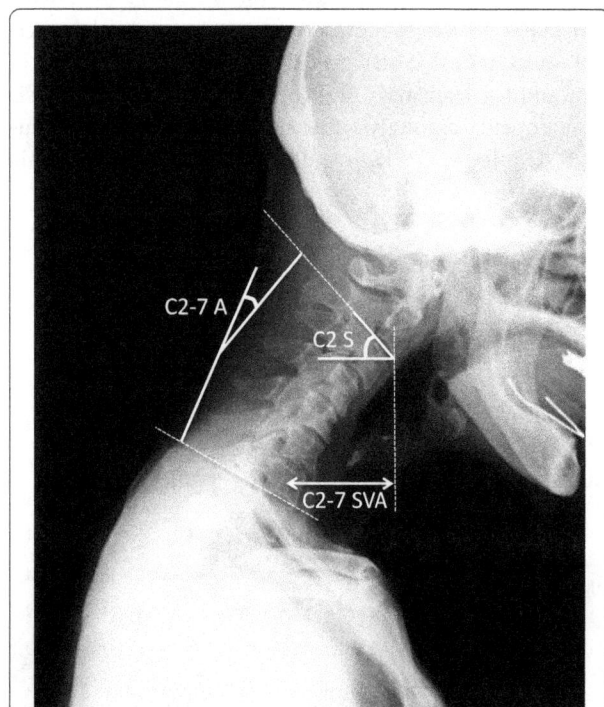

**Fig. 1** Cervical sagittal plane alignment. C2–7 sagittal vertical axis (C2–7 SVA), C2–7 angle (C2–C7 A), and C2 slope (C2 S) were measured. C2–7 A was minus in the kyphotic direction and positive in the lordotic direction

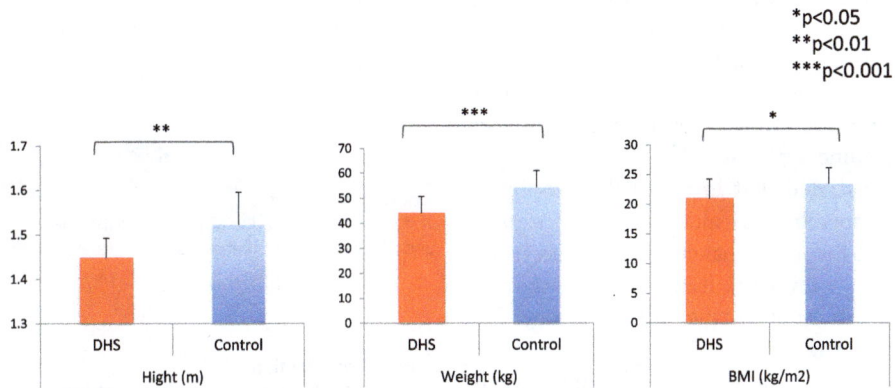

**Fig. 2** Height, weight, and BMI results. Height, weight, and BMI were significantly lower in the DHS group

In a report on sarcopenia and spinal diseases, Miyakoshi et al. [12] reported 20% of Japanese patients with osteoporosis suffer complications due to sarcopenia, while only 10% of healthy individuals have sarcopenia. However, no studies have clearly defined the relationship between sarcopenia and DHS.

In the present study, a large proportion of DHS cases had sarcopenia compared to controls: 70 versus 25%. Muscle mass decrease was noted not only in the neck muscles but also throughout the entire body. Involvement of trunk and upper limb muscles

in particular suggests a disuse atrophy of the upper body and spinal muscles. These results match those reported by Katz et al. for the shoulder blade and upper arm.

The pathogenesis of idiopathic DHS has not been elucidated. Regarding mechanisms of DHS, the spinal support muscles atrophy with age, resulting in sarcopenia. Furthermore, in cases of thoracolumbar kyphosis, due to decreases in spine flexibility, the load-bearing axis of the head shifts excessively forward, and mechanical load on the neck extensor muscle group is increased through the

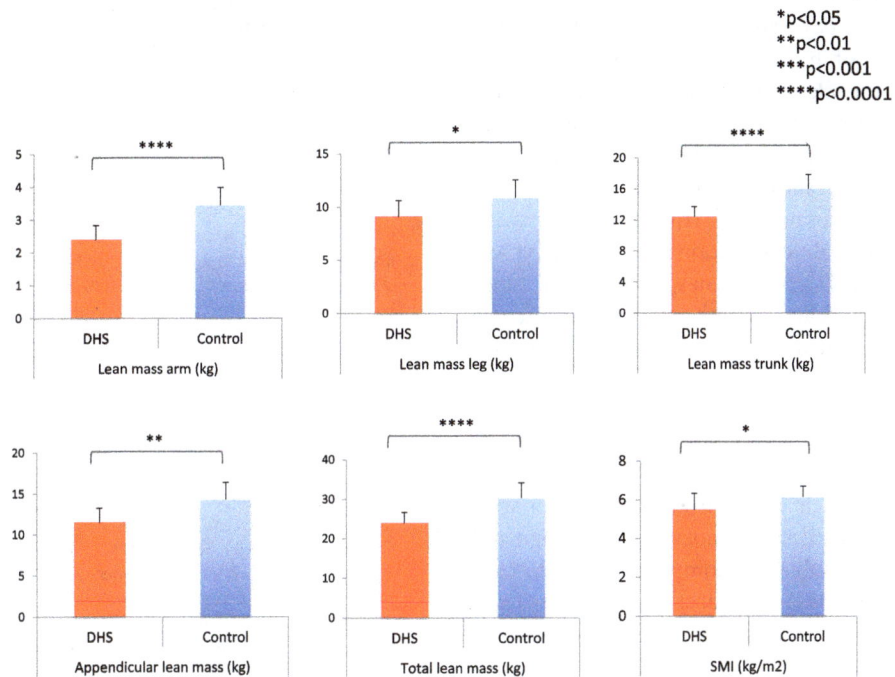

**Fig. 3** Skeletal muscle mass results. Lean mass arm was 2.39 kg for the DHS group and 3.45 kg for controls ($p < 0.0001$), lean mass leg was 9.11 kg for DHS and 10.86 kg for controls ($p < 0.05$), lean mass trunk was 12.44 kg for DHS and 16.02 kg for controls ($p < 0.0001$), appendicular lean mass was 11.50 kg for DHS and 14.31 kg for controls ($p < 0.01$), total lean mass was 23.94 kg for DHS and 30.33 kg for controls ($p < 0.0001$), and SMI was 5.49 kg/m$^2$ for DHS and 6.15 kg/m$^2$ for controls ($p < 0.05$). All items were significantly lower in the DHS group

action of the lever arm. As a result, the extensor muscle group is continually extended, and a nonspecific inflammation occurs. Over time, changes in muscle quality take place; further irreversible decline of extensor muscle group strength is thought to occur, resulting in additional cervical spine kyphosis.

This study demonstrated that in the DHS, atrophy of upper limbs and upper truncal muscle become significant, suggesting that the maintenance of lean mass trunk and arm perhaps may prevent to lean due to a failure in functional cervical extensors. Further studies are needed to clarify the mechanism.

Our study has several limitations. (1) The first is that a small number of subjects were investigated, requiring confirmation of our findings in a larger population. (2) We did not conduct comprehensive measurements of whole spine alignment. (3) We did not evaluate muscles using MRI. (4) The study is a cross-sectional analysis, not a longitudinal one. (5) Dual-energy X-ray absorptiometry (DXA) seems to be the most reliable tool to evaluate body composition and is often considered the gold standard in clinical practice. BIA could provide a simpler, portative, and less expensive alternative. BIA has a tendency to overestimate muscle mass compared to DXA, but agreement between DXA and BIA is high for lean mass arm and for axial lean mass [13]. In the future, results should be compared to DXA and MRI measurements of muscle mass. (5) The appreciation of muscle mass has limits because BIA does not appreciate some qualities of muscle tissue such as fat infiltration and the muscle functionality. Moreover, this method underestimates the prevalence of sarcopenia in obese subjects and overestimates in lean subjects. (6) We evaluated only slim Japanese women with low BMI; therefore, the amount of truncal fat is much less likely to affect their calculations than in a typical western population. (7) Sometimes, there is a more rapid decline in muscle strength relative to muscle mass. However, we did not evaluate muscle strength.

## Conclusions

We examined the role of sarcopenia in DHS. We measured skeletal muscle mass in elderly women with idiopathic DHS using BIA. Sarcopenia was recognized in 70% of our DHS subjects, compared with 25% of controls. Total lean mass was decreased in the DHS group, especially lean mass trunk and lean mass arm, suggesting a disuse atrophy of the upper body and spinal support musculature. BIA can easily evaluate whole-body skeletal muscle mass. We expect it to contribute to further elucidating the pathogenesis of DHS in the future.

## Abbreviations

BIA: Bioelectrical impedance analyzer; DHS: Dropped head syndrome; DXA: Dual-energy X-ray absorptiometry; SMI: Skeletal muscle mass index; SVA: Sagittal vertical axis

## Acknowledgements

The authors acknowledge all the staff at the Shimoshizu National Hospital and Chiba Qiball clinic for providing the support in carrying out this study.

## Authors' contributions

YE conducted the data collection and data entry and wrote the manuscript. TT developed the data collection. MK participated in the design of the study and performed the statistical analysis. MunetakaS, HY, HT, TK, SOrita, KY, MiyakoS, KI, KF, YA, HK, KA, KT, and SOhtori were responsible for the study design and manuscript preparation. All authors contributed to and have approved the final manuscript.

## Competing interests

The authors declare that they have no competing interests.

## Author details

[1]Department of Orthopeadic Surgery, Shimoshizu National Hospital, 934-5, Shikawatashi, Yotsukaido, Chiba 284-0003, Japan. [2]Department of Orthopaedic Surgery, Chiba Qiball Clinic, 4-5-1, Chuo-ku, Chiba 260-0013, Japan. [3]Department of Orthopaedic Surgery, Graduate School of Medicine, Chiba University, 1-8-1 Inohana, Chuo-ku, Chiba 260-8670, Japan. [4]Department of Orthopaedic Surgery, Eastern Chiba Medical Center, 3-6-2, Okayamadai, Togane, Chiba 283-8686, Japan.

## References

1. Petheram TG, Hourigan PG, Emran IM, Weatherley CR. Dropped head syndrome: a case series and literature review. Spine. 2008;33(1):47–51.
2. Martin AR, Reddy R, Fehlings MG. Dropped head syndrome: diagnosis and management. Evid Based Spine Care J. 2011;2(2):41–7.
3. Fujimoto K. Dropped head in Parkinson's disease. J Neurol. 2006;253(Suppl 7): VII21–6. Review.
4. Quinn N. Disproportionate antecollis in multiple system atrophy. Lancet. 1989;1(8642):844.
5. Katz JS, Wolfe GI, Burns DK, Bryan WW, Fleckenstein JL, Barohn RJ. Isolated neck extensor myopathy: a common cause of dropped head syndrome. Neurology. 1996;46(4):917–21.
6. Gaeta M, Mazziotti S, Toscano A, Rodolico C, Mazzeo A, Blandino A. "Dropped-head" syndrome due to isolated myositis of neck extensor muscles: MRI findings. Skeletal Radiol. 2006;35(2):110–2.
7. Cruz-Jentoft AJ, Landi F, Schneider SM, Zúñiga C, Arai H, Boirie Y, Chen LK, Fielding RA, Martin FC, Michel JP, Sieber C, Stout JR, Studenski SA, Vellas B, Woo J, Zamboni M, Cederholm T. Prevalence of and interventions for sarcopenia in ageing adults: a systematic review. Report of the International Sarcopenia Initiative (EWGSOP and IWGS). Age Ageing. 2014;43(6):748–59.
8. Wu IC, Lin CC, Hsiung CA, Wang CY, Wu CH, Chan DC, Li TC, Lin WY, Huang KC, Chen CY, Hsu CC. Sarcopenia and Translational Aging Research in Taiwan Team. Epidemiology of sarcopenia among community-dwelling older adults in Taiwan: a pooled analysis for a broader adoption of sarcopenia assessments. Geriatr Gerontol Int. 2014;14(Suppl 1):52–60.
9. Morley JE. Sarcopenia: diagnosis and treatment. J Nutr Health Aging. 2008;12:452–6.

10. Sanada K, Miyachi M, Tanimoto M, Yamamoto K, Murakami H, Okumura S, Gando Y, Suzuki K, Tabata I, Higuchi M. A cross-sectional study of sarcopenia in Japanese men and women: reference values and association with cardiovascular risk factors. Eur J Appl Physiol. 2010;110:57–65.

11. Janssen I, Baumgartner RN, Ross R, Rosenberg IH, Roubenoff R. Skeletal muscle cutpoints associated with elevated physical disability risk in older men and women. Am J Epidemiol. 2004;159(4):413–21.

12. Miyakoshi N, Hongo M, Mizutani Y, Shimada Y. Prevalence of sarcopenia in Japanese women with osteopenia and osteoporosis. J Bone Miner Metab. 2013;31(5):556–61.

13. Buckinx F, Reginster JY, Dardenne N, Croisiser JL, Kaux JF, Beaudart C, Slomian J, Bruyère O. Concordance between muscle mass assessed by bioelectrical impedance analysis and by dual energy X-ray absorptiometry: a cross-sectional study. BMC Musculoskelet Disord. 2015;16:60.

# 12

# Schroth physiotherapeutic scoliosis-specific exercises for adolescent idiopathic scoliosis: how many patients require treatment to prevent one deterioration?

Sanja Schreiber[1]* ⓘ, Eric C Parent[2], Doug L Hill[3], Douglas M Hedden[3], Marc J Moreau[3] and Sarah C Southon[3]

**Abstract**

**Background:** Recent randomized controlled trials (RCTs) support using physiotherapeutic scoliosis-specific exercises (PSSE) for adolescents with idiopathic scoliosis (AIS). All RCTs reported statistically significant results favouring PSSE but none reported on clinical significance. The number needed to treat (NNT) helps determine if RCT results are clinically meaningful. The NNT is the number of patients that need to be treated to prevent one bad outcome in a given period. A low NNT suggests that a therapy has positive outcomes in most patients offered the therapy. The objective was to determine how many patients require Schroth PSSE added to standard care (observation or brace treatment) to prevent one progression (NNT) of the Largest Curve (LC) or Sum of Curves (SOC) beyond 5° and 10°, respectively over a 6-month interval.

**Methods:** This was a secondary analysis of a RCT. Fifty consecutive participants from a scoliosis clinic were randomized to the Schroth PSSE + standard of care group ($n = 25$) or the standard of care group ($n = 25$). We included males and females with AIS, age 10–18 years, all curve types, with curves 10°- 45°, with or without brace, and all maturity levels. We excluded patients awaiting surgery, having had surgery, having completed brace treatment and with other scoliosis diagnoses. The local ethics review board approved the study (Pro00011552). The Schroth intervention consisted of weekly 1-h supervised Schroth PSSE sessions and a daily home program delivered over six months in addition to the standard of care. A prescription algorithm was used to determine which exercises patients were to perform. Controls received only standard of care.
Cobb angles were measured using a semi-automatic system from posterior-anterior standing radiographs at baseline and 6 months.
We calculated absolute risk reduction (ARR) and relative risk reduction (RRR). The NTT was calculated as: NNT = 1/ ARR. Patients with missing values (PSSE group; $n = 2$ and controls; $n = 4$) were assumed to have had curve progression (worst case scenario). The RRR is calculated as RRR = ARR/CER

(Continued on next page)

* Correspondence: sanja.schreiber@ualberta.ca
[1]Faculty of Rehabilitation Medicine, University of Alberta, Edmonton, Alberta, Canada
Full list of author information is available at the end of the article

(Continued from previous page)

**Results:** For LC, NNT = 3.6 (95% CI 2.0–28.2), and for SOC, NNT = 3.1 (95% CI 1.9–14.2). The corresponding ARR was 28% for LC and 32% for the SOC. The RRR was 70% for LC and 73% for the SOC. Patients with complete follow-up attended 85% of prescribed visits and completed 82.5% of the home program. Assuming zero compliance after dropout, 76% of visits were attended and 73% of the prescribed home exercises were completed.

**Conclusions:** The short term of Schroth PSSE intervention added to standard care provided a large benefit as compared to standard care alone. Four (LC and SOC) patients require treatment for the additional benefit of a 6-month long Schroth intervention to be observed beyond the standard of care in at least one patient.

**Keywords:** Physiotherapeutic scoliosis specific exercises, Number needed to treat, Clinical significance, Schroth, Exercise, Radiography, Cobb angle, Scoliosis, Adolescents, Spinal curvatures

## Background

The evidence on physiotherapeutic scoliosis specific exercises (PSSE) is rapidly growing and getting stronger. Several randomized controlled trials (RCT) investigating the effect of PSSE in adolescents with idiopathic scoliosis (AIS) have been published. Monticone et al., in their long-term RCT found that PSSE consisting of active self-correction and task-oriented exercises, consistent with Scientific Exercise Approach to Scoliosis (SEAS) [1, 2] improved Cobb angles by 5.3° at skeletal maturity in patients with AIS, while traditional exercises were associated with stable curves. [3] Kuru et al., in their 6-month long RCT [4] in patients with AIS concluded that Schroth PSSE improved the Cobb angle by 2.5° in the supervised group, while the patients who were not supervised deteriorated by 3.3° which was similar to controls (deteriorate by 3.1°) receiving no treatment [4]. Our RCT found that patients with AIS receiving Schroth PSSE for six months in conjunction with standard of care consisting of observation or bracing improved curves by 1.2°, while the controls receiving only standard of care deteriorated by 2.3°. [5] Monticone et al. in an RCT conducted on adults with idiopathic scoliosis with childhood onset undergoing a 20-week long SEAS PSSE or usual physiotherapy, found that the Cobb angle in the experimental group improved by 2.9° and in the control group deteriorated by 2.1° [6]

All these RCTs reported statistically significant results favouring PSSE but none reported on clinical significance. Assessing the clinical significance is important to interpret the results in a way, which is understandable to the end users (clinicians and patients), as well as to facilitate appropriate knowledge transfer. [7–10]

Reporting statistical test results should be supplemented with methods for determining clinically significant change [11–14]. The concept of "clinical significance" basically consists of determining whether "this matters in the real world of clinical medicine." [9] Several definitions have been proposed for "clinically meaningful effect". One

definition is "the extent to which therapy moves someone outside the range of scores typical of the dysfunctional population or within the range of the functional population" [12]. Another one states that "a clinically significant change is a difference score that is large enough to have an implication for the patient's treatment or care" [15]. These definitions are not associated with a definite statistic to determine the meaningfulness of an observed improvement or deterioration over time with clinical treatment. Therefore, in an effort to evaluate whether the treatment has had a clinically significant effect on a patient's outcome variable, several approaches have been proposed.

Researchers most commonly assess the minimal clinically important difference (MCID), and use it as a threshold for determining if a patient experienced meaningful change. The MCID is "the smallest difference in score in the domain of interest that patients perceive as important, either beneficial or harmful, and which would lead the clinician to consider a change in the patient's management" [7]. Two methods are used to establish the MCID: anchor- and distribution-based. Anchor-based methods use an external indicator (anchor) to assign participants into several groupings reflecting the importance/magnitude of their changes in outcome measurement (target). [16] The most commonly used anchor is the Global Rating of Change (GRC) [17]. Distribution-based methods rely on statistical properties of the outcome tool of interest to quantify how much change is deemed clinically important.

There is still no consensus as to which method is the most appropriate. [15, 18] Anchor-based methods because of their reliance on the GRC can be affected by recall bias. [18] Patients often do not remember accurately their health status before the treatment. Distribution-based methods depend only on the reliability of the measurement tool and generally ignore whether outcome changes are perceived as important. [18]

The number needed to treat (NNT) is the number of patients that need to be treated to prevent one bad outcome in a period. A low NNT indicates that a therapy has a positive outcome in most patients offered the therapy. The NNT is easier to interpret by the public than probabilities, and is therefore a useful measurement of the clinical effect.

Therefore, the objective of this secondary analysis of data from a RCT [5, 19, 20]study was to determine how many patients require Schroth PSSE added to standard care (observation or brace treatment) to prevent one progression of the Largest Curve (LC) by more than 5° or of the Sum of Curves (SOC) by more than 10° over a 6-month interval.

## Methods

### Design

This was a secondary analysis of a parallel group RCT on the effect of 6-month long Schroth PSSE intervention added to standard of care compared to standard of care alone (observation or bracing) on the change in Cobb angle in patients with AIS.

### Setting and participants

Fifty consecutive participants with AIS were recruited from a local scoliosis clinic by an independent research coordinator. We included male and female adolescents with AIS, age 10–18 years, all curve types, with curve magnitudes 10° - 45°Cobb angle, with or without brace, and all maturity levels (Risser = 0–5). Surgical candidates, adolescents who had had surgery, had completed a brace treatment and patients with diagnosis other than AIS were excluded. The local ethics review board approved the study, participants provided assent and parents' provided consent.

### Randomization

Participants were randomized using a computer-generated sequence in pre-sealed envelopes into the experimental or the control group, so that each group included 25 participants. Random block sizes varying between 4 and 8 and stratification for curve types were used. The sequence was prepared by an independent research assistant.

### Intervention

The Schroth intervention consisted of weekly 1-h long supervised Schroth exercises sessions combined with a 30–45-min long daily home exercise program delivered over six months in addition to the standard of care. An exercise prescription algorithm was used to determine which exercises patients were to perform [21]. Schroth PSSE, consist of passive and active postural auto-correction exercises done repeatedly. Exercises are progressed from lying, sitting, or standing positions and from most to least passive support per a review of the quality of the performance demonstrated during supervised visits. Controls received only standard of care (observation or bracing) during the trial time. A detailed description of the intervention has been published previously. [5, 19, 20]

### Outcomes and follow-up

Radiographic measurements included the largest curve (LC) and sum of the curves (SOC) measured by the Cobb angle. The *Cobb angle* is the angle between the upper endplate of the most tilted upper end vertebrae and lower endplate of the lower end vertebrae of the scoliosis curvature observed on a posterior-anterior radiograph [22]. Our semi-automated digital measurement demonstrated excellent reliability with a standard error of measurement (SEM) of ≤2.5°, which is better than most published values for Cobb angle measurements. [23] The intra- class correlation coefficient for estimating the intra-rater reliability was ICC = 0.99 (CI 0.987–0.992). One evaluator extracted all Cobb angles larger than 10° while blinded to groupings, image time points, prior measurements and subject identity. The largest Cobb angle measured was used as the LC and the sum of all Cobb angles exceeding 10° was used as the SOC outcome in the analyses.

### Statistical analysis

Numbers needed to treat (NTT) were calculated as: $NNT = \frac{1}{CER-EER}$, where CER is the control event rate and EER the experimental event rate. The CER and EER are the proportion of patients in the control and experimental group, respectively, who deteriorated by >5° for the LC or by >10° for the SOC. The Wilson score method was used for calculating the 95% CI for the NNT. This was justified because the most frequently used Wald method has several documented shortcomings, including dependency on sample size and producing unreliable and theoretically impossible results when event probabilities are close to 0 and 1 [24, 25]. The Wilson score method provides improved CI and interpretation compared to the Wald method. Tandberg's calculator for confidence intervals for the NNT was used [26].

We also provided absolute risk reduction (ARR) and relative risk reduction (RRR). ARR is calculated as the difference between the CER and the EER and describes how much better or worse one treatment is at preventing a curve progression by >5° (LC) or 10° (SOC). The RRR, calculated as the ARR divided by the CER, represents how much the treatment reduced the risk of curve deterioration by >5° (LC) or 10° (SOC) relative to the observations in the control group. [27] Intent to treat analysis was used. Patients with missing values were assumed to have had curve progression (worst case scenario).

*Sample size calculation*

This RCT was powered to detect a 0.50 effect size when comparing the change in the primary outcome between two groups with 80% power using a two-tailed 0.05 hypothesis test, and considering a 0.6 correlation between repeated measures in two time points, 50 patients per group were needed. [28] However, the study ended after recruiting 50 participants when funding was received to continue the study as a multicenter RCT with slightly different participants' criteria. [5]

## Results

The 25 participants in each group were recruited between April 2011 and November 2013. Patients in both groups had similar baseline characteristics and calculated risk of progression by Lonstein and Carlson formula [29] (Table 1). Two participants from the Schroth PSSE group and four from the control group dropped out, due to time constraint (PSSE group), relocation (one control) and travelling for a long time during the trial (one control). Patients with complete follow-up attended 85% of prescribed visits and completed 82.5% of the home program. Assuming zero compliance after dropout, 76% of visits were attended and 73% of the prescribed home exercises were completed. No adverse events were observed in this RCT.

Baseline and 6-month mean scores for LC and SOC are presented in Table 2.

There were 4 (16%) patients in the experimental and 1 (4%) in the control group who improved their LC by >5°. The LC remained within 5° for 18 (72%) participants in the experimental and 14 (56%) in the control group; and there were 3 (12%) participants in the experimental and 10 (40%) in the control group whose LC deteriorated by >5° (Table 3). For the LC, the NNT was 3.6 with a 95% CI 2.0 to 28.2.

One (4%) participant in the experimental and 1 (4%) in the control group improved their SOC by >10°. The SOC remained within 10° for 21 (84%) participants in

the experimental and 13 (52%) in the control group; and there were 3 (12%) participants in the experimental and 11 (44%) in the control group for whom the SOC deteriorated by >10° (Table 3). For the SOC, the NNT was 3.1 with a 95% CI 1.9 to 14.2. (Table 4).

The ARR indicated that, with the Schroth intervention, there was a 28% and 32% absolute reduction in the risk of curve progression over the respective clinically important thresholds associated with the LC and SOC, respectively (Table 4). Further, the RRR indicated that the Schroth intervention reduced the risk of curve deterioration in excess of 5° for the LC by 70% and exceeding 10° for the SOC by 73% (Table 4).

## Discussion

This first study to assess the NNT in patients with AIS undergoing Schroth exercise intervention demonstrated the clinically important effect of the Schroth intervention. We calculated that over a 6-months period one additional person will avoid LC deterioration by >5° or SOC deterioration by >10°, respectively, for every four participants undergoing Schroth PSSE intervention in addition to standard of care compared to receiving standard of care only.

While the health consequences of progression of LC by >5° or of the SOC by >10° over six months are not fully documented, it is clear that the goal of every scoliosis therapy is to stop the curves from progression into a range where a change in care would be warranted. For a patient under observation, progression of the LC by >5° might lead to a brace prescription, and for a participant in brace, progression might warrant a modification of the brace prescription or a recommendation for surgery. Therefore, avoiding a more aggressive treatment even if only for six months is clinically meaningful.

Monticone et al. [2] also reported results favouring SEAS PSSE at maturity. None of the patients from the SEAS PSSE group deteriorated by >5°, 62% improved, and 38% remained stable suggesting that 100% were

**Table 1** Baseline characteristics of the study participants

| | Schroth exercises + Standard of care (95% Confidence interval), n = 25 | Standard of care (95% Confidence interval), n = 25 |
|---|---|---|
| Age (years) | 13.5 (12.7–14.2) | 13.3 (12.7–13.9) |
| Girls n (%) | 23 (92) | 24 (96) |
| Braced participants n (%) | 17 (68) | 17 (68) |
| Height (m) | 1.60 (1.6–1.6) | 1.60 (1.6–1.6) |
| Weight (kg) | 45.9 (42.6–49.1) | 50.5 (47.1–54.0) |
| Largest curve (°) | 29.1 (25.4–32.8) | 27.9 (24.3–31.5) |
| Sum of curves (°) | 48.1 (39.1–57.2) | 54.3 (44.9–63.6) |
| Risser sign (0 to 5) | 1.76 (1.10 to 2.45) | 1.44 (0.77 to 2.11) |
| Lonstein and Carlson Risk of progression [29] (%) | 65 | 65 |

**Table 2** Mean scores for each outcome at baseline and 6-month follow-up

| Outcome | Group | Mean | Standard Deviation | 95% Confidence Interval | Minimum | Maximum |
|---|---|---|---|---|---|---|
| Largest Cobb at Baseline (°) | Control* | 27.9 | 8.8 | 24.3–31.5 | 11.7 | 42.0 |
| | Experimental* | 29.1 | 8.9 | 25.4–32.8 | 11.3 | 44.3 |
| | Total | 28.5 | 8.8 | 26.0–31.0 | 11.3 | 44.3 |
| Sum of Curves at Baseline (°) | Control | 54.3 | 22.6 | 44.9–63.6 | 11.7 | 95.1 |
| | Experimental | 48.2 | 21.9 | 39.1–57.2 | 11.3 | 86.0 |
| | Total | 51.2 | 22.3 | 44.9–57.5 | 11.3 | 95.1 |
| Largest Cobb at 6-months | Control | 29.1 | 8.8 | 25.0–33.3 | 12.1 | 44.7 |
| | Experimental | 27.7 | 8.9 | 23.8–31.5 | 14.4 | 43.9 |
| | Total | 28.4 | 8.8 | 25.7–31.0 | 12.1 | 44.7 |
| Sum of Curves at 6-months | Control | 57.5 | 24.9 | 45.8–69.1 | 15.8 | 102.4 |
| | Experimental | 45.7 | 21.4 | 36.4–54.9 | 14.4 | 80.6 |
| | Total | 51.2 | 23.6 | 43.9–58.4 | 14.4 | 102.4 |

*Control = Standard of care group; Experimental = "Schroth + standard of care group

treated successfully [2]. In the control group receiving general physiotherapy, none improved, 4 (8%) deteriorated, and 47 (92%) remained stable. We calculated NNT based on those results as 12.8 with CI containing "0", suggesting that the treatment effect was not significant. However, there were 61.5% more patients who improved beyond 5° in the PSSE group, clearly suggesting the benefit of PSSE over the long term. This lack of clinical importance in the treatment effect in this study is not clinically significant in terms of prevention of deterioration by >5°, could be contributed to the fact that the girls under investigation had low risk of progression (35% risk of progression according to Lonstein and Carlson's formula) [30], and the comparator was an active therapy.

While ours was the first study reporting NNT for exercise treatment, NNTs have been reported for brace management. The Bracing in Adolescent Idiopathic Scoliosis Trial (BrAIST) study, which was partly a randomized and partly a patient-preference trial, reported that 3.0

(95% CI, 2.0 to 6.2) patients needed to be treated in order to prevent one case of curve progression warranting surgery based on the results from the randomized cohort and applying intention-to-treat methodology. [31] This is not in line with Sanders et al. [32] results in a prospective follow-up of a cohort of 126 immature patients (Risser 0–2) with AIS and curves between 25° and 45° treated with a Boston brace and brace wear to the end point of progression to surgery. The noncompliant patients were compared both with highly compliant patients and with the entire cohort. The authors reported a NNT of 7 to avoid surgery. However, the 95% CI included "0", indicating that the treatment effect was not significant, so the NNT cannot be directly interpreted. For the highly compliant patients (bracewear >14 h) compared with non-compliant patients, the NNT (3.0; 95% CI, 2.0 to 7.0) was similar to that reported in the BrAISt and the present study.

Nachemson and Peterson multicenter study compared observation and bracing for girls with thoracic major

**Table 3** Number of participants improved, stable and deteriorated at the 6-month follow-up

| | Improved (Cobb angle reduced by ≥5°) number (%) | Stable (Cobb angle within 5°) number (%) | Deteriorated (Cobb angle increased by ≥5°) number (%) |
|---|---|---|---|
| Largest Cobb | | | |
| Schroth + standard of care | 4 (16) | 18 (72) | 3 (12) |
| Standard of Care | 1 (4) | 14 (56) | 10 (40) |
| | Improved (Cobb angle reduced by ≥10°) number (%) | Stable (Cobb angle within 10°) number (%) | Deteriorated (Cobb angle increased by ≥10°) number (%) |
| Sum of Curves | | | |
| Schroth + standard of care | 1 (4) | 21 (84) | 3 (12) |
| Standard of care | 1 (4) | 13 (52) | 11 (44) |

**Table 4** Numbers needed to treat (NNT) with 95% confidence intervals (CI), Absolute risk reduction (ARR) and Relative risk reduction (RRR)

|  | NNT (n, 95% CI) | Absolute Risk Reduction (%) | Relative Risk Reduction (%) |
|---|---|---|---|
| Largest Cobb Angle | 3.6 (2.0 to 28.2) | 28 | 70 |
| Sum of curves | 3.1 (1.9 to 14.2) | 32 | 73 |

curves and Cobb angles of 25° to 35°. [33] In their study they found that 17 of 88 braced patients with full follow-up deteriorated by >6°, and 58 of 120 observed patients, which gives NNT of 3.4 (95% CI 2.5 to 6.2). However, in the worst-case analysis when the dropouts are considered failures, there were 36% failures among braced patients and 56% among observed cohort, producing the NNT of 6.3 (3.6 to 30.3).

Danielsson et al. used some of the subjects from Nachemson and Peterson study, and determined the treatment failure at a mean of 16-year follow-up, found that none of the 41 initially braced patients progressed by >6°, whereas 40% of those initially under observation progressed. However, there was no difference in progression between the two groups after maturity (5.7° in the braced group and 7.0° in the observed patients). The authors concluded that since "70% of the observed patients during the original study period did not require any other treatment, 70% of the initially braced patients can therefore be regarded as having been treated unnecessarily." [34] Of the remaining observed patients, who needed a treatment, only 10% required surgery, meaning that 10 patients need to be brace-treated to avoid 1 surgery (NNT = 10; 95% CI 5.7 to 23.9).

In our sample, 17 (68%) patients wore a brace in each group. When a good compliance was assumed as brace wear of >16 h, there were 8 (47%) compliant patients in the Schroth PSSE group and 7 (41%) in the control group. There were 20 (80%) patients in the experimental group with >75% compliance with daily home exercise program. Of those who wore a brace in the Schroth PSSE group, 8 (47%) non-compliant and 7 (41%) compliant patients with brace had improved or stable curves. There was 1 (6%) compliant and 1 (6%) non-compliant patient with a brace who deteriorated. Of the 5 (20%) patients with <75% compliance with the home exercise program, 3 (60%) did not have a brace; of 2 that did have a brace, 1 (50%) was compliant with it and 1 (50%) was not. Of the eight patients in the Schroth PSSE group who did not wear a brace 7 (88%) improved, and 1 (12%) deteriorated.

While our sample size was relatively small, the distribution of compliant and non-compliant patients with a brace between the groups was similar. In addition, there was a similar number of compliant and non-compliant

patients with brace who improved or deteriorated in the experimental group. Therefore, the compliance with a brace did not have a direct influence on the effect of the intervention, as long as the patients were compliant with the exercises. However, this study did not compare Schroth PSSE with bracing alone, so this should be interpreted with caution.

There is a general consensus that current brace indications lead to overtreatment. [32, 34] Many patients wearing a brace do not need to wear one because their curves would naturally not increase to the surgical range, and only estimated 10% of braced patients would avoid surgery. [34] We showed that four participants undergoing Schroth PSSE intervention in addition to standard of care and not standard of care only would need to be treated in order to see one additional curve improvement over a 6-months period.

We observed that adding Schroth PSSE might address a need and offer a treatment complement in patients who are not fully compliant with brace treatment. In our sample, despite promoting both exercise and brace compliance, of nine patients reporting wearing their a brace less than 16 h a day in the exercise group, 8 (89%) were highly compliant with exercises.

Our study was designed to determine whether adding Schroth PSSE to standard of care (observation and bracing) would lead to better outcomes, as compared to standard of care alone. To assess the differences between brace vs. exercises alone, we would need to deny the brace treatment to the patients who meet the SRS bracing criteria, which would raise ethical concerns. Despite the clinically significant results in our study, the overarching question of who will benefit from wearing a brace, who from doing the Schroth PSSE, and who from a combined treatment still remains.

### Limitations

A limitation of this study is its short-term follow-up. Therefore, we cannot draw conclusions regarding the effects of a longer period of treatment, and cannot answer the question "how many patients need to be treated with Schroth PSSE added to standard of care to prevent one surgery or prevent the need for a brace?" However, our study shows that the Schroth PSSE intervention added to standard care consisting of bracing or observation can delay the time where a more aggressive scoliosis management is indicated.

The small sample size precluded us from conducting subgroup analysis related to compliance, curve type, baseline severity or maturity. Interestingly, of 25 patients in the exercise group, 20 reported >75% compliance with home exercise program. In the control group, there were 17 patients who wore braces. Of those, only seven were considered compliant as they wore their braces >16 h/

day. This might have resulted in a larger number of deteriorated patients in the control group as compared to the exercise group.

Small sample size also affected confidence intervals of the NNTs. Regardless, of the wide CI, the treatment was clinically important, because the CI were not disjointed (did not contain "0").

While the patients and therapists could not be blinded to treatment, our outcomes' assessors were blinded.

Participation in the Schroth intervention may have had an effect on brace wear compliance likely illustrating the importance of team-work.

## Conclusions

The short-term Schroth PSSE intervention added to standard care provided a clinically important benefit illustrated by low NNT when compared to standard care alone. Results suggest that four (LC, SOC) patients require treatment for the additional benefit of a 6-month long Schroth PSSE intervention added to standard of care to be observed beyond the standard of care in at least one patient.

## Abbreviations

AIS: Adolescent Idiopathic Scoliosis; ARR: Absolute Risk Reduction; BrAIST: Bracing Adolescent Idiopathic Scoliosis Trial; CER: Control Event Rate; CI: Confidence Interval; EER: Experimental Event Rate; ICC: Intra-class Correlation Coefficient; LC: Largest Curve; MCID: Minimal Clinical Important Difference; n: Number; NNT: Numbers Needed to Treat; PSSE: Physiotherapeutic Scoliosis-Specific Exercises; RCT: Randomized Controlled Trial; RRR: Relative Risk Ratio; SEAS: Scientific Exercise Approach for Scoliosis; SEM: Standard Error of Measurement; SOC: Sum of Curves

## Acknowledgements

Thanks to Kathleen Shearer for coordinating the study recruitment, Alan Richter for helping with the data entry and acting as an assessor, the participants and their parents for their commitment.

## Funding

This study was funded by: Scoliosis Research Society 2010 Small Exploratory Grant (US$ 10,000), Glenrose Rehabilitation Hospital Foundation, Glenrose Clinical Research Fund (CAD$ 10,000). An Interdepartmental Graduate Studentship jointly awarded by the Faculty of Medicine and Dentistry and Faculty of Rehabilitation Medicine supported the PhD work of Sanja Schreiber (CAD$ 92,000). The funders had no role in study design, data collection and analysis, decision to publish, or preparation of the manuscript. Dr. Parent is supported by a new investigator grant from the SickKids Foundation of Canada – CIHR Institute of Human Development, Child and Youth Health.

## Authors' contributions

Conceptualization: SS. Analysis: SS. Funding acquisition: SS ECP DMH DLH MM SCS. Investigation: SS ECP. Methodology: SS ECP DMH DLH MM SCS. Supervision: ECP. Visualization: SS. Writing – original draft: SS. Writing – review & editing: SS ECP DMH DLH MM SCS. All authors read and approved the final manuscript.

## Competing interests

SS owns a private clinic providing Schroth exercises opened after completing the research.
The authors declare that they have no other competing interests

## Author details

¹Faculty of Rehabilitation Medicine, University of Alberta, Edmonton, Alberta, Canada. ²Department of Physical Therapy, University of Alberta, Edmonton, Alberta, Canada. ³Department of Surgery, University of Alberta, Edmonton, Alberta, Canada.

## References

1. Negrini S, Bettany-Saltikov J, de Mauroy JC, Durmala J, Grivas TB, Knott P, Kotwicki T, Maruyama T, O'Brien JP, Parent E, Rigo M, Romano M, Stikeleather L, Villagrasa M, Zaina F: Letter to the Editor concerning: "Active self-correction and task-oriented exercises reduce spinal deformity and improve quality of life in subjects with mild adolescent idiopathic scoliosis. Results of a randomised controlled trial" by Monticone M, Ambrosini E, Cazzaniga D, Rocca B, Ferrante S (2014). Eur Spine J; DOI:10.1007/s00586-014-3241-y. Eur Spine J 2014, 23:2218–2220.
2. Monticone M. Answer to the letter to the editor of S. Negrini et al. concerning "active self-correction and task-oriented exercises reduce spinal deformity and improve quality of life in subjects with mild adolescent idiopathic scoliosis. Results of a randomised controlled trial" by Monticone M, Ambrosini E, Cazzaniga D, Rocca B, Ferrante S (2014) Eur spine J. Eur Spine J. 2014;23:2221–2. doi:10.1007/s00586-014-3241-y.
3. Monticone M, Ambrosini E, Cazzaniga D, Rocca B, Ferrante S. Active self-correction and task-oriented exercises reduce spinal deformity and improve quality of life in subjects with mild adolescent idiopathic scoliosis. Results of a randomised controlled trial. Eur Spine J. 2014;23:1204–14.
4. Kuru T, Yeldan İ, Dereli EE, Özdinçler AR, Dikici F, Çolak İ. The efficacy of three-dimensional Schroth exercises in adolescent idiopathic scoliosis: a randomised controlled clinical trial. Clin Rehabil. 2016;30:181–90.
5. Schreiber S, Parent EC, Moez EK, Hedden DM, Hill DL, Moreau M, Lou E, Watkins EM, Southon SC: Schroth Physiotherapeutic Scoliosis-Specific Exercises Added to the Standard of Care Lead to Better Cobb Angle Outcomes in Adolescents with Idiopathic Scoliosis – an Assessor and Statistician Blinded Randomized Controlled Trial. PLoS ONE, 11:e0168746.
6. Monticone M, Ambrosini E, Cazzaniga D, Rocca B, Motta L, Cerri C, Brayda-Bruno M, Lovi A. Adults with idiopathic scoliosis improve disability after motor and cognitive rehabilitation: results of a randomised controlled trial. Eur Spine J. 2016;25:3120–9.
7. Guyatt GH, Osoba D, Wu AW, Wyrwich KW, Norman GR. Clinical significance consensus meeting group: methods to explain the clinical significance of health status measures. Mayo Clin Proc. 2002;77:371–83.
8. Carreon LY, Sanders JO, Diab M, Sucato DJ, Sturm PF, Glassman SD. Spinal deformity study group: the minimum clinically important difference in Scoliosis Research Society-22 appearance, activity, and pain domains after surgical correction of adolescent idiopathic scoliosis. Spine. 2010;35:2079–83.
9. Sloan JA. Assessing the minimally clinically significant difference: scientific considerations, challenges and solutions. COPD. 2005;2:57–62.
10. Musselman KE. Clinical significance testing in rehabilitation research: what, why, and how? Phys Ther Rev. 2007;12:287–96.
11. Jacobson NS, Truax P. Clinical significance: a statistical approach to defining meaningful change in psychotherapy research. J Consult Clin Psychol. 1991;59:12–9.
12. Jacobson NS, Follette WC, Revenstorf D. Psychotherapy outcome research: methods for reporting variability and evaluating clinical significance. Behav Ther. 1984;15:336–52.
13. ScienceDirect - Behavior Therapy, Volume 17, Issue 3, Pages 197–312 (June 1986) [http://www.sciencedirect.com.login.ezproxy.library.ualberta.ca/science?_ob=PublicationURL&_tockey=%23TOC%2329681%231986%23999829996%23625529%23FLP%23&_cdi=29681&_pubType=J&_auth=y&_acct=C000051251&_version=1&_urlVersion=0&_userid=1067472&md5=fe78da66b4218f9977de028d13b6fd40].
14. Kazdin AE. The meanings and measurement of clinical significance. J Consult Clin Psychol. 1999;67:332–9.

15. Wyrwich KW, Bullinger M, Aaronson N, Hays RD, Patrick DL, Symonds T. Group TCSCM: estimating clinically significant differences in quality of life outcomes. Qual Life Res. 2005;14:285–95.

16. Revicki D, Hays R, Cella D, Sloan J. Recommended methods for determining responsiveness and minimally important differences for patient-reported outcomes. J Clin Epidemiol. 2008;61:102–9.

17. Kamper SJ, Maher CG, Mackay G. Global rating of change scales: a review of strengths and weaknesses and considerations for design. J Man Manip Ther. 2009;17:163–70.

18. Crosby RD, Kolotkin RL, Williams GR. Defining clinically meaningful change in health-related quality of life. J Clin Epidemiol. 2003;56:395–407.

19. Schreiber S, Parent EC, Hedden DM, Moreau M, Hill D, Lou E. Effect of Schroth exercises on curve characteristics and clinical outcomes in adolescent idiopathic scoliosis: protocol for a multicentre randomised controlled trial. J Phys. 2014;60:234.

20. Schreiber S, Parent EC, Moez EK, Hedden DM, Hill D, Moreau MJ, Lou E, Watkins EM, Southon SC: The effect of Schroth exercises added to the standard of care on the quality of life and muscle endurance in adolescents with idiopathic scoliosis-an assessor and statistician blinded randomized controlled trial: "SOSORT 2015 Award Winner". 2015, 10:1–12.

21. Watkins EM. Bosnjak S. Parent EC: Algorithms to prescribe Schroth exercises for each of four Schroth curve types. 2012;7:P22.

22. Adolescent Idiopathic Scoliosis - Treatment [http://www.srs.org/professionals/education/adolescent/idiopathic/treatment.php].

23. Zhang J, Lou E, Shi X, Wang Y, Hill DL, Raso JV, Le LH, Lv L. A computer-aided cobb angle measurement method and its reliability. J Spinal Disord Tech. 2010;23:383–7.

24. Bender R. Calculating confidence intervals for the number needed to treat. Control Clin Trials. 2001;22:102–10.

25. Newcombe RG. Interval estimation for the difference between independent proportions: comparison of eleven methods. Stat Med. 1998;17:873–90.

26. Tandberg D. Improved confidence intervals for the difference between two proportions and number needed to treat (NNT). Center for Evidence Based Medicine - cebmnet. 2009;

27. Portney LG, Watkins MP: Foundations of clinical research: applications to practice. Prentice Hall; 2009.

28. Fitzmaurice GM, Laird NM, Ware JH: *Applied Longitudinal Analysis*. 2nd edition. John Wiley & Sons; 2011.

29. Lonstein JE, Carlson JM. The prediction of curve progression in untreated idiopathic scoliosis during growth. J Bone Joint Surg Am. 1984;

30. Lonstein J, Carlson J. The prediction of curve progression in untreated idiopathic scoliosis during growth. J Bone Joint Surg. 1984;66:1061.

31. Weinstein SL, Dolan LA, Wright JG, Dobbs MB. Effects of bracing in adolescents with idiopathic scoliosis. N Engl J Med. 2013;369:1512–21.

32. Sanders JO, Newton PO, Browne RH, Katz DE, Birch JG, Herring JA. Bracing for idiopathic scoliosis: how many patients require treatment to prevent one surgery? J Bone Joint Surg Am. 2014;96:649.

33. Nachemson AL, Peterson LE. Effectiveness of treatment with a brace in girls who have adolescent idiopathic scoliosis : a prospective, controlled study based on data from the brace study of the Scoliosis Research Society. J Bone Joint Surg Am. 1995;77:815–22.

34. Danielsson AJ, Hasserius R, Ohlin A, Nachemson AL. A prospective study of brace treatment versus observation alone in adolescent idiopathic scoliosis: a follow-up mean of 16 years after maturity. Spine. 2007;32:2198–207.

# 13

# An observational study on surgically treated adult idiopathic scoliosis patients' quality of life outcomes at 1- and 2-year follow-ups and comparison to controls

Jennifer C. Theis[1,2], Anna Grauers[2,3], Elias Diarbakerli[2], Panayiotis Savvides[2], Allan Abbott[1,4,5,6] and Paul Gerdhem[2*] ⓘ

## Abstract

**Background:** Prospective data on health-related quality of life in patients with idiopathic scoliosis treated surgically as adults is needed. We compared preoperative and 1- and 2-year follow-up data in surgically treated adults with idiopathic scoliosis with juvenile or adolescent onset. Results were compared to untreated adults with scoliosis and population normative data.

**Methods:** A comparison of preoperative and 1- and 2-year follow-up data of 75 adults surgically treated for idiopathic scoliosis at a mean age of 28 years (range 18 to 69) from a prospective national register study, as well as a comparison with age- and sex-matched data from 75 untreated adults with less severe scoliosis and 75 adults without scoliosis, was made. Outcome measures were EuroQol-5 dimensions (EQ-5D) and Scoliosis Research Society (SRS)-22r questionnaire.

**Results:** In the surgically treated, EQ-5D and SRS-22r scores had statistically significant improvements at both 1- and 2-year follow-ups (all $p \leq 0.015$). The effect size of surgery on EQ-5D at 1-year follow-up was large ($r = -0.54$) and small-medium ($r = -0.20$) at 2-year follow-up. The effect size of surgery on SRS-22r outcomes was medium-large at 1- and 2-year follow-ups ($r = -0.43$ and $r = -0.42$ respectively). At the 2-year follow-up, the EQ-5D score and the SRS-22r subscore were similar to the untreated scoliosis group ($p = 0.56$ and $p = 0.91$ respectively), but lower than those in the adults without scoliosis ($p < 0.001$ for both comparisons).

**Conclusions:** Adults with idiopathic scoliosis experience an increase in health-related quality of life following surgery at 2-year follow-up, approaching the health-related quality of life of untreated individuals with less severe scoliosis, but remain lower than normative population data.

**Keywords:** Scoliosis, Adults, Idiopathic, Surgery

## Background

Scoliosis in adults has two primary etiologies, degenerative scoliosis and idiopathic scoliosis, defined as a skeletal deformity with a coronal plane Cobb angle greater than 10° in the skeletally mature individual [1, 2]. Adult idiopathic scoliosis stems from a progression of adolescent or childhood idiopathic scoliosis often associated with secondary spinal degeneration [1, 2]. Regardless of pathogenesis, adult scoliosis is associated with back pain, radicular pain, claudication symptoms, and continued degenerative changes [1, 2].

Considering the suggested impact of scoliosis on health-related quality of life (HRQOL) [3, 4], in addition to correcting the deformity and halting curve progression, interventions for adult scoliosis should attempt to relieve pain, improve function, and thus improve patient HRQOL. Additionally, radiographic changes have been suggested to poorly correlate with HRQOL outcome measures for adults with scoliosis [3]. For this reason,

---

* Correspondence: paul.gerdhem@sll.se
[2]Department of Orthopaedics, Department of Clinical Science, Intervention and Technology (CLINTEC), Karolinska Institutet, Karolinska University Hospital, SE-141 86 Stockholm, Sweden
Full list of author information is available at the end of the article

both generic patient reported HRQOL instruments like the EuroQol-5 dimensions (EQ-5D) and the preferred disease-specific outcome measure, Scoliosis Research Society (SRS)-22r, are suggested to evaluate treatment effectiveness in this population [5].

Even though evidence for effectiveness of non-operative treatment are scarce, such attempts should be performed before surgical procedures [6–8]. Patients with less deformity are more likely to benefit from non-operative treatment [7, 9]. Studies suggest surgery has a positive impact on deformity and HRQOL in adults with scoliosis [6, 7, 10–13]. However, few studies with prospective designs reporting HRQOL pre- and post-operatively for adults with scoliosis exist in the literature [6, 7, 10–12]. In addition, few report data specifically for adults with idiopathic scoliosis [14].

The aim of this prospective study is to contribute to the research pertaining to surgically treated adults with idiopathic scoliosis by utilizing the Swedish Spine register (Swespine) to (1) assess the effect of surgery on patient's HRQOL comparing preoperative and 1- and 2-year follow-up EQ-5D and SRS-22r scores, (2) compare 2-year follow-up EQ-5D and SRS-22r scores for adults with idiopathic scoliosis to age- and sex-matched controls of untreated individuals with less severe scoliosis as well as individuals without scoliosis.

## Methods

### Participants

This is an analysis of prospectively collected data from the Swedish Spine register (Swespine). Surgical procedures for spinal deformity, such as scoliosis, have been included in the register since 2006 [15]. Surgeon reported variables included data on surgical procedures and complications. Incidences of reoperation were registered by the surgeon responsible for the procedure.

Patient-reported HRQOL outcome measures including the EQ-5D and, since 2008, the SRS-22r. Patients completed the questionnaires preoperatively and again via mail at 1 and 2 years. Patient-reported complications are gathered at 1-year follow-up and defined as thrombosis, pulmonary embolism, and infection treated with antibiotics within the first three months following surgery.

The EQ-5D contains a question in five dimensions including mobility, self-care, usual activities, pain/discomfort, and anxiety/depression, scored from 1 (no problem) to 3 (extreme problems) that is converted to an index score between 1 (perfect health) and –0.59 (a health state worse than death) representing the societal view of health [16].

The disease-specific SRS-22r contains 22 questions covering five domains: function/activity, pain, self-perceived image, mental health, and satisfaction with treatment, scored from 1 (worst) to 5 (best) [17]. The 20 questions

related to the first four domains were analyzed in this study and collated to make the SRS-22r subscore.

Inclusion criteria for this study was (1) surgery prior to June 30, 2011, (2) age ≥18 years at time of surgery, (3) primary diagnosis of idiopathic scoliosis with juvenile or adolescent onset, (4) preoperative and 2-year follow-up data reported for EQ-5D and/or SRS-22r, and (5) no prior surgical intervention. The participant extraction from the Swespine register is outlined in Fig. 1. The final study cohort included 75 patients.

### Controls

Controls were matched at a 1:1 ratio for (i) sex and (ii) age corresponding to the 2-year follow-up for the cases. We chose to use two control populations: untreated individuals with scoliosis and individuals without scoliosis.

Data on previously observed, untreated, individuals with juvenile or adolescent idiopathic scoliosis collected are continuously collected by our research group, parts of which have been presented earlier [18]. These individuals were asked to fill out the EQ-5D and SRS-22r questionnaires, and 75 controls were selected out of 347 available individuals with EQ-5D and SRS-22r data.

The Swedish population register was used to identify individuals without scoliosis, and the EQ-5D and SRS-22r questionnaires were mailed to 407 randomly selected adults (aged 18–70) with 229 respondents, from which we selected 75 individuals. These were not physically examined. Data from this cohort have been presented elsewhere [18, 19].

### Radiology

Preoperative radiological images were retrieved for all 75 patients, and postoperative images for 72 out of 75 patients and classified by two of the authors according to Cobb [2] and Lenke et al. [20].

### Statistics

The power calculation was based on the postoperative effect sizes observed in adults with scoliosis [13]. The priori sample size was calculated using G*Power 3.1.7 (Universität Kiel, Germany) [21] with a Wilcoxon signed-rank test, effect size of 0.8, type I error $\alpha = 0.05$, and power = 0.8, yielding a required sample size of 12. Due to non-parametric distributions, effect size was calculated using $r = z/\sqrt{N}$ ($z = z$ value, $N$ = total number of observations used to calculate $z$).

The Wilcoxon signed-rank test was used for paired samples, the Welch-Satterthwaite $t$ test for unpaired samples, and the Pearson chi-square test for differences in the different EQ-5D domains. To analyze age differences, the patients were divided into two age groups: ≥25 and <25 years. In case of missing data, cases were excluded analysis by analysis. Descriptive statistics were

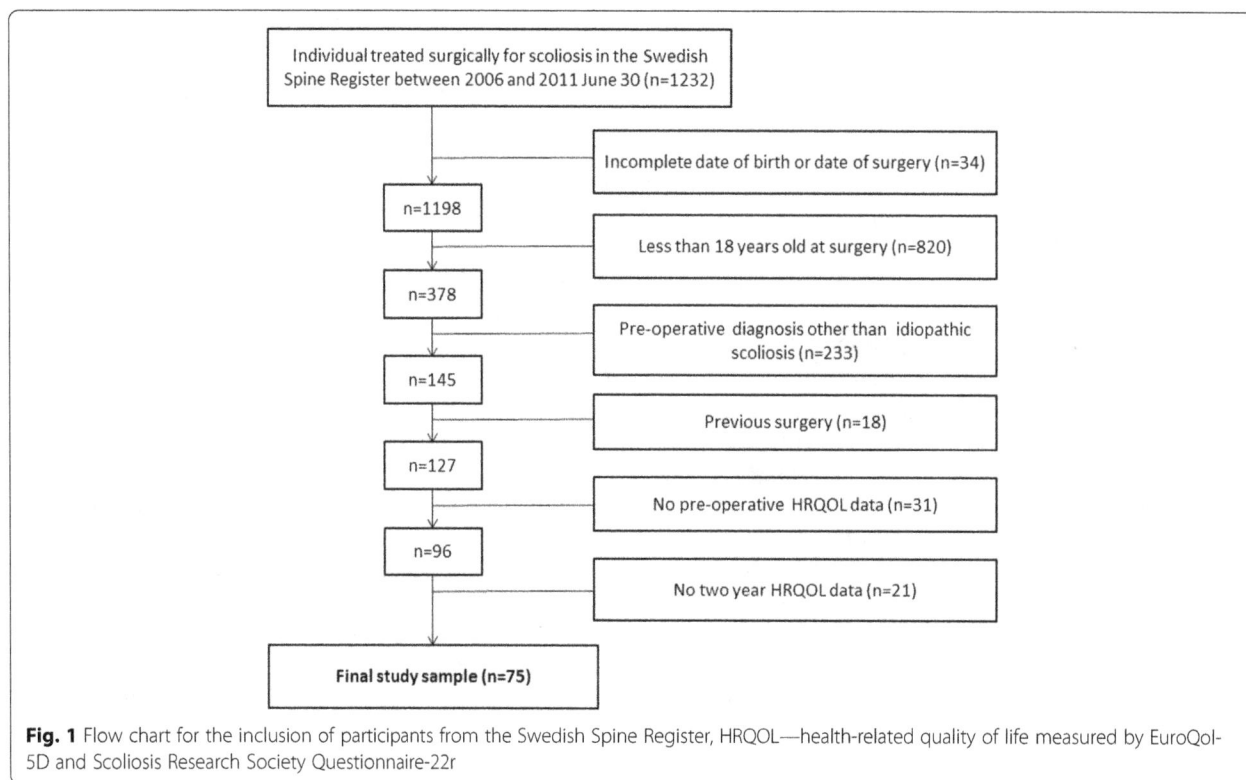

**Fig. 1** Flow chart for the inclusion of participants from the Swedish Spine Register, HRQOL—health-related quality of life measured by EuroQol-5D and Scoliosis Research Society Questionnaire-22r

reported as mean (SD), median (25th, 75th percentile), or number (%). A Bonferroni adjustment of significance was made from $p \leq 0.05$ to $p \leq 0.017$. IBM SPSS Statistics version 20 (Armonk, NY, 2011) was used for statistical analysis.

### Non-response analysis

The 31 participants without preoperative HRQOL data were not significantly different regarding age at surgery ($p = 0.56$), primary Cobb angle ($p = 0.26$), or number of fused vertebrae ($p = 0.03$) than the 96 individuals with preoperative HRQOL data (Fig. 1). The 21 participants lost to 2-year follow-up were not significantly different regarding preoperative age at time of surgery ($p = 0.99$), primary Cobb angle ($p = 0.50$), number of fused vertebrae ($p = 0.55$), EQ-5D index value ($p = 0.18$), or SRS-22r subscore ($p = 0.15$) to the 75 participants with 2-year follow-up data (Fig. 1). One patient died prior to 2-year follow-up. This death was not linked to the surgical event.

### Results

In each group of 75 individuals, there were 60 (80%) females. In the group of patients, mean age was 27 (18–69) years at the time of surgery. Of these, 54 patients were aged <25 years (mean age 20) and 21 were ≥25 years (mean age 46). Preoperative Cobb angle was 54 (8) degrees and postoperative 25 (10) degrees. Other descriptive data for the patients are outlined in Table 1. Regarding the

controls, the mean age of the untreated individuals with scoliosis was 30 (18–67) years, and their last available radiograph showed a mean Cobb angle of 28 (14) degrees. The mean age of the individuals without scoliosis was 32 (17–69) years.

There was a statistically significant improvement in EQ-5D index scores from preoperative to 1-year follow-up with 79% of respondent's scores improving while from preoperative to 2-year follow-up 53% of reported scores improved (Fig. 2). However, there was a statistically significant decrease in EQ-5D index scores from 1- to 2-year follow-up (Fig. 2). The effect size of surgery on 1-year follow-up EQ-5D index scores was large ($r = -0.54$) while at 2-year follow-up the effect was small towards medium ($r = -0.20$) [22]. The 2-year follow-up EQ-5D index was similar to the untreated individuals with scoliosis but continued to have statistically significant worse scores than the individuals without scoliosis (Table 2).

EQ-5D dimension scores for pain/discomfort and anxiety/depression demonstrated statistically significant improvement between preoperative and follow-up time points, with no significant differences noted for any other dimension between follow-ups (Fig. 3). At the 2-year follow-up, the EQ-5D dimension of pain/discomfort was significantly lower than that in both control groups, and the domain usual activities was lower than in individuals without scoliosis (Table 2).

**Table 1** Surgical, complication, and reoperation characteristics of study participants as reported in the Swedish Spine Registry. Complications reported by participants at 1-year follow-up; all other data reported by surgeon at time of initial surgery or reoperation. Data is shown as mean (SD) or number. $n = 75$ except where otherwise indicated

| Characteristic | |
| --- | --- |
| Lenke classification ($n = 70$) | |
|    Type 1 | 23 |
|    Type 2 | 7 |
|    Type 3 | 10 |
|    Type 4 | 2 |
|    Type 5 | 15 |
|    Type 6 | 13 |
| Procedure type, number of patients | |
|    Anterior | 6 |
|    Posterior | 68 |
|    Combined | 1 |
| Levels fused, number ($n = 74$) | 11 (3) |
| Fusion to sacrum, number ($n = 74$) | 4 |
| Intraoperative blood loss, L ($n = 71$) | 1.5 (1.0) |
| Hospital stay from operation to discharge, days ($n = 73$) | 8 (7, 10) |
| Complications | |
|    Nerve root injury, dural lesion, spinal cord injury, mortality | 0 |
|    Thrombosis | 1 |
|    Pulmonary embolism | 4 |
|    Surgical site infection treated with antibiotics | 2 |
| Reoperation, number of participants with reoperation, (indication) | 4 (1 implant replacement, 2 surgical site infection spine, 1 infection at bone graft harvest site) |

SRS-22r subscores had statistically significant improvement between preoperative and follow-up time points with no significant difference between follow-ups (Fig. 4). At 1- and 2-year follow-ups, 79 and 78% of participant's SRS-22r subscores improved compared to those of preoperative results. The overall medium to large ($r = -0.43$ and $r = -0.42$ respectively) effect of surgery on SRS-22r outcomes remained relatively constant from 1- to 2-year follow-ups. The over 25 years age group had significantly lower SRS-22r subscores preoperatively and at both 1- and 2-year follow-ups compared to the younger age group (Table 3), with corresponding results for the EQ-5D index (data not shown).

Statistically significant improvement in the SRS-22r pain domain occurred between preoperative and 1-year follow-up and continued at 2-year follow-up (Fig. 5). A similar statistically significant improvement was seen in the image domain between preoperative and 1- and 2-year follow-up (Fig. 5). At 2-year follow-up, all domains except for the image domain score was significantly lower in the older age group compared to the younger age group (Table 3). When comparing the surgically treated group and the untreated scoliosis group, the SRS-22r subscore and all domains were similar at the 2-year follow-up. However, the SRS-22r subscore and all domain scores, except the mental health domain, continued with statistically significant lower scores than normative population data at 2-year follow-up (Table 4).

Seven patients sustained at least one complication or reoperation (Table 1). The SRS-22r subscore and EQ-5D index at 1 and 2 years did not differ when compared to the patients without complications or reoperations (all $p \geq 0.19$).

## Discussion

This study found an overall significant improvement in HRQOL outcome measures at both 1 and 2-year follow-ups, potentially peaking at 1-year follow-up. HRQOL were similar to untreated scoliosis patients with smaller curves, but outcomes remained lower than population matched scores at 2-year follow-up.

The suggested positive HRQOL impact of surgery for adults with scoliosis is consistent with research summarized in recent reviews [10–13, 23]. In addition, the surgically treated individuals improved their HRQOL to a level comparable to untreated individuals with scoliosis. However, more than one fifth of the patients did not improve their HRQOL at all. Whether these achieve other benefits from surgery, such as better long-term pulmonary function, or later benefits in terms of HRQOL cannot be determined from the current study design.

The overall trend of postoperative HRQOL outcomes appears inconsistent in the current research. One study reported no change in SRS-22, Oswestry Disability Index (ODI), and Short Form-12 from 1 to 2-year follow-ups for surgically treated adult deformity patients [24]. Zimmerman et al. reported that in an adult scoliosis population, SRS-22 domain and subscores continued to significantly increase until 2-year follow-up while ODI and Short Form-36 components changed little after 6 months [25]. The SRS-22r results in our study follow the trend of improvement suggested by Glassman et al. [24] and Yoshida et al [14] with leveling off between 1- and 2-year follow-ups. Whether this is true also at longer follow-ups in adults is not known, necessitating further studies.

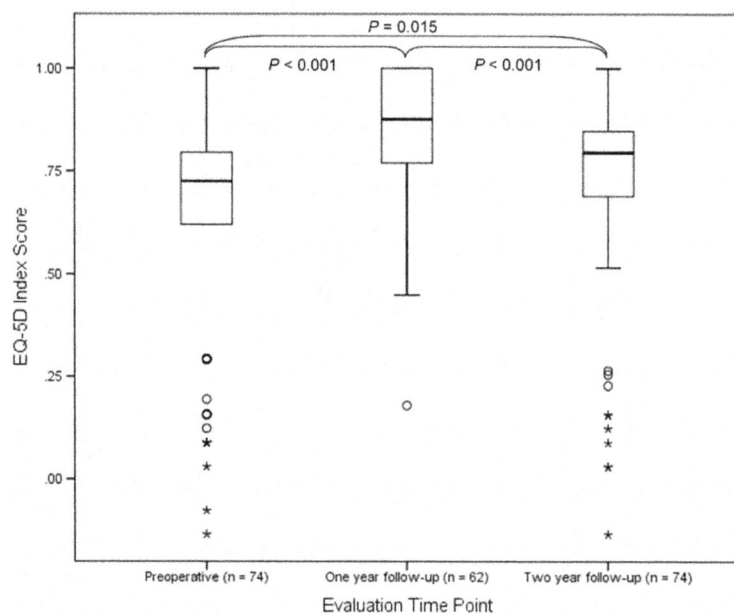

**Fig. 2** EuroQol-5 dimension (EQ-5D) questionnaire index scores, *boxes* represent inner quartile range (IQR) with median denoted by *horizontal line*, *inner fences* represent minimum and maximum values or 1.5 times IQR, *circles* outlier between 1.5 and 3 time IQR, *asterisks* far outlier greater than three times IQR. There was significant improvement in EQ-5D index scores from preoperative to 1- and 2-year follow-ups, with a significant decrease in index scores from 1- to 2-year follow-ups

**Table 2** EuroQol-5D-3L (EQ-5D) dimension and index scores for adult idiopathic scoliosis cohort at 2-year follow-up compared to untreated scoliosis patients and population matched scores. Percentage of participants reporting level of problem per dimension where level 1 indicates no problem, level 2 indicates some problems, and level 3 indicates extreme problems. UK Index reported as mean (SD)

| EQ-5D | | Number (%) of participants reporting level of problem | | | p* | p** |
|---|---|---|---|---|---|---|
| | | 2-year follow-up n = 74 | Untreated patients n = 75 | Matched normative n = 75 | | |
| Mobility | Level 1 | 64 (86%) | 69 (92%) | 72 (96%) | 0.28 | 0.04 |
| | Level 2 | 10 (14%) | 6 (8%) | 3 (4%) | | |
| | Level 3 | 0 | 0 | 0 | | |
| Self-care | Level 1 | 70 (96%) | 73 (97%) | 75 (100%) | 0.63 | 0.08 |
| | Level 2 | 3 (4%) | 2 (3%) | 0 | | |
| | Level 3 | 0 | 0 | 0 | | |
| Usual activities | Level 1 | 48 (66%) | 63 (84%) | 73 (97%) | 0.019 | <0.001 |
| | Level 2 | 22 (30%) | 12 (16%) | 2 (3%) | | |
| | Level 3 | 3 (4%) | 0 | 0 | | |
| Pain/discomfort | Level 1 | 23 (31%) | 22 (29%) | 52 (69%) | 0.003 | <0.001 |
| | Level 2 | 41 (55%) | 53 (71%) | 22 (29%) | | |
| | Level 3 | 10 (14%) | 0 | 1 (1%) | | |
| Anxiety/depression | Level 1 | 45 (61%) | 44 (59%) | 54 (72%) | 0.32 | 0.33 |
| | Level 2 | 27 (36%) | 31 (41%) | 19 (25%) | | |
| | Level 3 | 2 (3%) | 0 | 2 (3%) | | |
| EQ-5D index | | 0.72 (0.28) | 0.74 (0.25) | 0.88 (0.16) | 0.56 | <0.001 |

*p value for the comparison between surgically treated and untreated patients
**p value for the comparison between surgically treated patients and matched normative data

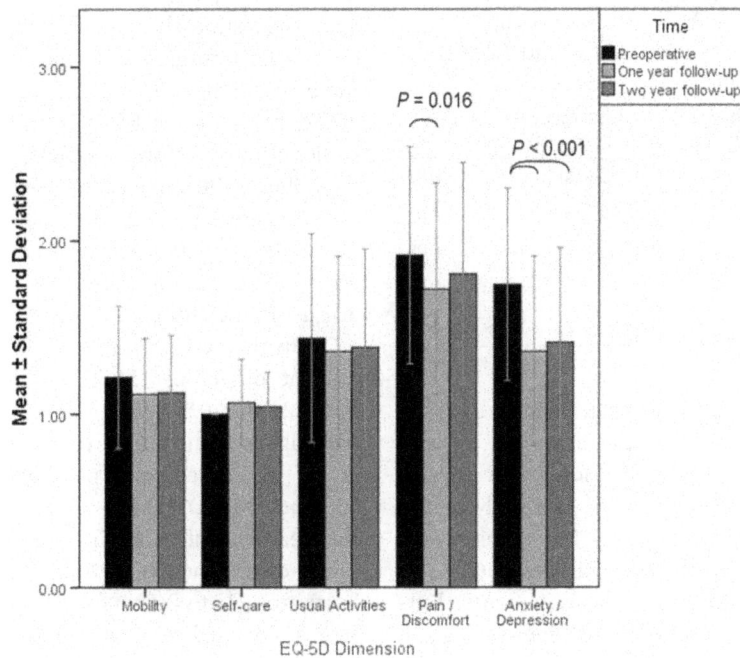

**Fig. 3** Preoperative and 1- and 2-year follow-up EQ-5D dimension scores, mean ± standard deviation. Significant difference found for pain/discomfort dimension between preoperative and 1-year follow-up and from preoperative to 1- and 2-year follow-ups for anxiety/depression dimension, significance levels indicated

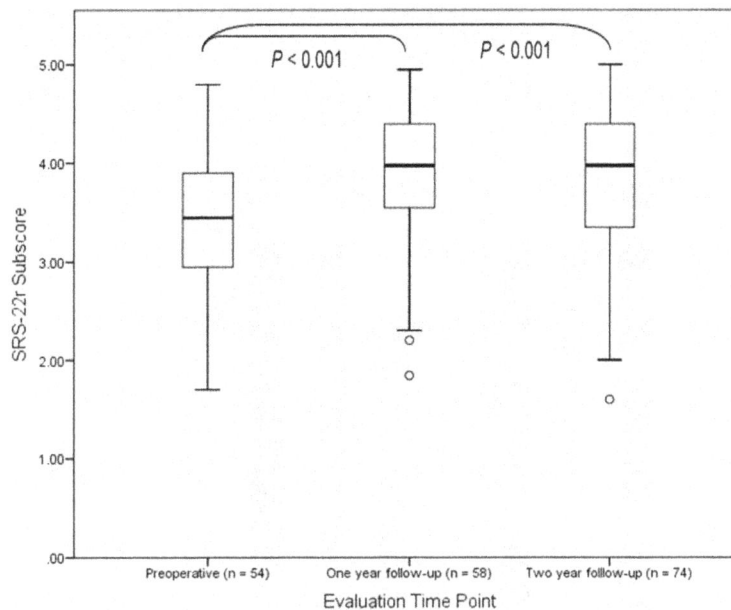

**Fig. 4** Scoliosis Research Society-22r (SRS-22r) questionnaire subscores, *boxes* represent inner quartile range (IQR) with median denoted by *horizontal line*, *inner fences* represent minimum and maximum values or 1.5 times IQR, *circles* outlier between 1.5 and 3 time IQR, *astersisks* far outlier greater than three times IQR. There was a significant increase in SRS-22r subscores from preoperative to 1- and 2-year follow-ups with no significant difference between follow-up scores

**Table 3** Scoliosis Research Society (SRS)-22r questionnaire domain and subscore at 2-year follow-up for adult idiopathic scoliosis participants 25 years or older compared to those under 25 years. Data shown as mean (SD)

| SRS-22r domain | At least 25 years old ($n = 21$) | Under 25 years old ($n = 54$) | $p$ |
|---|---|---|---|
| Function | 3.6 (0.8) | 4.3 (0.8) | 0.001 |
| Pain | 3.3 (1.2) | 4.0 (1.0) | 0.020 |
| Image | 3.5 (0.7) | 3.9 (0.9) | 0.052 |
| Mental health | 3.4 (0.9) | 3.9 (0.8) | 0.037 |
| SRS subscore | 3.4 (0.8) | 4.0 (0.7) | 0.006 |

$n$ number of participants

Even though the SRS-22r has been reported as the HRQOL outcome of choice in the surgically treated scoliosis population [26], the EQ-5D index is an important general HRQOL outcome measure, especially in discussion of cost utility. However, very few studies exist regarding EQ-5D results in the scoliosis population, especially adult surgically treated scoliosis patients. Burström et al. [16] suggested an EQ-5D index Swedish reference value of 0.89 for individuals 20–29 years old, comparable to this study's matched value and 1-year follow-up value (both 0.88) and higher than preoperative values (0.73). The suggested reference value is also higher than 2-year follow-up values reported in this study (0.80). In a surgically treated adolescent idiopathic scoliosis group, EQ-5D index values remained unchanged from 1- to 2-year follow-ups (0.82) [15].

Decreasing values were seen in the current study, possibly suggesting skeletal maturity at the time of surgery as a critical surgical consideration in regard to EQ-5D index outcomes. The behavior of specific dimensions and domains of the HRQOL tools highlight surgery as a positive intervention on critical aspects of quality of life including pain, anxiety, and image. Studies comparing non-operative to operative management of adult scoliosis suggests that surgical intervention is more effective on HRQOL outcomes and might be more cost-effective, at least in the short term [10, 23].

Of further consideration is the minimal clinical important difference (MCID). The median difference in SRS-22r was 0.5 from preoperative to 2-year follow-up and higher than the MCID (0.4) suggested by Crawford et al. [27], based on a population with a mean age of 53 years. MCID for EQ-5D has not been determined in the treatment of idiopathic scoliosis.

The discrepancy in the significant decline in the EQ-5D index from 1- to 2-year follow-ups while the SRS-22r subscores remained relatively similar might relate to reported poor concurrent validity between the two instruments found in the adolescent idiopathic scoliosis population [28].

The inclusion of the EQ-5D is a strength of this study as it expands the discussion of patient-reported HRQOL outcome measures applicable to the adult scoliosis population and introduces an index value. However, exclusion of the ODI, a commonly used HRQOL outcome measures in adult scoliosis research, and the

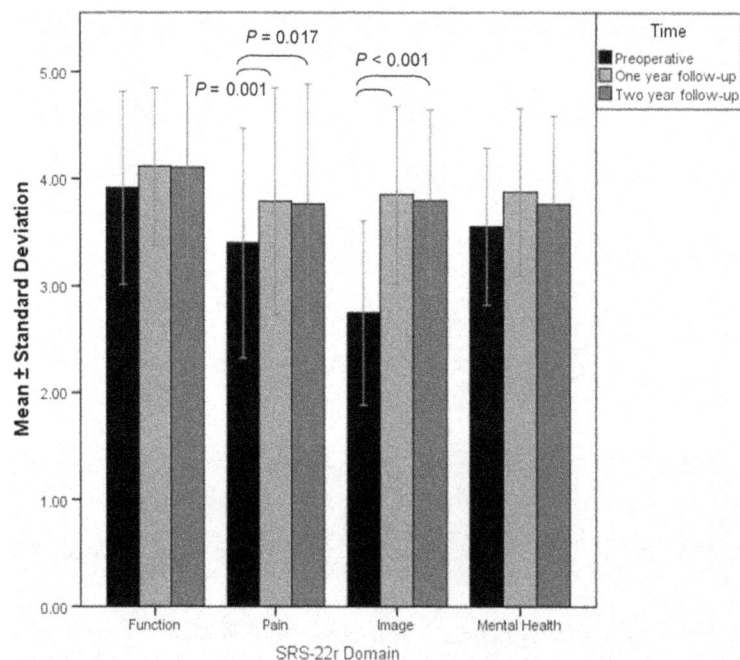

**Fig. 5** Preoperative and 1- and 2-year follow-up SRS-22r domain scores, mean ± standard deviation. Significant difference found for pain domain between preoperative and 1-year follow-up and image domain between preoperative and both 1- and 2-year follow-ups, significance levels indicated

**Table 4** SRS-22r domain scores and subscores shown as mean (SD) for surgically treated patients at 2-year follow-up, age-matched untreated individuals with less severe scoliosis, and age-matched individuals data from individuals without controls

| SRS-22r domain | 2-year follow-up (n = 74) | Untreated individuals with scoliosis (n = 75) | Individuals without scoliosis (n = 75) | p* | p** |
|---|---|---|---|---|---|
| Function | 4.1 (0.9) | 4.2 (0.8) | 4.7 (0.4) | 0.25 | <0.001 |
| Pain | 3.8 (1.1) | 3.9 (1.0) | 4.6 (0.6) | 0.61 | <0.001 |
| Image | 3.8 (0.9) | 3.7 (0.8) | 4.5 (0.5) | 0.71 | 0.001 |
| Mental health | 3.8 (0.8) | 3.7 (0.8) | 4.1 (0.8) | 0.45 | 0.018 |
| SRS subscore | 3.9 (0.8) | 3.9 (0.7) | 4.5 (0.5) | 0.91 | <0.001 |

*p value for the comparison between surgically treated and untreated patients
**p value for the comparison between surgically treated patients and matched normative data

availability of the SRS-22r scores only after 2008 are limitations of this study in the context of previous research.

Other limitations include the response rate and the comparably low age of the study group. The response rate is comparable to other studies using register data [29]. In the Norwegian spine register, non-respondents had similar outcome as respondents [30]. During the start of the deformity part of the SweSpine register, some clinics failed to handle pre- and postoperative questionnaires. However, non-response analyses indicated no substantial differences in baseline measures between participants and non-participants. We therefore do not believe the response rate indicate a selection bias.

The small subset of the cohort over age 25 years limited further analysis of the impact of age on HRQOL at the various time points; this small group could relate to Sweden's public health care system and school age screening resulting in surgical intervention for adolescent scoliosis. Another reason for the comparably low age in this study is that we specifically only included patients with idiopathic scoliosis with a juvenile or adolescent onset and treated as adults, and excluded adult degenerative spinal deformity. Whether treatment results in idiopathic and degenerative scoliosis differ may be an area of future studies. Nevertheless, the prospective, national register design of this study, meeting critical power calculations and reporting on the effect of surgery on two HRQOL outcome measures specifically in the adult surgically treated idiopathic scoliosis population at 2-year follow-up, represent strengths of this study and contribute to the literature in the discussion of evidence based treatment options.

## Conclusions

In conclusion, surgery has a positive effect on HRQOL outcomes, as reported by the EQ-5D index and SRS-22r subscore, at both 1- and 2-year follow-ups, potentially peaking at 1-year follow-up. The postoperative behavior of the different HRQOL outcome tools suggests the need for careful evaluation and interpretation both from a research and clinical perspective.

**Abbreviations**
EQ-5D: EuroQol-5 dimensions; HRQOL: Health-related quality of life; SRS-22r: Scoliosis Research Society-22r questionnaire; SweSpine: The Swedish Spine register

**Acknowledgements**
We would like to acknowledge all the surgeons, patients, and volunteers that have contributed with data to this study and Carina Blom at the Swespine registry for the assistance with data retrieval.

**Funding**
The study has received funds from the regional agreement on medical training and clinical research (ALF) between the Stockholm County Council and the Karolinska Institutet and the Karolinska Institutet research funds. The funding agencies had no involvement in the study design, collection of data, interpretation of data, writing of the report, or in the decision to submit the article for publication. The authors are independent from the funding agencies.

**Authors' contributions**
JT contributed to the study design, data analysis, and manuscript writing. AG, ED, PS, and AA were involved in the data collection and data analysis and commented on the manuscript. PG contributed to the study design, data collection, data analysis, manuscript writing, and financing. All authors read and approved the final manuscript.

**Competing interests**
The authors declare that they have no competing interests.

**Author details**
[1]Faculty of Health Science and Medicine, Bond Institute of Health and Sport, Bond University, 2 Promethean Way, Robina, Queensland 4226, Australia. [2]Department of Orthopaedics, Department of Clinical Science, Intervention and Technology (CLINTEC), Karolinska Institutet, Karolinska University Hospital, SE-141 86 Stockholm, Sweden. [3]Department of Orthopaedics, Sundsvall and Härnösand County Hospital, 85186 Sundsvall, Sweden. [4]Department of Physical Therapy, Karolinska University Hospital, SE-141 86 Stockholm, Sweden. [5]Division of Physiotherapy, Department of Neurobiology, Care Sciences and Society, Karolinska Institutet, SE-141 86 Stockholm, Sweden. [6]Department of Medical and Health Sciences, Division of Physiotherapy, Faculty of Health Sciences, Linköping University, SE-58183 Linköping, Sweden.

## References

1. Aebi M. The adult scoliosis. Eur Spine J. 2005;14(10):925–48.
2. Cobb J. Outline for the study of scoliosis. Instructional Course Lectures, The American Academy of Orthopaedic Surgeons (AAOS). Ann Arbor. 1948;5:261–75.
3. Berven S, Deviren V, Demir-Deviren S, Hu SS, Bradford DS. Studies in the modified Scoliosis Research Society Outcomes Instrument in adults: validation, reliability, and discriminatory capacity. Spine (Phila Pa 1976). 2003;28(18):2164–9. discussion 2169.
4. Baldus C, Bridwell KH, Harrast J, Edwards 2nd C, Glassman S, Horton W, Lenke LG, Lowe T, Mardjetko S, Ondra S, et al. Age-gender matched comparison of SRS instrument scores between adult deformity and normal adults: are all SRS domains disease specific? Spine (Phila Pa 1976). 2008; 33(20):2214–8.
5. Bago J, Climent JM, Perez-Grueso FJ, Pellise F. Outcome instruments to assess scoliosis surgery. Eur Spine J. 2013;22 Suppl 2:S195–202.
6. Smith JS, Lafage V, Shaffrey CI, Schwab F, Lafage R, Hostin R, O'Brien M, Boachie-Adjei O, Akbarnia BA, Mundis GM, et al. Outcomes of operative and nonoperative treatment for adult spinal deformity: a prospective, multicenter, propensity-matched cohort assessment with minimum 2-year follow-up. Neurosurgery. 2016;78(6):851–61.
7. Liu S, Diebo BG, Henry JK, Smith JS, Hostin R, Cunningham ME, Mundis G, Ames CP, Burton D, Bess S, et al. The benefit of nonoperative treatment for adult spinal deformity: identifying predictors for reaching a minimal clinically important difference. Spine J. 2016;16(2):210–8.
8. Everett CR, Patel RK. A systematic literature review of nonsurgical treatment in adult scoliosis. Spine (Phila Pa 1976). 2007;32(19 Suppl):S130–4.
9. Monticone M, Ambrosini E, Cazzaniga D, Rocca B, Motta L, Cerri C, Brayda-Bruno M, Lovi A. Adults with idiopathic scoliosis improve disability after motor and cognitive rehabilitation: results of a randomised controlled trial. Eur Spine J. 2016;25(10):3120–9.
10. Paulus MC, Kalantar SB, Radcliff K. Cost and value of spinal deformity surgery. Spine (Phila Pa 1976). 2014;39(5):388–93.
11. Liang CZ, Li FC, Li H, Tao Y, Zhou X, Chen QX. Surgery is an effective and reasonable treatment for degenerative scoliosis: a systematic review. J Int Med Res. 2012;40(2):399–405.
12. Yadla S, Maltenfort MG, Ratliff JK, Harrop JS. Adult scoliosis surgery outcomes: a systematic review. Neurosurg Focus. 2010;28(3):E3.
13. Theis J, Gerdhem P, Abbott A. Quality of life outcomes in surgically treated adult scoliosis patients: a systematic review. Eur Spine J. 2014;24(7):1343–55.
14. Yoshida G, Boissiere L, Larrieu D, Bourghli A, Vital JM, Gille O, Pointillart V, Challier V, Mariey R, Pellise F, et al. Advantages and disadvantages of adult spinal deformity surgery and its impact on health-related quality of life. Spine (Phila Pa 1976). 2016;42(6):411–9.
15. Ersberg A, Gerdhem P. Pre- and postoperative quality of life in patients treated for scoliosis. Acta Orthop. 2013;84(6):537–43.
16. Burstrom K, Johannesson M, Diderichsen F. Swedish population health-related quality of life results using the EQ-5D. Qual Life Res. 2001;10(7):621–35.
17. Danielsson AJ, Romberg K. Reliability and validity of the Swedish version of the Scoliosis Research Society-22 (SRS-22r) patient questionnaire for idiopathic scoliosis. Spine (Phila Pa 1976). 2013;38(21):1875–84.
18. Grauers A, Topalis C, Moller H, Normelli H, Karlsson M, Danielsson A, Gerdhem P. Prevalence of back problems in 1069 adults with idiopathic scoliosis and 158 adults without scoliosis. Spine (Phila Pa 1976). 2014; 39(11):886–92.
19. Diarbakerli E, Grauers A, Gerdhem P. Population-based normative data for the Scoliosis Research Society 22r questionnaire in adolescents and adults, including a comparison with EQ-5D. Eur Spine J. 2016 Epub Nov 11.
20. Lenke LG, Betz RR, Harms J, Bridwell KH, Clements DH, Lowe TG, Blanke K. Adolescent idiopathic scoliosis: a new classification to determine extent of spinal arthrodesis. J Bone Joint Surg Am. 2001;83-A(8):1169–81.
21. Faul F, Erdfelder E, Lang AG, Buchner A. G*Power 3: a flexible statistical power analysis program for the social, behavioral, and biomedical sciences. Behav Res Methods. 2007;39(2):175–91.
22. Cohen J. Statistical power analysis for the behavioral sciences. 2nd ed. Hoboken: Taylor and Francis; 2013.
23. Smith JS, Lafage V, Shaffrey CI, Schwab F, Lafage R, Hostin R, O'Brien M, Boachie-Adjei O, Akbarnia BA, Mundis GM, et al. Outcomes of operative and nonoperative treatment for adult spinal deformity: a prospective, multicenter, propensity-matched cohort assessment with minimum 2-year follow-up. Neurosurgery. 2015;78(6):851–61.
24. Glassman SD, Schwab F, Bridwell KH, Shaffrey C, Horton W, Hu S. Do 1-year outcomes predict 2-year outcomes for adult deformity surgery? Spine J. 2009;9(4):317–22.
25. Zimmerman RM, Mohamed AS, Skolasky RL, Robinson MD, Kebaish KM. Functional outcomes and complications after primary spinal surgery for scoliosis in adults aged forty years or older: a prospective study with minimum two-year follow-up. Spine (Phila Pa 1976). 2010;35(20):1861–6.
26. Bridwell KH, Berven S, Glassman S, Hamill C, Horton 3rd WC, Lenke LG, Schwab F, Baldus C, Shainline M. Is the SRS-22 instrument responsive to change in adult scoliosis patients having primary spinal deformity surgery? Spine (Phila Pa 1976). 2007;32(20):2220–5.
27. Crawford 3rd CH, Glassman SD, Bridwell KH, Berven SH, Carreon LY. The minimum clinically important difference in SRS-22R total score, appearance, activity and pain domains after surgical treatment of adult spinal deformity. Spine (Phila Pa 1976). 2015;40(6):377–81.
28. Adobor RD, Rimeslatten S, Keller A, Brox JI. Repeatability, reliability, and concurrent validity of the scoliosis research society-22 questionnaire and EuroQol in patients with adolescent idiopathic scoliosis. Spine (Phila Pa 1976). 2010;35(2):206–9.
29. Stromqvist B, Fritzell P, Hagg O, Jonsson B, Sanden B. Swespine: the Swedish spine register : the 2012 report. Eur Spine J. 2013;22(4):953–74.
30. Solberg TK, Sorlie A, Sjaavik K, Nygaard OP, Ingebrigtsen T. Would loss to follow-up bias the outcome evaluation of patients operated for degenerative disorders of the lumbar spine? Acta Orthop. 2011;82(1):56–63.

# 14

# Reproducibility of thoracic kyphosis measurements in patients with adolescent idiopathic scoliosis

Søren Ohrt-Nissen[1]* (iD), Jason Pui Yin Cheung[2], Dennis Winge Hallager[1], Martin Gehrchen[1], Kenny Kwan[2], Benny Dahl[1], Kenneth M. C. Cheung[2] and Dino Samartzis[2]*

## Abstract

**Background:** Current surgical treatment for adolescent idiopathic scoliosis (AIS) involves correction in both the coronal and sagittal plane, and thorough assessment of these parameters is essential for evaluation of surgical results. However, various definitions of thoracic kyphosis (TK) have been proposed, and the intra- and inter-rater reproducibility of these measures has not been determined. As such, the purpose of the current study was to determine the intra- and inter-rater reproducibility of several TK measurements used in the assessment of AIS.

**Methods:** Twenty patients (90% females) surgically treated for AIS with alternate-level pedicle screw fixation were included in the study. Three raters independently evaluated pre- and postoperative standing lateral plain radiographs. For each radiograph, several definitions of TK were measured as well as L1–S1 and nonfixed lumbar lordosis. All variables were measured twice 14 days apart, and a mixed effects model was used to determine the repeatability coefficient (RC), which is a measure of the agreement between repeated measurements. Also, the intra- and inter-rater intra-class correlation coefficient (ICC) was determined as a measure of reliability.

**Results:** Preoperative median Cobb angle was 58° (range 41°–86°), and median surgical curve correction was 68% (range 49–87%). Overall intra-rater RC was highest for T2–T12 and nonfixed TK (11°) and lowest for T4–T12 and T5–T12 (8°). Inter-rater RC was highest for T1–T12, T1-nonfixed, and nonfixed TK (13°) and lowest for T5–T12 (9°). Agreement varied substantially between pre- and postoperative radiographs. Inter-rater ICC was highest for T4–T12 (0.92; 95% CI 0. 88–0.95) and T5–T12 (0.92; 95% CI 0.88–0.95) and lowest for T1-nonfixed (0.80; 95% CI 0.72–0.88).

**Conclusions:** Considerable variation for all TK measurements was noted. Intra- and inter-rater reproducibility was best for T4–T12 and T5–T12. Future studies should consider adopting a relevant minimum difference as a limit for true change in TK.

**Keywords:** Adolescent idiopathic scoliosis, Thoracic, Kyphosis, Radiograph, Sagittal, Flexibility, Reproducibility, Reliability, Agreement, Intra-class correlation, Mixed effects model, Repeatability coefficient, Limits of agreement

## Background

Adolescent idiopathic scoliosis (AIS) is characterized by a lateral deviation of the spine in the coronal plane, vertebral rotation in the transverse plane, and often hypokyphosis in the sagittal plane [1, 2]. Current surgical treatment for AIS involves multisegmental pedicle screw

instrumentation, which results in considerable correction in the coronal plane with limited loss of correction over time [3, 4]. However, several studies have reported failure to restore the thoracic kyphosis (TK) to a normal range seen in non-scoliotic subjects, and in recent years, the importance of surgical correction of sagittal malalignment has gained increased focus [5, 6].

Although measuring TK in AIS patients on plain radiographs has become commonplace throughout the decades, considerable variation across studies in terms of defining TK exists and no consensus has been established on what

* Correspondence: ohrtnissen@gmail.com; dsamartzis@msn.com
[1]Spine Unit, Department of Orthopedic Surgery, Rigshospitalet, University of Copenhagen, Blegdamsvej 9, Copenhagen East 2100, Denmark
[2]Department of Orthopedics and Traumatology, The University of Hong Kong, Professorial Block, 5th Floor 102 Pokfulam Road, Hong Kong, SAR, China

should be regarded as an actual change in TK as opposed to expected measurement variation. For one, a recent meta-analysis evaluated the surgical correction of TK in AIS patients; however, the analysis included various studies with different definitions of TK, which made direct comparisons challenging [7]. Moreover, several studies have attempted to define the TK range in normal subjects but have used different definitions without addressing differences in measurement variation [8–10]. Furthermore, the Lenke classification [11] is widely used in preoperative planning; however, classification of the sagittal thoracic modifier has shown poor reliability and the measurement agreement for T2–T12 and T5–T12 kyphosis have been found to be reduced compared to the frontal Cobb angle [12, 13]. For T2–T5 regional kyphosis, reliability has been shown to be poor [13, 14] and other studies have shown that the upper part of the thoracic spine is inherently challenging to visualize due to structural overlap of the shoulder girdle [8, 15, 16]. As the clinical importance of the spinal sagittal profile becomes increasingly evident, there is a need to ensure that the measuring methods used to evaluate TK are both accurate and reproducible, especially since the rotational component of the curve may alter reproducibility depending on definitions of TK. Traditionally, TK is determined by a fixed limit Cobb technique (fixed TK, e.g., T4–T12); conversely, the definitions of fixed TK vary among studies [17–20]. A few authors have suggested applying a nonfixed approach where limits of TK are based on the individual sagittal shape of the spine as it has been shown that the cranial and caudal end vertebrae of the nonfixed TK vary among normal adolescents [8, 21–23].

Overall, the intra- and inter-rater reproducibility of these various TK measurements has not been established, and there is no consensus as to which measurements offer the least amount of variability. While a few studies have addressed the intra- and inter-rater correlation for certain TK measurements [24], it is of limited application on individual patients and it will be of great clinical and academic value to know the actual expected variation for repeated TK measurements on the same subject. As such, the objective of the following study was to determine intra- and inter-rater reproducibility of commonly used TK measurements.

## Methods

Plain radiographs of 20 patients who were at one point diagnosed with AIS and surgically treated at our institution with alternate-level pedicle screw fixation [25, 26] were examined. Institutional review board approval was obtained. Gender and patient age was recorded, and curve type was determined based on the Lenke classification [27]. On the coronal radiograph, pre- and postoperative main Cobb angle was measured and correction rate was calculated.

One spine research fellow (rater 1) and two spine surgeons (raters 2 and 3) independently evaluated 20 sets of pre- and postoperative standing lateral radiographs. For each radiograph, the following were determined (Fig. 1):

1. Fixed TK defined as the Cobb angle between the superior end plate and the inferior end plate of T1–T12, T2–T12, T4–T12, and T5–T12 [28]
2. T1-nonfixed TK: From the superior end plate of T1 to the inferior end plate of the most tilted vertebra in the thoracolumbar region [21, 22]
3. Nonfixed TK: From the superior end plate of the most tilted vertebra in the proximal thoracic region to the inferior end plate of the most tilted vertebra in the thoracolumbar region [8]
4. Fixed lumbar lordosis (LL): From the superior end plate of L1 to the superior end plate of S1 [29]
5. Nonfixed LL: From the superior end plate of the most tilted vertebra in the thoracolumbar region to the superior end plate of S1 [23]

Each rater independently performed all measurements twice 14 days apart. Before the second round of measurements, the sequence of the radiographs was randomly reassigned and the raters were blinded from the results of the first round. All raters were blinded to patient details. The total analysis produced 1920 data points for further analysis. All radiographs were measured on a high-resolution monitor using the Picture Archiving Communication system, and identification and labeling of individual vertebrae was based on the Radiographic Measurement Manual by the Spine Deformity Study Group [28]. Application of this manual was discussed among the raters, and consensus was established prior to the study. The protocol for the study was based on the Guidelines for Reporting Reliability and Agreement studies [30].

### Imaging details

For the scoliosis radiographs, all patients were positioned in erect position with the feet together and in the straightest posture possible. For lateral images, patients were in the clavicle position with flexed shoulders and elbows past 90° with hands pointing at the sternal notch to allow better spine visualization while preventing changes to the sagittal balance [31]. A computed detector was utilized to determine the position of the patient's skull and hip joints and also the length of the image required. The detector was 40 cm in length, and thus, image splitting was required. Up to 2–3 exposures were required depending on the patient's height. The postero-anterior radiographs were taken with 78-peak kilovoltage and 20 mAs of X-ray energy. The lateral radiographs were taken with 88-peak kilovoltage and

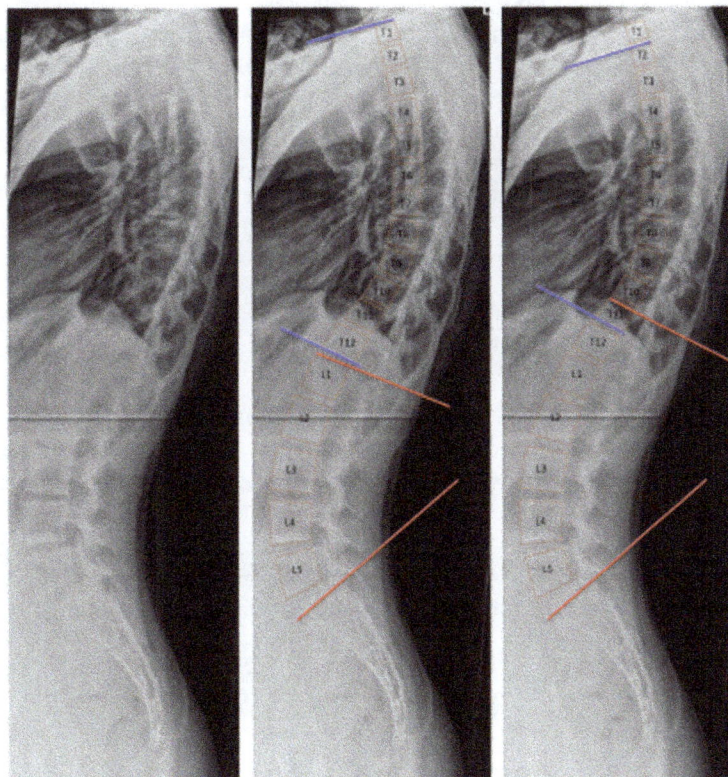

**Fig. 1** *Left*: Standing sagittal radiograph of a thoracic single curve with apex at T8. *Middle*: Fixed measurements of T1–T12 thoracic kyphosis (*blue*) and L1-S1 (*red*). *Right*: Nonfixed measurements of thoracic kyphosis (*blue*) and lumbar lordosis (*red*)

32 mAs of X-ray energy. For both images, the focus film distance was 180 cm.

## Statistical analysis

All statistical analyses were performed using R version 3.2.3 (R core team, 2014, Vienna, Austria). Data was reported as proportions (%), mean with standard deviation (SD), or median with range, and data distribution was assessed by histograms.

Reproducibility is a term that entails both measurement agreement and reliability. Intra- and inter-rater agreement is defined as the degree to which repeated measurements are identical whereas reliability is defined as the ability of a measurement to differentiate between subjects [30]. Intra- and inter-rater agreement per subject was estimated for each type of TK measurement using the repeatability coefficient (RC), which is the difference in measurements exceeded by only 5% of pairs of measurements on the same subject. Ninety-five percent limits of agreement were defined as ±RC, meaning that a high RC indicated a high variation (poor agreement) in repeated measurements.

Intra-rater agreement for each rater was calculated according to Bland and Altman [32]:

Single rater RC = 1.96 * SD of the difference between repeated measurements for each rater.

Overall, intra- and inter-rater RC was calculated using a linear mixed effects model with subjects and rater-within-subject variation as random effects and timing of radiograph (e.g., pre- or postoperative) as a fixed effect: [24]

Overall intra-rater RC = 2.77 * √(residual mean square)
Overall inter-rater RC = 2.77 * √(rater:subject mean square + residual mean square)

Inter-rater RC was further analyzed for pre- and postoperative radiographs separately.

Intra- and inter-rater reliability was estimated with intra-class correlation coefficient (ICC) with 95% confidence interval (CI). We considered an ICC of 0.0–0.24 to represent absent to poor, 0.25–0.49 low, 0.50–0.69 fair/moderate, 0.70–0.89 good, and 0.90–1.0 excellent reliability [33, 34].

## Results

Eighteen patients were female (90%), and the median age was 13.8 years (range 11.5–27.6 years). Eighty-five percent of curves were Lenke type 1 and 15% Lenke type

3, and the preoperative median coronal Cobb angle was 58° (range 41°–86°), which was corrected to a postoperative median Cobb angle of 20° (range 8°–27°) corresponding to a median curve correction of 68% (range 49–87%). Median number of fused levels was 9 (range 6–11 levels). The upper instrumented vertebra was T4, T5, T6, and T7 in one, 13, five, and one patient, respectively. Lowest instrumented vertebra (LIV) was T11, T12, L1, L2, and L3 in two, five, eight, three, and two patients, respectively. Summary of all measurements of both pre- and postoperative radiographs for each round is listed in Table 1 (Additional file 1).

### Intra- and inter-rater agreement
Single rater RC showed substantial differences among raters ranging from 5° to 13° (Table 2). Overall intra-rater RC was highest for T2–T12, T1-nonfixed, and nonfixed TK (11°) and lowest for T4–T12 and T5–T12 (8°). The overall inter-rater RC was highest for T1–T12, T1-nonfixed, and nonfixed TK (13°) and lowest for T5–T12

(9°) (Table 3). Inter-rater RC ranged between 7° and 14° across pre- and postoperative radiographs. For fixed LL and nonfixed LL, variation was similar to intra- and inter-rater RC ranging from 10° to 11° (Tables 2 and 3).

### Intra- and inter-rater reliability
Intra-rater ICC was highest for T4–T12 (0.94; 95% CI 0.92–0.96) and T5–T12 (0.94; 95% CI 0.91–0.96) and lowest for T2–T12 (0.84; 95% CI 0.79–0.85) (Fig. 2). Inter-rater ICC was highest for T4–T12 (0.92; 95% CI 0.88–0.95) and T5–T12 (0.92; 95% CI 0.88–0.95) and lowest for T1-nonfixed (0.80, 95% CI 0.72–0.88) (Fig. 3).

### Discussion
Our study noted a substantial measurement variation for all definitions of TK with the best reproducibility for T4–T12 and T5–T12 both in terms of intra- and inter-rater agreement as well as reliability. Only a few previous studies have addressed the variation of TK measurements in a systematic manner. For example, in a study by Ilharreborde

**Table 1** Summary of measurements for each rater for pre- and postoperative sagittal radiographs of both rounds of measurements

| Variable | Rater 1 Cobb angle, mean ± SD | | Rater 2 Cobb angle, mean ± SD | | Rater 3 Cobb angle, mean ± SD | |
|---|---|---|---|---|---|---|
| | Round 1 | Round 2 | Round 1 | Round 2 | Round 1 | Round 2 |
| T1–T12 | | | | | | |
| Preoperative | 29 ± 11 | 29 ± 11 | 30 ± 11 | 32 ± 10 | 34 ± 9 | 31 ± 10 |
| Postoperative | 26 ± 7 | 26 ± 8 | 30 ± 9 | 32 ± 8 | 31 ± 6 | 31 ± 7 |
| T2–T12 | | | | | | |
| Preoperative | 28 ± 12 | 28 ± 12 | 31 ± 13 | 30 ± 10 | 33 ± 14 | 28 ± 11 |
| Postoperative | 26 ± 8 | 26 ± 9 | 29 ± 8 | 31 ± 8 | 28 ± 6 | 28 ± 8 |
| T4–T12 | | | | | | |
| Preoperative | 24 ± 13 | 23 ± 12 | 26 ± 13 | 25 ± 12 | 29 ± 15 | 26 ± 13 |
| Postoperative | 19 ± 7 | 18 ± 6 | 21 ± 8 | 19 ± 7 | 21 ± 6 | 20 ± 6 |
| T5–T12 | | | | | | |
| Preoperative | 23 ± 12 | 21 ± 12 | 25 ± 12 | 23 ± 13 | 25 ± 14 | 24 ± 14 |
| Postoperative | 16 (6) | 16 ± 7 | 17 ± 7 | 16 ± 6 | 18 ± 6 | 18 ± 6 |
| T1-nonfixed | | | | | | |
| Preoperative | 30 ± 12 | 30 ± 11 | 30 ± 12 | 32 ± 10 | 35 ± 10 | 32 ± 11 |
| Postoperative | 27 ± 7 | 27 ± 8 | 31 ± 9 | 32 ± 7 | 32 ± 7 | 31 ± 7 |
| Nonfixed TK | | | | | | |
| Preoperative | 32 ± 11 | 31 ± 11 | 35 ± 12 | 35 ± 10 | 37 ± 11 | 34 ± 13 |
| Postoperative | 28 ± 8 | 28 ± 9 | 32 ± 10 | 34 ± 9 | 33 ± 7 | 32 ± 8 |
| L1–S1 | | | | | | |
| Preoperative | 58 ± 11 | 56 ± 10 | 55 ± 11 | 58 ± 12 | 55 ± 10 | 56 ± 10 |
| Postoperative | 55 ± 8 | 53 ± 9 | 51 ± 9 | 53 ± 9 | 49 ± 9 | 52 ± 8 |
| Nonfixed LL | | | | | | |
| Preoperative | 60 ± 11 | 60 ± 11 | 60 ± 12 | 62 ± 12 | 58 ± 12 | 59 ± 11 |
| Postoperative | 57 ± 9 | 55 ± 9 | 55 ± 9 | 57 ± 9 | 52 ± 9 | 54 ± 9 |

*SD* standard deviation, *TK* thoracic kyphosis, *LL* lumbar lordosis

**Table 2** Single rater RC for all three raters and overall intra-rater RC with pre- and postoperative subgroups

| Variable | Single rater RC, degrees | | | Intra-rater RC for all raters, degrees | | |
|---|---|---|---|---|---|---|
| | Rater 1 | Rater 2 | Rater 3 | Pre-OP | Post-OP | Overall |
| T1–T12 | 5 | 11 | 9 | 9 | 9 | 9 |
| T2–T12 | 6 | 12 | 13 | 12 | 9 | 11 |
| T4–T12 | 5 | 7 | 10 | 9 | 6 | 8 |
| T5–T12 | 5 | 7 | 10 | 10 | 5 | 8 |
| T1-nonfixed | 6 | 12 | 10 | 10 | 10 | 11 |
| Nonfixed TK | 6 | 12 | 13 | 12 | 10 | 11 |
| L1–S1 | 6 | 6 | 7 | 9 | 12 | 11 |
| Nonfixed LL | 6 | 9 | 14 | 9 | 11 | 10 |

RC reliability coefficient, TK thoracic kyphosis, LL lumbar lordosis

et al. [35], the authors found an intra-rater agreement of 6° and 4° for T1–T12 and T4–T12, respectively, and an inter-rater agreement of 7° and 6°, respectively. This study, however, utilized EOS-imaging, which is a slot-scanning device that may improve the agreement. Moreover, EOS is currently only available in selective centers. Similarly, Kuklo et al. [36] found that the intra-rater agreement for T2–T12 and T5–T12 was 5° and 6°, respectively. However, none of these studies addressed the issue of random effects, so these results are not directly comparable to the present study and likely to underestimate the overall variation seen between randomly chosen raters. Carman et al. [37] measuring nonfixed TK found 95% of the differences between raters to be within 7° and found a trend towards less variation with increased clarity on radiographs. The study also found that an 11° difference in TK was required to rule out measurement error with 95% confidence. Our results are in line with these findings showing that TK measurements have considerable intra- and inter-rater variation and a difference of 8° to 13° (depending on TK definition) may solely be produced by observer error alone.

In order to ensure clinical applicability of our results, our study included both pre- and postoperative radiographs.

**Table 3** Inter-rater RC between three raters with pre- and postoperative subgroups

| Variable | Inter-rater RC, degrees | | |
|---|---|---|---|
| | Pre-OP | Post-OP | Overall |
| T1–T12 | 11 | 14 | 13 |
| T2–T12 | 12 | 10 | 11 |
| T4–T12 | 12 | 7 | 10 |
| T5–T12 | 11 | 7 | 9 |
| T1-nonfixed | 12 | 14 | 13 |
| Nonfixed TK | 14 | 13 | 13 |
| L1–S1 | 9 | 12 | 11 |
| Nonfixed LL | 11 | 12 | 11 |

RC reliability coefficient, TK thoracic kyphosis, LL lumbar lordosis

Our analysis showed substantial differences in both intra- and inter-rater agreement between pre- and postoperative radiographs, showing markedly better agreement in postoperative radiographs for T4–T12 and T5–T12 (Tables 2 and 3). For the remaining TK measurements, analyses of pre- and postoperative subgroups were not conclusive but, generally, we found poorer or unchanged agreement. The reason for these changes may be that the variation seen in T4–12 and T5–T12 is mainly due to the lateral and rotational deformity of the curve which is surgically corrected whereas the variation seen in measurements including T1 and T2 is more likely due to structural overlap (e.g., of the humeral head) and therefore not affected by surgery. Interestingly, our analysis also showed considerable variation for the fixed and nonfixed LL, indicating that the sagittal radiograph, as a whole, is inherently difficult to analyze in a reproducible manner in AIS patients.

Our study focused on the overall TK because we found that a wide range of definitions exist in the literature. Establishing the respective reproducibility of these measurements was our main objective, but we would encourage future studies to include additional clinically important parameters, such as proximal TK (T2–T5) and thoracolumbar alignment (T10–L2) as well as several other clinically relevant measurements.

The ICC analysis showed good to excellent reliability for all measurements. However, while the ICC analysis is frequently reported in studies of this type, it holds limited practical value when assessing potential variation of individual measurements per subject, as it is a measure of the reliability for the measurement to differentiate between subjects. By applying a mixed effects model to our data, the observed variance is split into both the variability between the raters within subjects (inter-rater variation) and a residual error term (representing intra-rater variation). Ultimately, an RC is generated which represents the upper and lower 95% limits of agreement for an individual measurement. By using the rater as random effects, our results represent conservative estimates

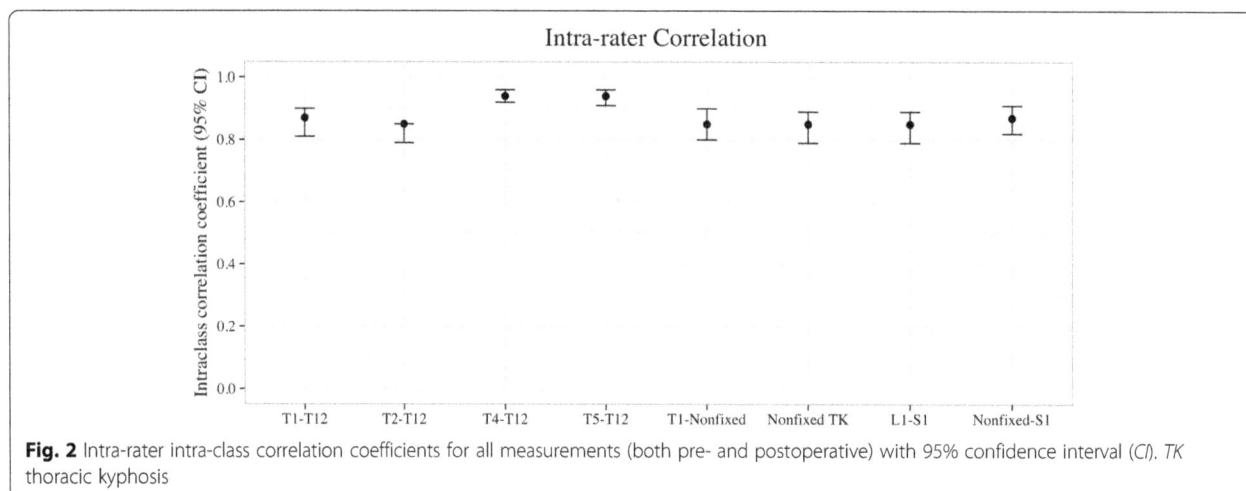

**Fig. 2** Intra-rater intra-class correlation coefficients for all measurements (both pre- and postoperative) with 95% confidence interval (*CI*). *TK* thoracic kyphosis

and we hypothesize that measurement variation found in our study would also apply for other raters.

Our results are limited by a substantial variation in single rater RC among raters, which was lowest for T4–T12 and highest for T2–T12 (Table 2). Several steps were taken before the initiation of the study to minimize bias in terms of discrepancies in labeling vertebra, handling of odd number of ribs, or definitions using the nonfixed approach. Rater 1 had more than 3 years of experience in evaluating radiographs from AIS patients, and raters 2 and 3 had 8 and 10 years of experience, respectively. It should be noted that all raters routinely use mainly T5–T12 or T2–12 when evaluating patients with AIS although rater 1 also uses the nonfixed approach on a regular basis. As such, we believe that our results reflect the expected variation between clinicians. In addition, our patient sample did not include lumbar curves, so we cannot infer that our results may be readily applied to this group. Also, the sample size in our study did not allow for analyzing individual curve types, but variation may be greater for

thoracic curves since TK has been found to depend on curve type [38]. Nonetheless, we hope that our study can form the foundation whereby future studies can further elaborate upon different curve types.

Our results may guide clinicians and researchers in the evaluation of the sagittal profile following surgery in defining the limits of actual improvement of worsening of TK as opposed to expected measurement variation. Applying such variation in clinical definitions of progression has previously been described in guidelines for evaluation of radiographic results of brace treatment [37, 39, 40]. Our results indicate that T4–T12 and T5–T12 offer the least amount of observer variation, and while measuring nonfixed TK may offer a more individualized assessment of the spine, we found considerable measurement variation using this approach that may limit the clinical applicability. It is outside the scope of this paper to determine how these various measurements correlate with clinical outcomes; however, we recommend that future studies specifically state the applied definition

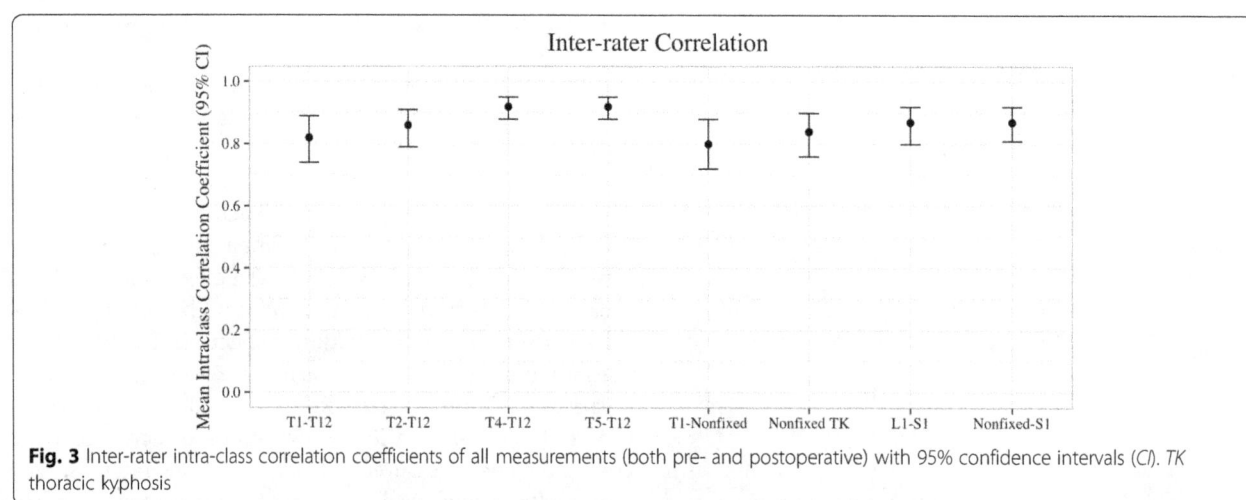

**Fig. 3** Inter-rater intra-class correlation coefficients of all measurements (both pre- and postoperative) with 95% confidence intervals (*CI*). *TK* thoracic kyphosis

of TK and also adequately address measurement variation when evaluating treatment results. This will further help with standardization of measurements between studies for comparative purposes.

## Conclusions

Our study addresses the intra- and inter-rater reproducibility of TK measurements in AIS patients, and we noted a considerable variation for all TK measurements. Both intra- and inter-rater reproducibility were best for T4–T12 and T5–12. Future studies should consider adopting a relevant minimum difference (depending on TK definition) as a limit for indication of true change in TK within a patient. As such, our findings have implications in the decision-making of the spine specialist.

## Abbreviations

AIS: Adolescent idiopathic scoliosis; CI: Confidence interval; ICC: Intra-class correlation coefficient; LL: Lumbar lordosis; RC: Reliability coefficient; SD: Standard deviation; TK: Thoracic kyphosis

## Acknowledgements

There are no further individuals or entities we wish to acknowledge that have played a role in the development and completion of our work.

## Funding

SO was supported by a grant from the Lundbeck foundation
The following grants were received outside the submitted work:
SO: Research grant from K2M
DWH: Research grant from Globus Medical
MG: Grant from Globus Medical, K2M, and Medtronic
BD: Grant from Globus Medical, K2M, and Medtronic

## Authors' contributions

SO, DS, DH, and JC participated in the conception and design of the study. SO, JC, and KK made radiographic measurements. SO and DH analyzed the data. SO, DS, DH, JC, and KK wrote the manuscript, and BD, MG, and KC made critical revisions. DS supervised the study and provided administrative support. All authors have read and approved the final manuscript.

## Competing interests

The authors declare that they have no competing interests.

## Disclosures

Søren Ohrt-Nissen was supported by a grant from the Lundbeck foundation and a research fellowship from K2M.

## References

1. Perdriolle R, Vidal J. Morphology of scoliosis: three-dimensional evolution. Orthopedics. 1987;10:909–15.
2. Fletcher ND, Jeffrey H, Anna M, et al. Residual thoracic hypokyphosis after posterior spinal fusion and instrumentation in adolescent idiopathic scoliosis. Spine (Phila Pa 1976). 2012;37:200–6.
3. Hwang SW, Samdani AF, Marks M, et al. Five-year clinical and radiographic outcomes using pedicle screw only constructs in the treatment of adolescent idiopathic scoliosis. Eur Spine J. 2013;22:1292–9.
4. Lykissas MG, Jain VV, Nathan ST, et al. Mid- to long-term outcomes in adolescent idiopathic scoliosis after instrumented posterior spinal fusion: a meta-analysis. Spine (Phila Pa 1976). 2013;38:E113–9.
5. Hwang S, Samdani A, Tantorski M, et al. Cervical sagittal plane decompensation after surgery for adolescent idiopathic scoliosis: an effect imparted by postoperative thoracic hypokyphosis. J Neurosurg Spine. 2011; 15:491–6.
6. Ilharreborde B, Morel E, Mazda K, et al. Adjacent segment disease after instrumented fusion for idiopathic scoliosis: review of current trends and controversies. J Spinal Disord Tech. 2009;22:530–9.
7. Cao Y, Xiong W, Li F. Pedicle screw versus hybrid construct instrumentation in adolescent idiopathic scoliosis: meta-analysis of thoracic kyphosis. Spine (Phila Pa 1976). 2014;39:E800–10.
8. Boseker EH, Moe JH, Winter RB, et al. Determination of "normal" thoracic kyphosis: a roentgenographic study of 121 "normal" children. J Pediatr Orthop. 2000;20:796–8.
9. Propst-Proctor SL, Bleck EE. Radiographic determination of lordosis and kyphosis in normal and scoliotic children. J Pediatr Orthop. 1983;3:344–6.
10. Gelb DE, Lenke LG, Bridwell KH, et al. An analysis of sagittal spinal alignment in 100 asymptomatic middle and older aged volunteers. Spine (Phila Pa 1976). 1995;20:1351–8.
11. Rose PS, Lenke LG. Classification of Operative Adolescent Idiopathic Scoliosis: Treatment Guidelines. Orthop Clin North Am. 2007;38:521-9.
12. Dang NR, Moreau MJ, Hill DL, et al. Intra-observer reproducibility and interobserver reliability of the radiographic parameters in the Spinal Deformity Study Group's AIS Radiographic Measurement Manual. Spine (Phila Pa 1976). 2005;30:1064–9.
13. Kuklo T, Potter B, Polly D et al. Reliability analysis for manual adolescent idiopathic scoliosis measurements. Spine (Phila Pa 1976). 2005;30:444–54.
14. Wu W, Liang J, Du Y, et al. Reliability and reproducibility analysis of the Cobb angle and assessing sagittal plane by computer-assisted and manual measurement tools. BMC Musculoskelet Disord. 2014;15:33.
15. Basques BA, Long WD, Golinvaux NS, et al. Poor visualization limits diagnosis of proximal junctional kyphosis in adolescent idiopathic scoliosis. Spine J. 2015. Epub ahead of print.
16. Cheung J, Wever DJ, Veldhuizen AG, et al. The reliability of quantitative analysis on digital images of the scoliotic spine. Eur Spine J. 2002;11:535–42.
17. Harrison DE, Cailliet R, Harrison DD, et al. Reliability of centroid, Cobb, and Harrison posterior tangent methods: which to choose for analysis of thoracic kyphosis. Spine (Phila Pa 1976). 2001;26:E227–34.
18. Crawford AH, Lykissas MG, Gao X, et al. All-pedicle screw versus hybrid instrumentation in adolescent idiopathic scoliosis surgery: a comparative radiographical study with a minimum 2-year follow-up. Spine (Phila Pa 1976). 2013;38:1199–208.
19. Yu C-H, Chen P-Q, Ma S-C, et al. Segmental correction of adolescent idiopathic scoliosis by all-screw fixation method in adolescents and young adults. Minimum 5 years follow-up with SF-36 questionnaire. Scoliosis. 2012;7:5.
20. Kadoury S, Cheriet F, Labelle H. Prediction of the T2-T12 kyphosis in adolescent idiopathic scoliosis using a multivariate regression model. Stud Health Technol Inform. 2008;140:269–72.
21. Voutsinas SA, MacEwen GD. Sagittal profiles of the spine. Clin Orthop Relat Res. 1986;210:235–42.
22. Mac-Thiong J-M, Pinel-Giroux F-M, de Guise JA, et al. Comparison between constrained and non-constrained Cobb techniques for the assessment of thoracic kyphosis and lumbar lordosis. Eur Spine J. 2007;16:1325–31.
23. Vaz G, Roussouly P, Berthonnaud E, et al. Sagittal morphology and equilibrium of pelvis and spine. Eur Spine J. 2002;11:80–7.
24. Dimar J, Carreon L, Labelle H, et al. Intra- and inter-observer reliability of determining radiographic sagittal parameters of the spine and pelvis using a manual and a computer-assisted methods. Eur Spine J. 2008;17:1373–9.

25. Cheung KMC, Frcs M, Fhkam F, et al. Predictability of the fulcrum bending radiograph in scoliosis correction with alternate-level pedicle screw fixation. J Bone Joint Surg Am. 2010;92:169–76.

26. Samartzis D, Leung Y, Shigematsu H, et al. Selection of fusion levels using the fulcrum bending radiograph for the management of adolescent idiopathic scoliosis patients with alternate level pedicle screw strategy: clinical decision-making and outcomes. PLoS One. 2015;10:e0120302.

27. Lenke LG, Betz RR, Harms J, et al. Adolescent idiopathic scoliosis: a new classification to determine extent of spinal arthrodesis. J Bone Joint Surg Am. 2001;83:1169–81.

28. O'Brien M, Kuklo T, Blanke T et al. Radiographic measurement manual. Spine Deformity Study Group. Minnesota: Medtronic Sofamor Danek USA Inc.; 2008.

29. Schwab F, Ungar B, Blondel B, et al. Scoliosis Research Society—Schwab adult spinal deformity classification. Spine (Phila Pa 1976). 2012;37:1077–82.

30. Kottner J, Audige L, Brorson S, et al. Guidelines for reporting reliability and agreement studies (GRRAS) were proposed. Int J Nurs Stud. 2011;48:661–71.

31. Horton WC, Brown CW, Bridwell KH, et al. Is there an optimal patient stance for obtaining a lateral 36″ radiograph? A critical comparison of three techniques. Spine (Phila Pa 1976). 2005;30:427–33.

32. Bland JM, Altman DG. Measuring agreement in method comparison studies. Stat Methods Med Res. 1999;8:135–60.

33. Munro B. Statistical methods for health care research. 3rd ed. Philadelphia: Lippincott-Raven; 1997. p. 224–45.

34. Kuklo TR, Potter BK, O'Brien MF, et al. Reliability analysis for digital adolescent idiopathic scoliosis measurements. J Spinal Disord Tech. 2005;18:152–9.

35. Ilharreborde B, Steffen JS, Nectoux E, et al. Angle measurement reproducibility using EOS three-dimensional reconstructions in adolescent idiopathic scoliosis treated by posterior instrumentation. Spine (Phila Pa 1976). 2011;36:E1306–13.

36. Kuklo TR, Potter BK, Schroeder TM, et al. Comparison of manual and digital measurements in adolescent idiopathic scoliosis. Spine (Phila Pa 1976). 2006;31:1240–6.

37. Carman DL, Browne RH, Birch JG. Measurement of scoliosis and kyphosis radiographs. Intraobserver and interobserver variation. J Bone Joint Surg Am. 1990;72:328–33.

38. Charlebois M, Mac-Thiong J-M, Huot M-P, et al. Relation between the pelvis and the sagittal profile in adolescent idiopathic scoliosis: the influence of curve type. Stud Health Technol Inform. 2002;91:140–3.

39. Richards BS, Bernstein RM, D'Amato CR, et al. Standardization of criteria for adolescent idiopathic scoliosis brace studies: SRS committee on bracing and nonoperative management. Spine (Phila Pa 1976). 2005;30:2068–75. discussion 2076–7.

40. Negrini S, Hresko TM, O'Brien JP, et al. Recommendations for research studies on treatment of idiopathic scoliosis: consensus 2014 between SOSORT and SRS non-operative management committee. Scoliosis. 2015;10:1–12.

# 15

# Analysis of instrumentation failures after three column osteotomies of the spine

Niranjan Kavadi[1], Richard A. Tallarico[1] and William F. Lavelle[1,2]*

## Abstract

**Background:** Correction of fixed spinal imbalance in a sagittal and/or coronal plane frequently needs a tricolumnar wedge resection when the deformity is rigid. Complications associated with deformity correction surgery are pseudoarthrosis and implant failure located along the construct. The purposes of this study were to assess comparative rates of pseudoarthrosis (implant failure) at weaker points along lumbosacral junction and level of osteotomy, estimate overall incidence of implant failure, and comparatively analyze failures at different points along the construct.

**Methods:** This was an IRB approved, single center study retrospective analysis. Twenty-six patients who underwent three column osteotomies were grouped according to procedure: pedicle subtraction osteotomy (PSO, ($n = 18$)); vertebral column resection (VCR, ($n = 4$)); hemivertebra excision (HE, ($n = 2$)); and extracavitary corpectomy (EC, ($n = 2$)). Follow-up data is presented on all of the study patients. Number of levels of fusion, anchors, percent saturation of fixation levels, type of bone graft and graft substitutes, and rod material and diameter were recorded. Radiographical data was reviewed preoperatively and postoperatively at 2 weeks and 3, 6, and 12 months and annually to determine sagittal and coronal balance, lumbopelvic parameters, presence or absence of interbody structural support, laterality or rod failure, and time to implant failure.

**Results:** Twenty-seven percent (7/26) patients demonstrated rod breakage either unilaterally ($N = 2$) or bilaterally ($N = 5$) during follow-up. Seventy-one percent had increasing back pain or worsening sagittal balance, while remaining failures found incidentally. No failures in children were seen.

**Conclusion:** Tricolumnar osteotomy by posterior approach is a valuable tool. Rod failures found approximately 1 year from surgery, with 86% located at level of osteotomy and 14% at lumbosacral junction. Possible reasons are increased stress in the rod at this point and relatively deficient bone stock secondary to wide laminectomy. The low rate of rod breakage at lumbosacral junction may be related to adoption of structural interbody graft and stronger iliac screws. Additional biomechanical studies needed to assess the importance of these factors. This was a level IV study.

**Keywords:** Spinal deformity, Fixed sagittal imbalance, Tricolumnar osteotomy, Pseudoarthrosis, Implant rod failure, Lumbosacral junction

## Background

Fixed sagittal imbalance can be defined as a syndrome in which the patient is unable to stand erect without flexing knees and hips [1]. With advancing age, progressive degenerative changes in the disc lead to gradual loss of lumbar lordosis. Over time distal lumbar segments and the lumbosacral junction fail to compensate for positive sagittal balance. Pelvic alignment changes with worsening posture finally lead to fixed changes in spinopelvic

parameters: lumbar lordosis, pelvic tilt, sacral slope, and sagittal vertical axis. Fixed sagittal imbalance with alteration in these spinopelvic parameters relates to increased energy expenditure resulting in declining quality of life [2, 3]. Hence, correction of these parameters while treating sagittal imbalance is critical.

Optimal sagittal balance can be achieved surgically with utilization of different types of osteotomies. Two broad groups are as follows: osteotomies involving only the posterior column of the spine and tricolumnar osteotomies achieving correction through all three columns of the spine. The Smith-Petersen [4–6] osteotomy involves resection of

* Correspondence: lavellew@upstate.edu
[1]Department of Orthopedic Surgery, SUNY Upstate Medical University, 750 E. Adams Street, Syracuse, NY 13210, USA
[2]6620 Fly Road, Suite 200, East Syracuse, NY 13057, USA

only posterior elements in a spinal segment with an intact mobile disc leading to shortening of posterior column and lengthening of the anterior column of the spine. Pedicle subtraction osteotomy (PSO) [7–10] entails removal of a tricolumnar wedge when more significant correction is required. Shortening of the posterior column is achieved without lengthening the anterior column with no risk to the anterior soft tissues. PSO outcomes to correct fixed sagittal malalignment have been well documented in literature [11]. Vertebral column resection (VCR) [12–15] involves complete resection of one or more vertebral segments and is applied for correction of moderate to severe spinal deformities, including large rigid curves and fixed trunk translation.

Successful outcomes of deformity correction require maintenance of the optimal sagittal and coronal balance over time. High rates of pseudoarthrosis have been reported secondary, due to a large number of segments fused [16, 17]. Implant failures are commonly located at weak points along the construct, the lumbosacral junction, and the area of previous laminectomies. Different strategies have utilized L5–S1 interbody graft and iliac screws to support weak S1 screws and have significantly reduced the rates of pseudoarthrosis at the lumbosacral junction [18, 19]. The purposes of this study were to assess the comparative rates of pseudoarthrosis at the weaker points along the construct, the lumbosacral junction, and the level of osteotomy; estimate overall incidence of implant failure in long fusions for spine deformity; and comparatively analyze failures at different points along the construct.

## Methods

After Institutional Review Board (IRB) approval, a single center, retrospective analysis from the spine patient database was undertaken to identify patients who underwent surgical spinal deformity correction. Twenty-six patients were identified who had undergone tricolumnar wedge resection for correction of fixed spinal imbalance. All patients were managed by three surgeons from 2008 to 2011. Demographic data was recorded. Radiographs were made prospectively and reviewed retrospectively. Postoperative follow-up ranged from 12 to 54 months (mean 30 months).

The study population consisted of 26 patients (19 adults (12 female, 7 male; mean age 61.3 years (range 37 to 76 years)) and 7 pediatric patients). In the adult population, 16 were diagnosed with idiopathic scoliosis with flat back with or without previous spine surgery, one presented with de novo scoliosis with coronal imbalance, one diagnosed with charcot spine, and one with secondary thoracolumbar kyphosis related to a T12 burst fracture. Diagnoses for pediatric patients included congenital or early onset scoliosis in four and neuromuscular scoliosis in three patients.

Surgical data was collected from review of operative notes and intraoperative radiographs. Patients included in the study were grouped according to type of tricolumnar resection procedure: pedicle subtraction osteotomy (PSO, $n = 18$); vertebral column resection (VCR, $n = 4$); hemivertebra excision (HE, $n = 2$); or extracavitary corpectomy (EC, $n = 2$). The surgical technique common to all procedures included subperiosteal dissection of the spine at desired levels followed by securing fixation points proximal and distal to the planned level of osteotomy. Wide laminectomy was carried out at the level of osteotomy to allow inspection of the dura and neural elements and to avoid dural impingement when corrective forces were applied. Laminectomy was extended from a level of pedicles of the vertebra above to a level of pedicles of the vertebra below the level of resection. PSO was performed in patients with scoliosis and kyphoscoliosis with rigid structural curves in accordance with the technique described by Bridwell et al. [1]. Four patients demonstrating severe structural curves with higher than expected angle of correction or with truncal translation needed a VCR procedure performed utilizing a technique described by Suk et al. [12]. Holte et al. [20] described an effective procedure for correction of a congenital scoliotic curve resulting from asymmetric growth of the spine due to a hemivertebra which was utilized for correction in two children with segmented hemivertebrae. Two patients underwent corpectomy by an extracavitary approach in the thoracic region.

The vertebral level undergoing osteotomy and number of levels resected was noted for each patient. The number of levels included in the fusion, anchors used at most proximal and distal points of fixation, and percent saturation of fixation levels were recorded. Also, type of bone graft, bone graft substitutes, and use of bone morphogenic protein (BMP) were documented. Implant characteristics, specifically rod material and diameter, were noted whenever available.

Long cassette standing anteroposterior and lateral radiographs were made preoperatively and postoperatively at 2 weeks and 3, 6, and 12 months and annually thereafter. Radiographs were analyzed to determine anchor type used at most proximal and distal points of fixation, percent saturation of fixation levels and level of the osteotomy, C7 sagittal plumb line [21] (measured from center of C7 body to the posterosuperior corner of S1 body), and coronal plumb line (measured from center of C7 body to center of S1 body on an anteroposterior radiograph). Presence or absence of interbody structural graft at the lumbosacral junction was noted. Implant related to findings of screw loosening and/or fracture of the rod if the present level and laterality of the rod failure were recorded. A note was made if pseudoarthrosis was obvious on plain radiographs.

## Statistical methods

Failures were classified according to location either at osteotomy site or at a remote site. Continuous data was compared by paired $t$ test. Chi-square analysis was used to compare demographic data of patients who had a failure of the hardware. Potential risk factors were also analyzed. $P$ values <0.05 were considered significant.

## Results

The predominant type of corrective osteotomy in the adult population was PSO (18/19). The mean number of levels fused was 11.2 (range 2 to 16). Fusion was extended to the pelvis to include the lumbosacral junction in 17 adult patients, while L5 was the last instrumented vertebra in two adult patients due to healthy L5–S1 disc with minimal signs of degeneration. Iliac screws [22] were used in 16 adult patients to protect S1 screws in the relatively weak cancellous bone of the sacrum. Structural interbody graft was used in eight of the 17 patients with extension across lumbosacral junction. Transverse process hooks were used in eight patients as proximal most points of fixation, while pedicle screws were used in 18 patients supported by sublaminar wires in one patient with severely osteoporotic bone. A titanium rod was used to achieve and maintain correction in all adults. A stainless steel rod was utilized to hold correction in two children for better maintenance of correction due to the higher stiffness of the metal. Twenty-five patients had bilateral pedicle screws as fixation anchors two levels above and below the level of osteotomy. One patient with PSO at L3 level had only one screw at the adjacent L4 level as the other screw was removed due to fracture of the pedicle in osteoporotic bone during a compression maneuver. Autogenous bone graft obtained locally and from the iliac crest mixed with crushed cancellous allograft was used in all adults, and BMP was also utilized in seven adults who were either smokers or demonstrated pseudoarthrosis from previous surgery.

The level of the osteotomy was chosen based on a number of factors. The osteotomy was preferably done caudad to the level of conus medullaris wherever possible and at previously fused segments. Angular correction resulting from resection at one level was adequate for 22 patients, two patients needed more extensive osteotomy at two adjacent levels due to severe deformity, one patient needed unilateral decancellation of one adjacent segment in addition to the level of osteotomy to achieve coronal plane correction, and one patient underwent bone-disc-bone type of osteotomy to achieve optimal balance. Table 1 depicts the frequency of levels of osteotomy.

Thirty-seven percent of adults (7/19), i.e., 27% of patients overall (7/26 patients) demonstrated rod breakage either unilaterally or bilaterally during the follow-up. One failure (4%) was at the lumbosacral junction and six (23%)

**Table 1** Frequency of levels of osteotomy

| Level of osteotomy | Number of patients |
| --- | --- |
| T8 | 1 |
| T9 | 1 |
| T10 | 1 |
| T12 | 1 |
| L1 | 3 |
| L2 | 10 |
| L3 | 3 |
| L4 | 2 |
| L5 | 2 |
| L2 and L3 | 2 |

occurred at the osteotomy level having accompanying same level previous laminectomy ($P = 0.014$) (Figs. 1, 2, and 3). A broken rod was noted at the L2 level in three patients, L4 in two patients, and L3 in one patient (Table 2).

Failure of both rods was evident in five patients while two patients demonstrated a unilateral broken rod. A titanium rod was used in all patients with rod failures.

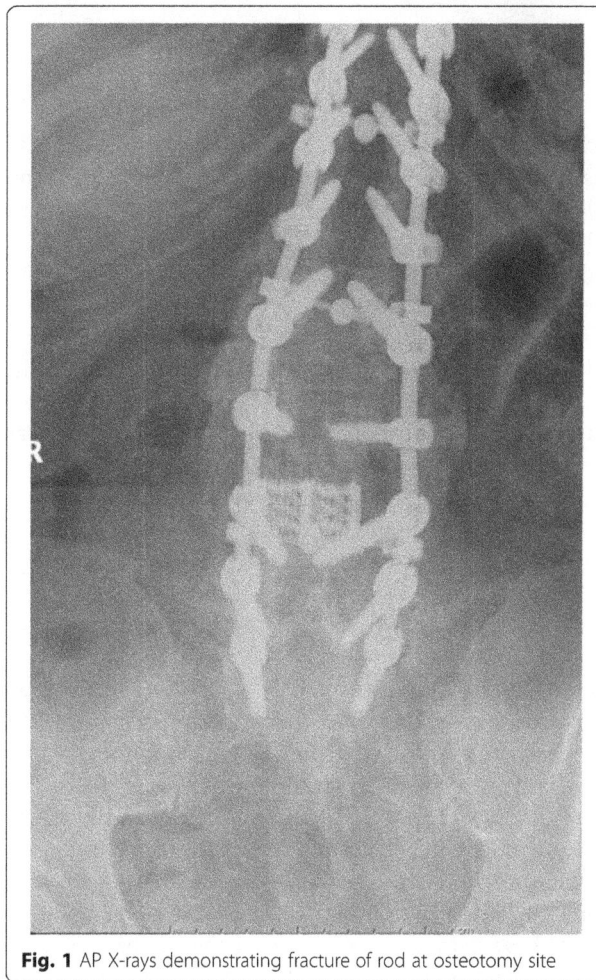

**Fig. 1** AP X-rays demonstrating fracture of rod at osteotomy site

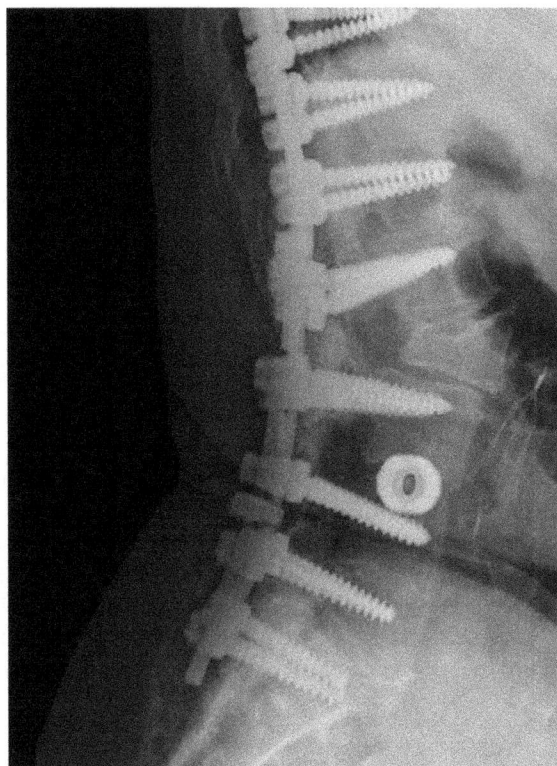

**Fig. 2** Lateral X-rays demonstrating fracture of rod at osteotomy site

Failure of the formation of bony trabeculae resulting in pseudoarthrosis was evident at the respective levels on plain radiographs. All patients who demonstrated implant failure at the level of osteotomy were between 6 and 12 months post surgery. Symptomatic rod failure occurred at 24 months in a patient with L5–S1 failure. There were no failures in patients with thoracic location of wedge resection and no failures in pediatric patients. Junctional kyphosis was apparent on follow-up radiographs in seven patients while only one patient was symptomatic with increased upper back pain. None developed any neurological symptoms as a result of worsening angulation due to a failure. This radiographic finding whenever evident was noted during midterm follow-ups frequently between 3 and 6 months after corrective surgery. Three patients with radiographic evidence of rod failure were symptomatic with increasing back pain, two experienced a steady decline in function due to worsening standing balance and back pain, and two with rod failure were completely asymptomatic. All symptomatic patients chose to have revision of failed implant addressed with exploration of pseudoarthrosis, replacement of the broken rod, and autogeneous iliac crest bone graft. BMP was used in three patients with revision after reviewing the benefits and possible adverse effects with these patients. A CT scan of the lumbar spine or flexion/extension views demonstrated solid arthrodesis

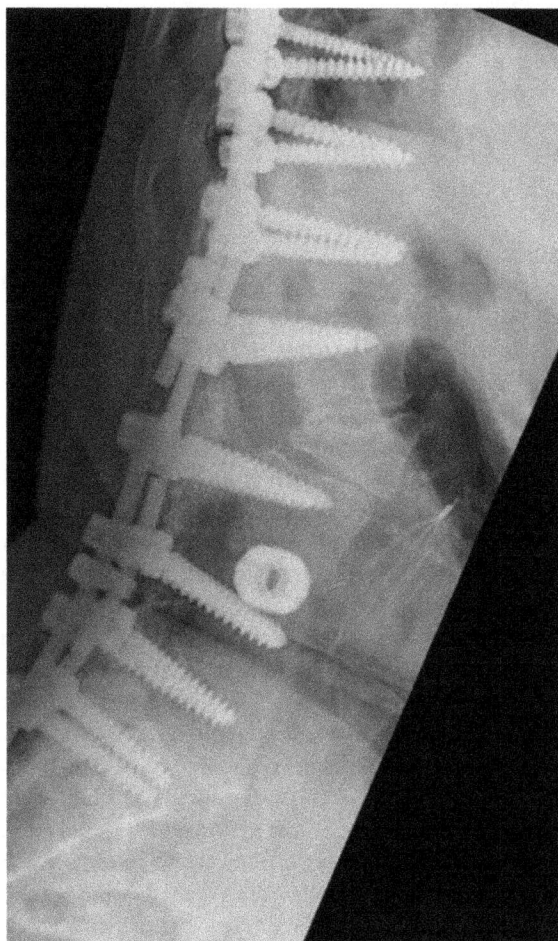

**Fig. 3** Flexion views demonstrate clear motion at the osteotomy

in three of five patients (patients 5, 14, and 19) at 1 year follow-up. The other two patient revision surgeries did not demonstrate any evidence of implant failure at the latest visit; however, their follow-up was less than 1 year from surgery (Table 3) (Figs. 4 and 5).

## Discussion

Tricolumnar osteotomy by posterior approach is a valuable tool in the spine surgeon's armamentarium. PSO and VCR deal with more severe structural deformities with rigid curves where only posterior column osteotomy like Smith-Peterson or Ponte's osteotomy may not be sufficient to achieve correction. Another advantage of these osteotomies is the ability to shorten the posterior column while achieving angular correction without lengthening of the anterior column, thus avoiding injury to major anterior visceral structures. Implant failures and pseudoarthrosis are common long-term complications associated with long fusions in spine deformities. The purposes of our study were to estimate the incidence of implant failures in deformity patients undergoing tricolumnar osteotomies and

**Table 2** Data of implant failure

| Patient no. | Type of osteotomy | Level of osteotomy | Rod material | Level of rod failure |
|---|---|---|---|---|
| Patient 5 | PSO | L1 | Titanium | L5–S1 |
| Patient 11 | PSO | L2 | Titanium | L2–L3 |
| Patient 14 | PSO | L4 | Titanium | L4 |
| Patient 19 | PSO | L2 | Titanium | L2 |
| Patient 20 | PSO | L2 and L3 | Titanium | L2–L3 |
| Patient 21 | PSO | L4 | Titanium | L4–L5 |
| Patient 25 | PSO | L2 | Titanium | L2 on left, L3 on right |

determine relative rates of failures at different points along the construct with analysis of possible factors leading to these failures.

Pseudoarthrosis rates have been reported to range from 17 to 24% in long fusions in a series by Kim et al. [23, 24]. In their analysis of 144 patients, 34 patients demonstrated pseudoarthrosis on follow-up radiographs. Almost all patients demonstrated this nonunion at junctional segments (17 at T10–L2 and 15 at L5–S1) in their study. High rates of implant failure have been reported at the osteotomy level in patients with PSO by Bridwell et al. and Yang et al. in their analysis of 33 and 35 patients, respectively [16, 25]. Our study demonstrated implant failure in 37% of adults and 27% of the overall study population. Six of seven (86%) of these failures were located at the level of osteotomy with accompanying previous laminectomies, whereas 14% (1/7) were located at the lumbosacral junction. This is comparable to 89% rod failure rate at the osteotomy site in patients undergoing PSO reported by Smith et al. in a multicenter retrospective review of 442 patients by the International Spine Study Group [26]. In our study, all patients had rod failures approximately 1 year from their surgery qualifying as "early" failures correlating with the International Spine Study Group's findings. Interestingly, all of our failures of the osteotomy site occurred in PSO patients. Those patients were older as compared to the

VCR and HE patients, and as such may have simply been more at risk patients with a higher potential for a non-union.

A comparatively low rate of rod breakage at the lumbosacral junction site seen in our study may be related to adopting the use of structural interbody graft and stronger iliac screws. This may have indirectly reflected a relatively higher rate at the previous laminectomy sites. Another caveat may be deficient posterior bone stock as a result of wide laminectomy essential to assess and prevent dural impingement during osteotomy closure. This is particularly relevant when the osteotomy is done through previously unfused segments and a surgeon must rely predominantly on anterior elements for arthrodesis. Complete closure of posterior elements or the base of the wedge by different maneuvers is ideal and desirable but may not always be practically possible, particularly in osteoporotic bone where balance needs to be achieved between adequate closure and preventing screw cutout or pullout. Optimal closure of the osteotomy wedge to achieve maximum bone surface contact as allowed by bone quality along with generous use of autograft to bridge the gap between two adjacent posterior elements is suggested. Efficacy of the bone morphogenic protein (RhBMP-2) and even its superiority over the iliac crest bone graft to enhance the rates of fusion has been well documented in long-term follow-up studies [27].

**Table 3** Patients with rod failures

| Patient no. | Symptoms | Intervention | Outcome |
|---|---|---|---|
| Patient 5 | Increasing back pain | Replacement of rod and use of lateral connectors Iliac crest bone graft | Fusion at the nonunion site |
| Patient 11 | Increasing back pain | Rod replacement Use of BMP | Follow up less than 1 year No implant failure noted |
| Patient 14 | Worsening posture Increasing back pain | Rod replacement Use of BMP | Fusion at the nonunion site |
| Patient 19 | Worsening standing balance Back discomfort and muscle fatigue | Replacement of rod with lateral connectors Use of BMP | Fusion at the nonunion site |
| Patient 20 | Asymptomatic | None | – |
| Patient 21 | Increasing back pain | Rod replacement Iliac crest bone graft | Follow-up less than 1 year No implant failure noted |
| Patient 25 | Asymptomatic | None | – |

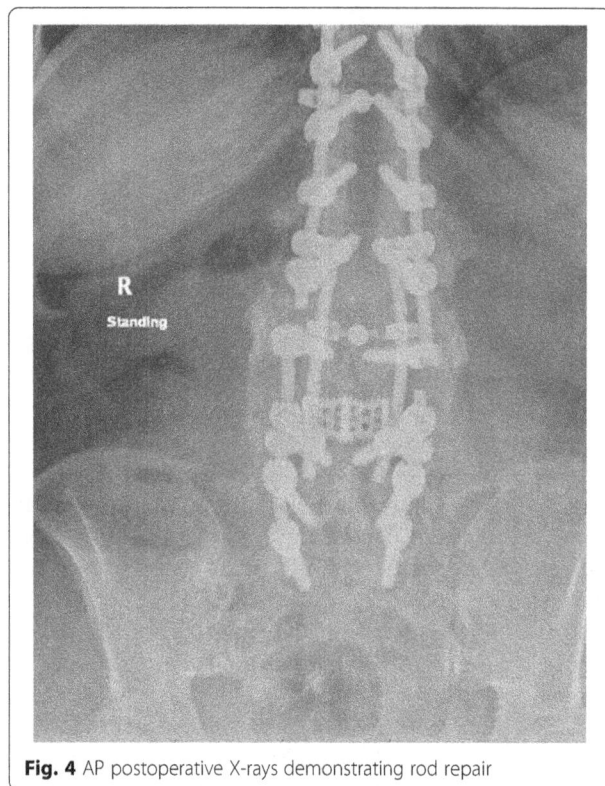

**Fig. 4** AP postoperative X-rays demonstrating rod repair

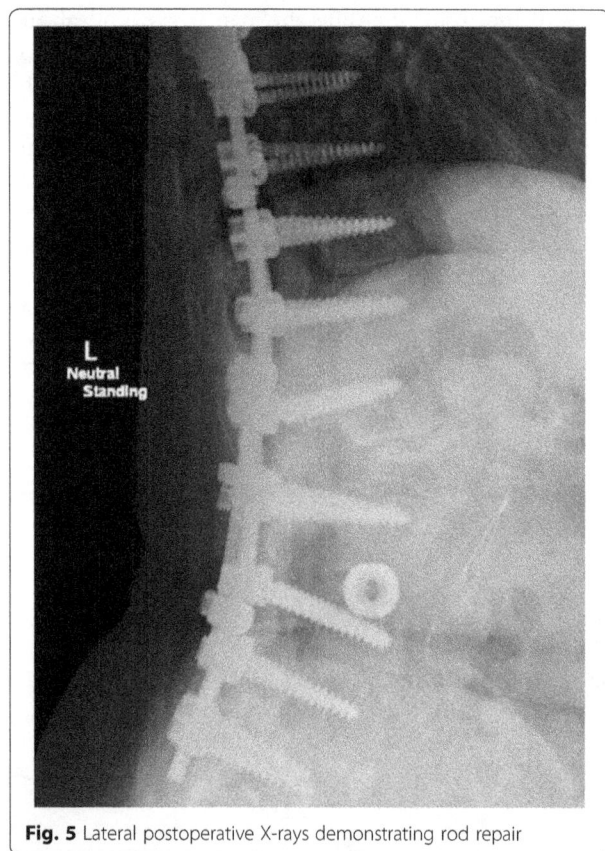

**Fig. 5** Lateral postoperative X-rays demonstrating rod repair

However, its use around the laminectomy site is limited in view of adverse effects over exposed neural elements and should be used judiciously. Finally, an apex of the new spinal curvature will be located at the osteotomy site, and maximum stress borne by the implants and maximum rod contouring at this point compounded by high notch sensitivity of titanium, especially during the early postoperative period until fusion occurs, and may be cited as one possible reason for relatively high implant failure rates at this location [28].

Another important finding was that 71% (5/7 patients) with an implant failure had increasing back pain or worsening sagittal balance or a combination of both, while two patients (29%) were asymptomatic and failure was an incidental finding on follow-up radiographs. Considering revision surgery is a significant endeavor for the patient both physically and mentally, a choice was offered to them to have it fixed surgically versus close observation. Being asymptomatic, both made an informed decision against surgical intervention but understood the possible need for revision surgery in the future if symptoms appear or function worsens.

The strength of our study is being one of the few studies attempting to analyze failures after three column osteotomy of the spine with direct comparison of failures at the osteotomy site and junctional levels. It highlights that maintenance of the correction, obtained through an osteotomy over time by optimizing rates of fusion through the segment, is as crucial to the success of deformity surgery as achieving this correction with intraoperative maneuvers. The primary limitation of our study is its retrospective nature. Also, longer follow-ups may increase the number of rod failures recorded. A prospective study with randomization of patients is warranted but may not be feasible due to ethical issues and expected high rates of crossover based on intraoperative decisions. Nonetheless, this study was an attempt to directly compare rates of implant failure at different points along the construct and highlight possible factors which may be related to differences in the rates of failure.

## Conclusion

The overall incidence of rod/implant failure noted after three column osteotomies for deformity correction was 27%. Among these, 86% occurred at the level of osteotomy as compared to 14% at the junctional level. Possible reasons for this significant difference are increased stress in the rod at this point as a result of maximum contouring and relatively deficient posterior bone stock secondary to wide laminectomy. The observation is also likely a result of improved fusion rates at the lumbosacral junction consequent to adoption of interbody structural graft and strong iliac screws. However, additional biomechanical studies are needed to assess the importance of these factors.

## Abbreviations
BMP: Bone morphogenic protein; EC: Extracavitary corpectomy; HE: Hemivertebra excision; IRB: Institutional Review Board; PSO: Pedicle subtraction osteotomy; VCR: Vertebral column resection

## Acknowledgements
There is no one to acknowledge.

## Funding
We did not receive support or payment of any kinds for any aspect of this submitted work. NK has nothing to declare. RT has consulting, speaking arrangements and trips/travel arrangements with Stryker Spine and does research support for Vertiflex. WL received grants(money paid to the institution) from DePuy, Medtronic, IntegraLife, Sigmus, Inc., Spinal Kinetics, Inc., K2M, Inc., Providence Technologies, Stryker Spine and Vertebral Technologies, Inc.

## Authors' contributions
NK carried out the conception and design, acquisition of data, analysis and interpretation of data, and drafting of the manuscript. RT carried out the conception and design, acquisition of data, critical revision of the manuscript, and administrative support. WL carried out the conception and design, acquisition of data, analysis and interpretation of data, drafting of the manuscript, critical revision of the manuscript, statistical analysis, administrative support, and supervision of the project. All authors have read and approved the final manuscript.

## Competing interests
The authors declare that they have no competing interests.

## References
1. Bridwell KH, Lewis SJ, Lenke LG, Baldus C, Blanke K. Pedicle subtraction osteotomy for the treatment of fixed sagittal imbalance. J Bone Joint Surg Am. 2003;85-A(3):454–63.
2. Wang TP, Zheng ZM, Liu H, Zhang KB, Wang H. Correlation of adult spinal sagittal imbalance and life quality. Zhonghua Yi Xue Za Zhi. 2012;92(21):1481–5.
3. Glassman SD, Berven S, Bridwell K, Horton W, Dimar JR. Correlation of radiographic parameters and clinical symptoms in adult scoliosis. Spine (Phila Pa 1976). 2005;30(6):682–8.
4. Lagrone MO, Bradford DS, Moe JH, Lonstein JE, Winter RB, Oglivie JW. Treatment of symptomatic flatback after spinal fusion. J Bone Joint Surg Am. 1988;70(4):569–80.
5. Farcy JP, Schwab FJ. Management of flatback and related kyphotic decompensation syndromes. Spine (Phila Pa 1976). 1997;22(20):2452–7.
6. Shufflebarger HL, Clark CE. Thoracolumbar osteotomy for postsurgical sagittal imbalance. Spine (Phila Pa 1976). 1992;17(8 Suppl):S287–90.
7. Gertzbein SD, Harris MB. Wedge osteotomy for the correction of post-traumatic kyphosis. A new technique and a report of three cases. Spine (Phila Pa 1976). 1992;17(3):374–9.
8. Thiranont N, Netrawichien P. Transpedicular decancellation closed wedge vertebral osteotomy for treatment of fixed flexion deformity of spine in ankylosing spondylitis. Spine (Phila Pa 1976). 1993;18(16):2517–22.
9. Lehmer SM, Keppler L, Biscup RS, Enker P, Miller SD, Steffee AD. Posterior transvertebral osteotomy for adult thoracolumbar kyphosis. Spine (Phila Pa 1976). 1994;19(18):2060–7.
10. Berven SH, Deviren V, Smith JA, Emami A, Hu SS, Bradford DS. Management of fixed sagittal plane deformity: results of the transpedicular wedge resection osteotomy. Spine (Phila Pa 1976). 2001;26(18):2036–43.
11. Kim KT, Lee SH, Suk KS, Lee JH, Jeong BO. Outcome of pedicle subtraction osteotomies for fixed sagittal imbalance of multiple etiologies: a retrospective review of 140 patients. Spine (Phila Pa 1976). 2012;37(19):1667–75.
12. Suk SI, Kim JH, Kim WJ, et al. Posterior vertebral column resection for severe spinal deformities. Spine (Phila Pa 1976). 2002;27(21):2374–82.
13. Suk SI, Chung ER, Kim JH, Lee SM, Chung ER, Nah KH. Posterior vertebral column resection for severe rigid scoliosis. Spine (Phila Pa 1976). 2005; 30(14):1682–7.
14. Smith JS, Wang VY, Ames CP. Vertebral column resection for rigid spinal deformity. Neurosurgery. 2008;63(3 Suppl):177–82.
15. Lenke LG, Sides BA, Koester LA, Hensley M, Blanke KM. Vertebral column resection for the treatment of severe spinal deformity. Clin Orthop Relat Res. 2010;468(3):687–99.
16. Bridwell KH, Lewis SJ, Edwards C, Lenke LG, Iffrig TM, Berra A, et al. Complications and outcomes of pedicle subtraction osteotomies for fixed sagittal imbalance. Spine (Phila Pa 1976). 2003;28(18):2093–101.
17. Kim YJ, Bridwell KH, Lenke LG, Cheh G, Baldus C. Results of lumbar pedicle subtraction osteotomies for fixed sagittal imbalance: a minimum 5-year follow-up study. Spine (Phila Pa 1976). 2007;32(20):2189–97.
18. Kostuik JP, Anderson DG, Kebaish KM. Surgery for adult spinal deformity. In: Heary H, Albert T, editors. Spinal deformities: the essentials 2nd edition. New York: Thieme Medical Publishers, Inc; 2007. p. 224.
19. Tsuchiya K, Bridwell KH, Kuklo TR, Lenke LG, Baldus C. Minimum 5-year analysis of L5-S1 fusion using sacropelvic fixation (bilateral S1 and iliac screws) for spinal deformity. Spine (Phila Pa 1976). 2006;31(3):303–8.
20. Holte DC, Winter RB, Lonstein JE, Denis F. Excision of hemivertebrae and wedge resection in the treatment of congenital scoliosis. J Bone Joint Surg Am. 1995;77(2):159–71.
21. Bernhardt M, Bridwell KH. Segmental analysis of the sagittal plane alignment of the normal thoracic and lumbar spines and thoracolumbar junction. Spine (Phila Pa 1976). 1989;14(7):717–21.
22. Kuklo TR, Bridwell KH, Lewis SJ, Baldus C, Blanke K, Iffrig TM, et al. Minimum 2-year analysis of sacropelvic fixation and L5-S1 fusion utilizing S1 and iliac screws. Spine (Phila Pa 1976). 2001;26(18):1976–83.
23. Kim YJ, Bridwell KH, Lenke LG, Rhim S, Cheh G. Pseudarthrosis in long adult spinal deformity instrumentation and fusion to the sacrum: prevalence and risk factor analysis of 144 cases. Spine (Phila Pa 1976). 2006;31(20):2329–36.
24. Kim YJ, Bridwell KH, Lenke LG, Rinella AS, Edwards 2nd C. Pseudarthrosis in primary fusions for adult idiopathic scoliosis: incidence, risk factors, and outcome analysis. Spine (Phila Pa 1976). 2005;30(4):468–74.
25. Yang BP, Ondra SL, Chen LA, Jung HS, Koski TR, Salehi SA. Clinical and radiographic outcomes of thoracic and lumbar pedicle subtraction osteotomy for fixed sagittal imbalance. J Neurosurg Spine. 2006;5(1):9–17.
26. Smith JS, Shaffrey CI, Ames CP, Demakakos J, Fu KM, Keshavarzi S, et al. Assessment of symptomatic rod fracture after posterior instrumented fusion for adult spinal deformity. Neurosurgery. 2012;71(4):862–7.
27. Kim HJ, Buchowski JM, Zebala LP, Dickson DD, Koester L, Bridwell KH. RhBMP-2 is superior to iliac crest bone graft for long fusions to the sacrum in adult spinal deformity: 4- to 14-year follow-up. Spine (Phila Pa 1976). 2013;38(14):1209–15.
28. Lindsey C, Deviren V, Xu Z, Yeh RF, Puttlitz CM. The effects of rod contouring on spinal construct fatigue strength. Spine (Phila Pa 1976). 2006;31(15):1680–7.

# Radiographic indices for lumbar developmental spinal stenosis

Jason Pui Yin Cheung*, Karen Ka Man Ng, Prudence Wing Hang Cheung, Dino Samartzis and Kenneth Man Chee Cheung

## Abstract

**Background:** Patients with developmental spinal stenosis (DSS) are susceptible to developing symptomatic stenosis due to pre-existing narrowed spinal canals. DSS has been previously defined by MRI via the axial anteroposterior (AP) bony spinal canal diameter. However, MRI is hardly a cost-efficient tool for screening patients. X-rays are superior due to its availability and cost, but currently, there is no definition of DSS based on plain radiographs. Thus, the aim of this study is to develop radiographic indices for diagnosing DSS.

**Methods:** This was a prospective cohort of 148 subjects consisting of patients undergoing surgery for lumbar spinal stenosis (patient group) and asymptomatic subjects recruited openly from the general population (control group). Ethics approval was obtained from the local institutional review board. All subjects underwent MRI for diagnosing DSS and radiographs for measuring parameters used for creating the indices. All measurements were performed by two independent investigators, blinded to patient details. Intra- and interobserver reliability analyses were conducted, and only parameters with near perfect intraclass correlation underwent receiver operating characteristic (ROC) analysis to determine the cutoff values for diagnosing DSS using radiographs.

**Results:** Imaging parameters from a total of 66 subjects from the patient group and 82 asymptomatic subjects in the control group were used for analysis. ROC analysis suggested sagittal vertebral body width to pedicle width ratio (SBW:PW) as having the strongest sensitivity and specificity for diagnosing DSS. Cutoff indices for SBW:PW were level-specific: L1 (2.0), L2 (2.0), L3 (2.2), L4 (2.2), L5 (2.5), and S1 (2.8).

**Conclusions:** This is the first study to define DSS on plain radiographs based on comparisons between a clinically relevant patient group and a control group. Individuals with DSS can be identified by a simple radiograph using a screening tool allowing for better cost-saving means for clinical diagnosis or research purposes.

**Keywords:** Developmental spinal stenosis, Radiological indices, MRI, X-ray

## Background

Lumbar spinal stenosis is a constriction of the spinal canal that can cause compression of the neural tissue. Patients can experience symptoms of leg pain, radiculopathy, and claudication [1]. The cause of lumbar spinal stenosis can be grossly classified as developmental, degenerative, or a combination of both [2–5]. The degree of constriction required to cause symptoms is unclear, but with a developmentally narrowed spinal canal, patients are more susceptible to canal compression.

Lumbar developmental spinal stenosis (DSS) is likely a result of abnormal fetal and postnatal development of the lumbar vertebrae [6–8]. The definition of developmental narrowing has been suggested by Verbiest [7] to be an abnormally short anteroposterior (AP) canal diameter. The proposed absolute value of less than 10 mm is commonly accepted as canal narrowing [5, 8], but the method for coming up with this value is based on intraoperative measurements in a small number of operated cases and hence cannot be directly translated to imaging. In addition, magnification errors are common for radiographs, and these measurements should be standardized to other parameters such as an individual's vertebral body size

* Correspondence: cheungjp@hku.hk
Department of Orthopaedics and Traumatology, Queen Mary Hospital, The University of Hong Kong, Pokfulam Road, Hong Kong, SAR, China

[9]. Other imaging-based criteria have been suggested in the past [7, 8, 10–17] but were based on inconsistent imaging modalities [8, 10, 13, 16, 17], heterogeneous populations [8, 10, 11, 13, 16, 18, 19], lacked control groups [8, 10, 11, 13, 19], and generalized measurements of the entire lumbar spine [8, 10, 11, 13, 16–19].

Cheung et al. [2] previously defined the lumbar DSS phenotype in a large-scale homogenous group of southern Chinese with standardized measurements based on magnetic resonance imaging (MRI). The axial AP bony spinal canal diameter translated to the pedicle width and generally decreased from cranially to caudally. Its cutoff values were defined using data derived from both symptomatic and asymptomatic subjects with high sensitivity and specificity values. The results from this study suggest that DSS plays an important role in the pathogenesis of symptomatic lumbar spinal stenosis. However, no similar study has been conducted on plain radiographs.

MRI is the gold standard for the assessment of patients with spinal stenosis. As a diagnostic imaging tool, it has no equal in assessment of intervertebral disc abnormalities and canal stenosis [20, 21]. Despite the advantages of using MRI for the diagnosis of lumbar DSS, there are cost concerns for overuse. If MRI is used in all suspected cases of spinal stenosis for either clinical management or research, the financial burden is astronomical. Therefore, MRI is not a cost-efficient tool for screening patients for lumbar DSS. Alternatively, plain radiographs are superior for screening due to low cost and availability.

In the eyes of experienced clinicians, radiographs with short pedicles suggestive of DSS may be identified (Figs. 1 and 2). Several studies [22–25] have discussed canal narrowing and its measurements in the past, but these analyses were not based on a derived radiographic index and thus are subject to influence by body size. In addition, it is difficult to determine from a simple visual inspection whether pedicles are short or not because pedicle widths reduce from cranial to caudally. An attempt in creating radiographic indices has been performed in the past [26], but this was based on the comparison of MRI dural sac diameters which is affected by degenerative changes and cannot be contributed to developmental malformation. Moreover, no description has been made regarding how radiographic measurements were performed limiting relevance of their findings to actual developmental narrowing of the bony spinal canal. Therefore, there is a need for an easily used radiographic definition for lumbar DSS. As such, the aim of this study is to develop practical radiographic indices for diagnosing DSS.

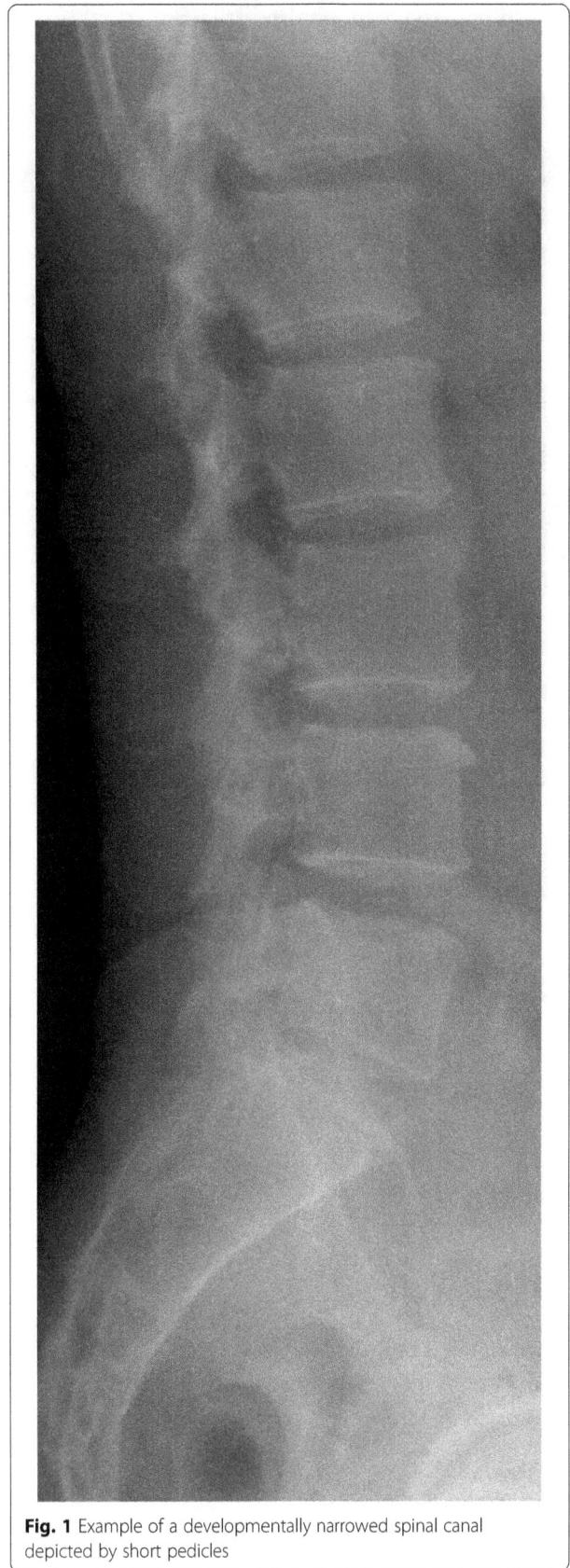

**Fig. 1** Example of a developmentally narrowed spinal canal depicted by short pedicles

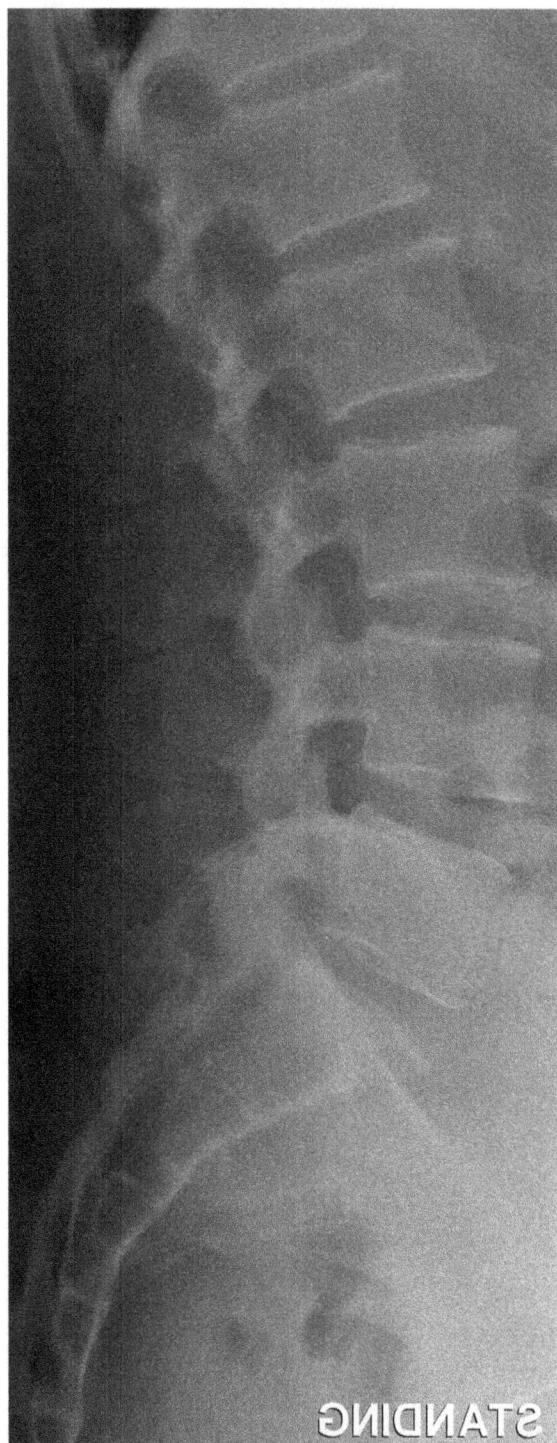

**Fig. 2** Example of a normal sized spinal canal

## Methods

### Study design and population

This was a prospectively collected cohort of 66 patients who underwent surgery for lumbar spinal stenosis (patient group) and 82 asymptomatic subjects who were openly recruited from the general population via advertisement (control group) as part of the Hong Kong Disc Degeneration Cohort study [27–30]. There were 34 females (51.5%) and 32 males (48.5%) in the patient group with mean age of 65.9 years (±SD 10.9). There were 31 males (38.3%) and 50 females (61.7%) in the control group with mean age of 56.4 years (±SD 6.8). Ethics review was performed by a local institutional review board. All subjects were of Chinese ethnicity and were recruited via written consent since December 2012. Subject recruitment ended on December 2014. Subjects with congenital deformities, previous infections, tumors, trauma, or spondylolisthesis were excluded from the study. Various patient demographics and clinical profile were noted, including age and sex and, for the patient group, symptomatology, operation performed, and number of operated levels. All subjects underwent MRI and standing AP and lateral radiographs of the lumbosacral spine. For the patient group, all imaging were performed preoperatively.

### MRI measurements

Axial T1-weighted MRI images of the lumbar spine from L1 to S1 were utilized for all subjects. 1.5 or 3 T HD MRI machines were used for imaging. The field of view was 18 × 18 cm, slice thickness was 4 mm, and slice spacing was 0 mm. The imaging matrix was 288 × 192. The repetition time (TR) was 700–800 ms, and the echo time (TE) was 8–10 ms for the T1 images. There were 11 slices per vertebral level, and parallel slices were made according to the disc and pedicle levels. The axial image used for measurement was the cut with the thickest pedicle diameter and could also visualize the whole bony ring at the pedicle level. The midline AP bony spinal canal diameter was used to diagnose DSS (L1 <20 mm, L2 <19 mm, L3 <19 mm, L4 <17 mm, L5 <16 mm, S1 <16 mm) [2, 31]. Only the AP bony spinal canal diameter (Fig. 3) was used because it was most representative of DSS. The subjects in the control group were all confirmed to have normal sized spinal canals by the MRI cutoff values discussed.

### Plain radiographic assessment

All subjects underwent lumbar AP and lateral standing radiographs of the lumbosacral spine (view of the thoracolumbar region to sacrum) extracted to measure parameters including interpedicular distance (IPD) and axial vertebral body height and width (ABW) on AP views (Fig. 4) and foraminal width (FW), pedicle width (PW), posterior pedicle margin (PPM), and sagittal vertebral body height and width (SBW) on lateral views (Fig. 5). The FW was taken at the widest diameter below the pedicle and above the intervertebral disc. The PW was measured from the posterior

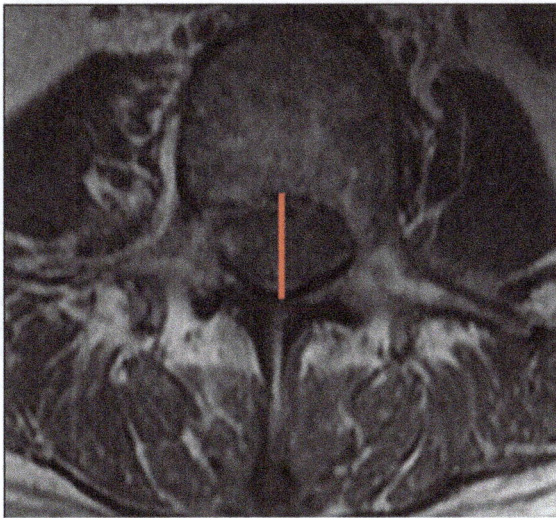

**Fig. 3** Axial T1 MRI image showing the measurement for the anteroposterior bony spinal canal diameter

border of the vertebral body to the line connecting the cranial and caudal facet joints. The PPM was measured from the posterior vertebral body to the base of the spinous process. These were the most consistent landmarks visible on lateral radiographs. The IPD on the AP view was taken at the narrowest horizontal diameter between the two pedicles. The vertebral body height and width measurements were taken at the midpoint of the vertebral body in both AP and lateral radiographs from the superior endplate to the inferior endplate. In case of any film rotation, there will be a "double feature" of the landmarks. For these cases, the midpoint between the more proximal and more distal landmarks was taken as the correct measurement point.

## Image analysis

All measurements were performed independently by two investigators, and all clinical information was blinded to the investigators during measurements. For reliability testing, 20 subjects were randomly selected from both groups for intra- and interobserver reliability assessments. The first and second round of measurements was performed at least 1 month apart. Radiographs and MRIs were measured separately and not consecutively for any single subject to avoid bias during measurements. The blinding and reliability procedures were arranged by a third independent investigator who performed scrambling of the images and order of subjects prior to the measurements. All images were measured using the Centricity Enterprise Web V3.0 (GE Medical Systems, 2006).

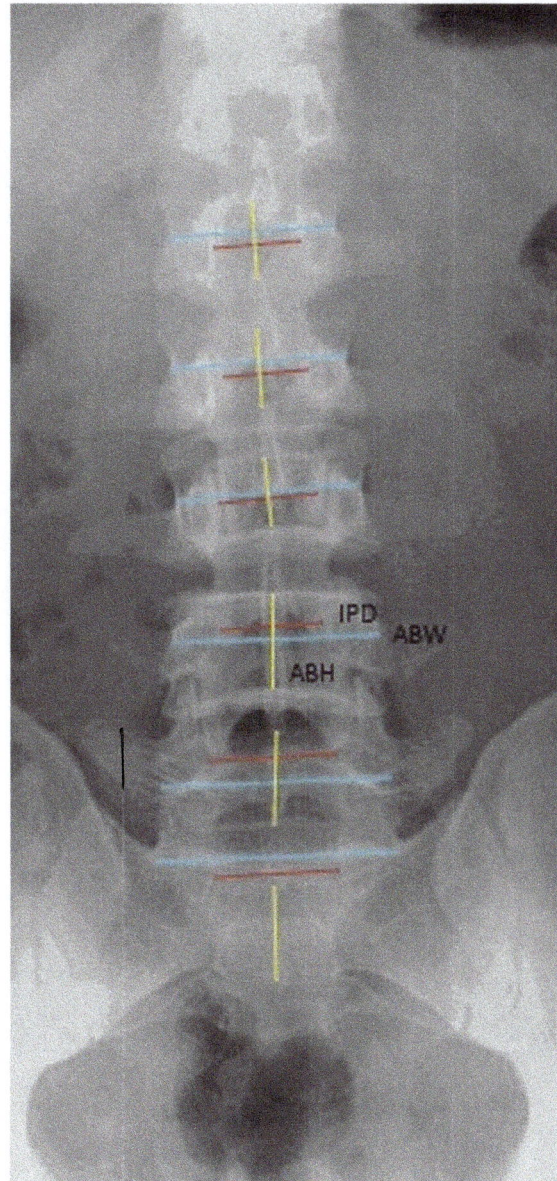

**Fig. 4** Measurement scheme for the anteroposterior standing radiograph: axial vertebral body width (*ABW: light blue*), axial vertebral body height (*ABH: yellow*), and interpedicular distance (*IPD: red*)

## Statistical analysis

Descriptive and frequency statistics were performed of the data. Median values were used for analysis of the different parameters and ratios to avoid skewing of the data. Reliability assessment was based on intraclass correlation (ICC) analysis. ICC could be interpreted based on the following alpha values: 0–0.29 indicated poor agreement, 0.30–0.49 indicated fair agreement, 0.50–0.69 indicated moderate agreement, 0.70–0.80 indicated strong agreement, and >0.80 indicated almost perfect agreement [32, 33]. The 95%

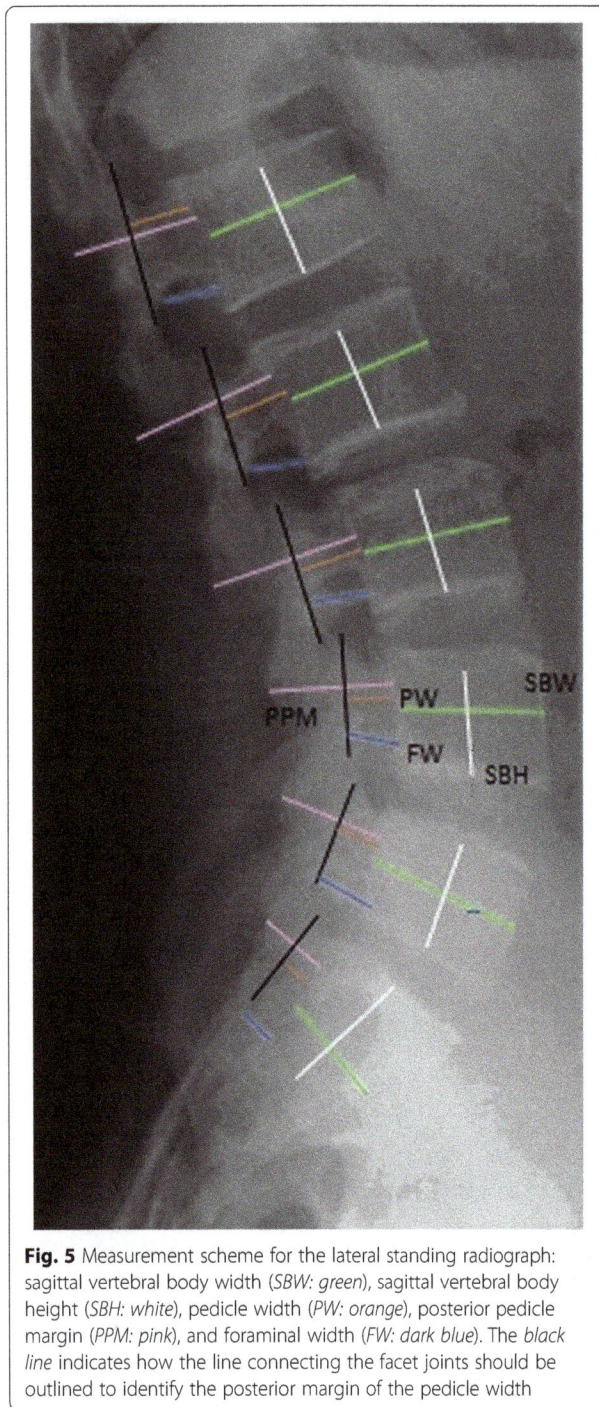

**Fig. 5** Measurement scheme for the lateral standing radiograph: sagittal vertebral body width (*SBW: green*), sagittal vertebral body height (*SBH: white*), pedicle width (*PW: orange*), posterior pedicle margin (*PPM: pink*), and foraminal width (*FW: dark blue*). The *black line* indicates how the line connecting the facet joints should be outlined to identify the posterior margin of the pedicle width

confidence interval (CI) bounds were assessed for precision. A *p* value of <0.05 was considered significant. Only radiographic parameters with near-perfect agreement were used for radiographic indices and underwent receiver operating characteristic (ROC) analysis to identify the cutoff values that diagnose subjects with DSS. Cutoff values with the highest sensitivity and specificity results were chosen.

## Results

The MRI diameters and reliability assessment of both groups were listed in Table 1. The median AP bony spinal canal diameters of the patient group gradually decreased from cranial to caudally while the normal subjects were generally similar throughout the levels. According to the criteria for diagnosing DSS on MRI, all 66 subjects in the patient group had DSS while none of the 82 asymptomatic subjects had developmental canal narrowing. Both intra- and interobserver reliability for the AP bony spinal canal diameter on MRI were near perfect using ICC analysis. Only clinical symptomatic levels from L3 to S1 were observed in the patient group.

Almost perfect ICC agreement was found for PW, PPM, SBW, ABW, and IPD (Table 2). The PW and PPM measurements gradually decreased from cranial to caudally for the patient group, but this trend only existed for PW in the control group. The ABW and IPD gradually increased from cranial to caudally for both groups. According to the ICC agreement, three radiographic indices were created (two from lateral radiographs and one from AP radiographs). For the lateral radiograph, SBW:PW and SBW:PPM ratios were calculated. Similarly, ABW:IPD was calculated for the AP radiograph (Table 3).

ROC analysis (Table 4) suggested that the SBW:PW ratio had the highest area under the curve analysis and strongest sensitivity and specificity results. In addition, the overall median values for SBW:PW had a wider difference in margin value between patient and control groups while the indices for SBW:PPM and ABW:IPD did not have a significant difference between groups to represent a clinically useful cutoff value. For SBW:PW, level-specific cutoff values were suggested: L1 (2.0), L2 (2.0), L3 (2.2), L4 (2.2), L5 (2.5), and S1 (2.8). As a simple guideline, developmental canal narrowing could be defined as an index greater than 2.8 for SBW:PW. This was a general statement of the calculated results using the largest index (S1) for SBW:PW. This was an attempt to avoid over-diagnosis of DSS since the indices were level-specific and some of the lumbosacral levels had smaller indices than others.

## Discussion

With these radiographic indices, patients with lumbar DSS can be identified on either the AP or lateral lumbar spine radiographs, which can produce the same diagnostic purpose as MRI. From the results, absolute measurements of PW generally decrease from cranial to caudally in both groups. These measurements mirror that of the AP bony spinal canal diameter and are thus a good representation of the actual MRI findings. SBW and PPM appears to differ between the groups as there is a gradual change in size for the patient group while they stay

**Table 1** MRI measurements of lumbar developmental spinal stenosis

| Measurement<br>AP bony spinal canal diameter | Median, mm (±SD) | | Intraobserver reliability | 95% CI | Interobserver reliability | 95% CI |
|---|---|---|---|---|---|---|
| | Patient | Control | | | | |
| L1 | 18.2 (1.4) | 19.3 (2.3) | 0.94* | 0.75–0.99 | 0.91* | 0.70–0.97 |
| L2 | 17.3 (1.5) | 19.1 (2.3) | 0.97* | 0.87–0.99 | 0.96* | 0.87–0.98 |
| L3 | 16.5 (2.0) | 18.8 (2.9) | 0.98* | 0.94–1.00 | 0.97* | 0.88–0.99 |
| L4 | 14.8 (1.9) | 19.1 (2.1) | 0.97* | 0.89–0.99 | 0.94* | 0.82–0.99 |
| L5 | 14.2 (1.3) | 19.4 (3.8) | 0.98* | 0.91–0.99 | 0.99* | 0.87–0.99 |
| S1 | 14.1 (1.6) | 17.4 (2.1) | 0.96* | 0.82–0.99 | 0.89* | 0.78–0.99 |

Abbreviations: SD standard deviation, AP anteroposterior, CI confidence interval
*$p < 0.001$

similar across levels in the control group. In addition, the measurements of the ABW and IPD increase from cranial to caudally in both groups. These findings further support the fact that the AP bony spinal canal diameter (or the PW in this study) is most predictive of DSS since it is likely to be independent from the patient size which is something that cannot be derived from the IPD. Hence, it is likely that the cutoff values provided by the SBW:PW radio is more predictive of DSS. Whether this is true or not requires further investigation.

Previously, there has been no agreement on the clinical or radiological definition of lumbar canal stenosis despite many imaging and cadaveric studies [7, 10, 11, 14–17, 23, 34, 35]. Reasons for these discrepancies are based on the lack of a uniformed method of measurement for the bony spinal canal diameter. DSS can now be defined based on a standardized method for the assessment of spinal canal MRI phenotypes [2]. In this study, patients with DSS are diagnosed by the AP bony spinal canal diameter phenotype on MRI, which is the parameter determined to be the most representative of DSS and can be obtainable from axial MRI images [2, 31]. However, due to the obvious cost-related concerns of MRI, this study is conducted to develop new phenotypes of DSS on radiographs using easily measurable radiographic parameters. In terms of radiation exposure, only two standing radiographs are required for assessment, and these are usually required prior to any treatment to assess the loaded spine since MRIs are performed in supine. Thus, the clinical risk of these radiographs is minimal. Use of scanning systems like the EOS® will require further study to assess feasibility and reliability of measurements.

It is important to note that these indices are created based on a cohort of both symptomatic patients requiring surgical decompression and asymptomatic subjects recruited from the general population. Interestingly, none of the subjects in the control group has DSS on MRI measurements. This suggests that DSS is likely an important parameter that differentiates subjects who become symptomatic requiring surgery and those that

may remain asymptomatic. Although this can be theorized from our results, at present, these indices can only serve as reference for identifying subjects with narrowed spinal canals without further longitudinal follow-up of these asymptomatic individuals. These radiographic indices are not meant to be a guide to whether a patient deserves decompression or not. Symptomatology is not a parameter we used to define these indices, and not all developmentally narrowed levels may be symptomatic. The overall denominator of subjects with DSS is unknown in the general population, and thus, what is considered "healthy" or "normal" is unknown without large-scale population studies.

Developmentally, the pedicle is the main reason for a narrowed spinal canal. Applying the knowledge from patients with achondroplasia, a disorder in endochondral ossification leads to fusion of pedicles to vertebral bodies; formation of abnormally short pedicles and narrowed IPD gives rise to inadequate spinal canal sizes and risk of neurological compromise [36]. In the general population, a widening of the IPD is observed from cranial to caudal spinal segments [37, 38]. This finding is echoed by our study results. As radiographic parameters of pedicle sizes and IPD are more consistent in our subjects, our indices are derived from the PW, PPM, and IPD. Although it is impossible to measure the exact width of the pedicle depicted on lateral radiographs, two consistent landmarks (facet joints and posterior vertebral body) are used to help guide us to where the pedicle should be. The exact location of our measurement parameter is of little concern because we only require a consistent parameter that can reflect a short pedicle. This value is then compared to the vertebral body width to create a ratio. The IPD is another consistent landmark since the well-defined pedicle is usually seen clearly on AP radiographs. However, this is likely not as representative as the PW as the pedicle sizes are more directly related to the AP bony spinal canal diameter measured on MRI. This is supported by our study results which proves that SBW:PW is the most significant index

**Table 2** Radiograph measurements and reliability analysis

| Measurement | Median, mm (±SD) | | Interobserver reliability | 95% CI[*] | Intraobserver reliability | 95% CI[*] |
|---|---|---|---|---|---|---|
| | Patient | Control | | | | |
| Foraminal width | | | | | | |
| L1 | 11.8 (1.8) | 13.1 (1.5) | 0.84 | 0.59–0.94 | 0.96 | 0.91–0.99 |
| L2 | 11.1 (1.6) | 13.2 (1.8) | 0.78 | 0.43–0.92 | 0.89 | 0.71–0.96 |
| L3 | 10.5 (1.9) | 12.8 (1.6) | 0.86 | 0.64–0.95 | 0.93 | 0.83–0.97 |
| L4 | 9.5 (1.9) | 11.1 (1.7) | 0.84 | 0.58–0.94 | 0.89 | 0.70–0.96 |
| L5 | 8.0 (1.9) | 9.3 (1.6) | 0.72 | 0.27–0.89 | 0.88 | 0.70–0.96 |
| S1 | 6.6 (2.0) | 7.5 (1.5) | 0.92 | 0.55–0.99 | 0.86 | 0.63–0.95 |
| Pedicle width | | | | | | |
| L1 | 16.5 (2.5) | 17.9 (2.2) | 0.95 | 0.87–0.98 | 0.95 | 0.88–0.98 |
| L2 | 16.7 (2.5) | 17.7 (1.8) | 0.97 | 0.93–0.99 | 0.91 | 0.78–0.97 |
| L3 | 15.0 (1.9) | 18.3 (1.8) | 0.96 | 0.90–0.99 | 0.89 | 0.72–0.96 |
| L4 | 14.6 (2.8) | 17.4 (2.1) | 0.97 | 0.92–0.99 | 0.90 | 0.75–0.96 |
| L5 | 11.3 (1.9) | 16.0 (2.5) | 0.95 | 0.86–0.98 | 0.95 | 0.88–0.98 |
| S1 | 8.2 (2.3) | 11.2 (3.8) | 0.98 | 0.93–0.99 | 0.93 | 0.81–0.97 |
| Posterior pedicle margin | | | | | | |
| L1 | 27.6 (3.8) | 28.0 (3.1) | 0.97 | 0.93–0.99 | 0.98 | 0.95–0.99 |
| L2 | 28.5 (4.0) | 27.7 (2.6) | 0.99 | 0.96–0.99 | 0.97 | 0.91–0.99 |
| L3 | 29.7 (3.5) | 29.3 (2.4) | 0.98 | 0.94–0.99 | 0.93 | 0.81–0.97 |
| L4 | 28.5 (4.4) | 29.7 (2.7) | 0.97 | 0.93–0.99 | 0.93 | 0.81–0.97 |
| L5 | 25.6 (4.4) | 27.5 (2.9) | 1.00 | 0.99–1.00 | 0.97 | 0.93–0.99 |
| S1 | 20.6 (4.2) | 21.9 (4.0) | 0.99 | 0.98–1.00 | 0.95 | 0.86–0.98 |
| Sagittal vertebral body width | | | | | | |
| L1 | 35.6 (4.7) | 35.0 (3.9) | 0.97 | 0.92–0.99 | 0.94 | 0.85–0.98 |
| L2 | 37.3 (5.3) | 35.8 (4.3) | 0.97 | 0.91–0.99 | 0.95 | 0.87–0.98 |
| L3 | 39.3 (4.6) | 37.2 (4.0) | 0.97 | 0.91–0.99 | 0.96 | 0.90–0.99 |
| L4 | 39.7 (3.9) | 36.5 (3.9) | 0.95 | 0.86–0.98 | 0.93 | 0.82–0.97 |
| L5 | 39.3 (3.8) | 36.5 (3.7) | 0.97 | 0.92–0.99 | 0.96 | 0.90–0.99 |
| S1 | 27.9 (4.0) | 29.4 (3.9) | 0.91 | 0.77–0.97 | 0.90 | 0.75–0.96 |
| Sagittal vertebral body height | | | | | | |
| L1 | 29.0 (3.4) | 28.6 (3.6) | 0.97 | 0.91–0.99 | 0.94 | 0.83–0.98 |
| L2 | 29.6 (3.4) | 29.9 (2.4) | 0.96 | 0.90–0.99 | 0.87 | 0.67–0.95 |
| L3 | 29.3 (3.3) | 30.2 (2.5) | 0.90 | 0.75–0.96 | 0.62 | 0.01–0.85 |
| L4 | 28.3 (3.7) | 30.3 (2.3) | 0.95 | 0.88–0.98 | 0.94 | 0.84–0.98 |
| L5 | 27.6 (3.9) | 30.0 (2.5) | 0.93 | 0.81–0.97 | 0.94 | 0.85–0.98 |
| S1 | 31.6 (3.5) | 32.2 (3.6) | 0.82 | 0.53–0.93 | 0.98 | 0.94–0.99 |
| Interpedicular distance | | | | | | |
| L1 | 24.5 (2.3) | 25.9 (2.7) | 0.94 | 0.84–0.97 | 0.96 | 0.89–0.98 |
| L2 | 24.8 (2.2) | 26.2 (2.6) | 0.92 | 0.79–0.97 | 0.96 | 0.91–0.99 |
| L3 | 26.2 (3.0) | 27.7 (2.1) | 0.97 | 0.92–0.99 | 0.98 | 0.95–0.99 |
| L4 | 27.7 (4.0) | 29.7 (2.7) | 0.97 | 0.92–0.99 | 0.98 | 0.94–0.99 |
| L5 | 30.7 (4.2) | 34.2 (3.3) | 1.00 | 0.99–1.00 | 0.95 | 0.88–0.98 |
| S1 | 34.4 (4.9) | 37.5 (3.2) | 0.99 | 0.96–1.00 | 0.94 | 0.84–0.98 |

**Table 2** Radiograph measurements and reliability analysis *(Continued)*

| Axial vertebral body width | | | | | | |
|---|---|---|---|---|---|---|
| L1 | 43.0 (4.2) | 41.6 (4.3) | 0.98 | 0.96–0.99 | 1.00 | 0.99–1.00 |
| L2 | 45.7 (4.3) | 42.2 (4.6) | 0.98 | 0.96–0.99 | 0.99 | 0.98–1.00 |
| L3 | 47.1 (4.5) | 44.1 (4.8) | 0.99 | 0.97–1.00 | 0.98 | 0.94–0.99 |
| L4 | 50.6 (5.0) | 48.2 (4.9) | 0.98 | 0.96–0.99 | 0.94 | 0.84–0.98 |
| L5 | 53.7 (5.9) | 55.4 (5.7) | 0.98 | 0.95–0.99 | 0.94 | 0.84–0.98 |
| Axial vertebral body height | | | | | | |
| L1 | 25.3 (4.1) | 29.1 (3.1) | 0.98 | 0.96–0.99 | 0.68 | 0.19–0.87 |
| L2 | 27.0 (3.9) | 29.9 (2.8) | 0.98 | 0.95–0.99 | 0.98 | 0.95–0.99 |
| L3 | 27.2 (3.3) | 30.0 (2.4) | 0.95 | 0.87–0.98 | 0.93 | 0.81–0.97 |
| L4 | 26.7 (3.6) | 30.6 (2.7) | 0.92 | 0.80–0.97 | 0.82 | 0.55–0.93 |
| L5 | 28.1 (4.4) | 28.1 (4.3) | 0.95 | 0.86–0.98 | 0.78 | 0.43–0.91 |

*Abbreviations*: *SD* standard deviation, *CI* confidence interval
*Statistical significance (all *p* values <0.05)

that has strong sensitivity and specificity in identifying DSS especially for L3–S1 which are clinically the more commonly affected levels by lumbar spinal stenosis.

Since all ratios have a component of the vertebral body width, the confounding effect of body size and magnification error can be accounted for. One of the key issues with measurement of the vertebral body width is to avoid measuring any osteophytes anterior to the vertebral body. This can be discerned by locating the most vertical tangential line lateral (for AP radiographs) to or anterior (for lateral radiographs) to the vertebral body using adjacent vertebral bodies as a reference. This is important to avoid a false positive result of narrowed canal due to overestimation of the vertebral body width. In addition, these ratios are based on static bony parameters which are unlikely to be subjected to change with posture or movement as compared to other dynamic measurements. Hence, we can expect these ratios to be consistent even on flexion-extension dynamic radiographs.

The vertebral body height and FW have large variability among the radiographs because they are dependent on a neutral view. Any tilt in the view exposes a double endplate contour because there is no longer overlap between the two sides of the endplate (anterior/posterior

**Table 3** Radiographic indices for lumbar developmental spinal stenosis

| Measurement | Median (±SD) | | Median (±SD) | | Median (±SD) | |
|---|---|---|---|---|---|---|
| | SBW:PW | | SBW:PPM | | ABW:IPD | |
| | Patient | Control | Patient | Control | Patient | Control |
| L1 | 2.2 (0.4) | 2.0 (0.4) | 1.3 (0.2) | 1.2 (0.2) | 1.8 (0.2) | 1.6 (0.2) |
| L2 | 2.4 (0.5) | 2.0 (0.3) | 1.3 (0.3) | 1.3 (0.2) | 1.8 (0.2) | 1.6 (0.2) |
| L3 | 2.6 (0.5) | 2.0 (0.2) | 1.4 (0.2) | 1.2 (0.2) | 1.8 (0.2) | 1.6 (0.2) |
| L4 | 2.8 (0.8) | 2.1 (0.3) | 1.4 (0.4) | 1.2 (0.1) | 1.8 (0.3) | 1.6 (0.2) |
| L5 | 3.5 (1.4) | 2.3 (0.4) | 1.6 (0.3) | 1.3 (0.2) | 1.7 (0.2) | 1.6 (0.2) |
| S1 | 3.5 (1.7) | 2.8 (0.9) | 1.4 (0.4) | 1.4 (0.2) | 1.8 (0.4) | 1.5 (0.1) |

*Abbreviations*: *SD* standard deviation, *SBW* sagittal vertebral body width, *PW* pedicle width, *PPM* posterior pedicle margin, *ABW* axial vertebral body width, *IPD* interpedicular distance

**Table 4** Cutoffs for lumbar developmental spinal stenosis

| | Cutoff | Sensitivity | Specificity | Area under curve | *p* value | 95% CI |
|---|---|---|---|---|---|---|
| SBW:PW | | | | | | |
| L1 | 2.0 | 0.76 | 0.50 | 0.67 | 0.18 | 0.53–0.81 |
| L2 | 2.0 | 0.78 | 0.67 | 0.73 | 0.06 | 0.58–0.89 |
| L3 | 2.2 | 0.90 | 0.83 | 0.92 | 0.001 | 0.83–1.00 |
| L4 | 2.2 | 0.92 | 0.83 | 0.94 | <0.001 | 0.88–1.00 |
| L5 | 2.5 | 0.90 | 0.99 | 0.96 | <0.001 | 0.91–1.00 |
| S1 | 2.8 | 0.81 | 0.99 | 0.91 | 0.001 | 0.84–0.99 |
| SBW:PPM | | | | | | |
| L1 | 1.2 | 0.64 | 0.50 | 0.57 | 0.56 | 0.42–0.73 |
| L2 | 1.2 | 0.68 | 0.67 | 0.58 | 0.54 | 0.36–0.79 |
| L3 | 1.2 | 0.76 | 0.67 | 0.66 | 0.20 | 0.45–0.87 |
| L4 | 1.3 | 0.70 | 0.83 | 0.77 | 0.03 | 0.64–0.91 |
| L5 | 1.4 | 0.71 | 0.83 | 0.81 | 0.01 | 0.68–0.94 |
| S1 | 1.4 | 0.56 | 0.67 | 0.58 | 0.53 | 0.45–0.71 |
| ABW:IPD | | | | | | |
| L1 | 1.6 | 0.81 | 0.50 | 0.70 | 0.11 | 0.49–0.90 |
| L2 | 1.6 | 0.95 | 0.67 | 0.71 | 0.09 | 0.44–0.99 |
| L3 | 1.6 | 0.90 | 0.67 | 0.77 | 0.03 | 0.60–0.95 |
| L4 | 1.7 | 0.78 | 0.83 | 0.83 | 0.01 | 0.72–0.94 |
| L5 | 1.7 | 0.61 | 0.83 | 0.72 | 0.09 | 0.58–0.85 |
| S1 | 1.7 | 0.68 | 0.99 | 0.83 | 0.01 | 0.72–0.94 |

*Abbreviations*: *SD* standard deviation, *SBW* sagittal vertebral body width, *PW* pedicle width, *PPM* posterior pedicle margin, *ABW* axial vertebral body width, *IPD* interpedicular distance for AP view; medial/lateral for lateral view). Similar problem can be seen with scoliosis. Readers would have difficultly deciding on which endplate to measure, hence resulting in poorer reliability between the readers. Furthermore, deformities of vertebral body height are well documented and can be due to age-related effects, congenital problems, or osteoporotic fractures [39]. This will lead to age-dependent variations in measurements. Similar problems are observed with the FW measurements.

The limitation of this study is the lack of longitudinal data. Impactful clinical applications cannot be generated at this stage unless longitudinal follow-up of the patient group with DSS shows recurrence of stenosis at nonoperated levels and the control group without DSS shows no development of stenosis symptoms. This is an important follow-up study since our control group is generally younger than our patient group. The lack of age matching and random selection of subjects are also limitations. Nevertheless, the aim of this study is to present clinically useful indices for diagnosis, and the values were based on clearly distinct groups. A potential limitation of our upper level (L1–L2) indices is the lack of patients with upper level stenosis symptoms. Although these are reference indices based on patients and controls, further correlation analysis between symptoms and canal size is required to better understand its relationship in future studies. As the results of our study are based on MRI and X-ray image assessments, at this stage, these radiographic measurements are useful for classifying a subject as having normal or developmentally narrowed spinal canals but they cannot be used for influencing clinical decision and outcomes of surgery. In addition, there is an inherent bias with open recruitment as the possible underlying reason for these "normal" subjects to actively engage us for imaging may be because they experience, however mild, some sort or spinal disorder or symptom.

## Conclusions

To our knowledge, this is the first study to identify easy-to-use radiological indices for DSS. Subject identification can be based on a simple radiograph which, as a screening tool, is more cost-efficient and is more readily available than MRI. The radiographic indices created here are sufficient for case identification since they are based on MRI-diagnosed phenotypes and standardized measurement methods. To understand how a developmentally narrowed spinal canal correlates with symptoms requires further understanding of phenotypic differences between symptomatic and asymptomatic DSS as well as longitudinal follow-up studies to determine any age-related effects on

measurement parameters. There is also value in comparing measurements in the loaded and the unloaded spine and in other populations and ethnic groups for validation. Future study should further determine the clinical significance of DSS especially with the risk of symptom recurrence and reoperation.

## Abbreviations
ABW: Axial vertebral body width; AP: Anteroposterior; CI: Confidence interval; DSS: Developmental spinal stenosis; FW: Foraminal width; ICC: Intraclass correlation; IPD: Interpedicular distance; MRI: Magnetic resonance imaging; PPM: Posterior pedicle margin; PW: Pedicle width; ROC: Receiver operating characteristic; SBW: Sagittal vertebral body width; TE: Echo time; TR: Repetition time

## Acknowledgements
Nil

## Funding
No funding source supported this study.

## Authors' contributions
JPYC conceived and designed the study, performed data collection and statistical analysis, and wrote the manuscript. KKMN and PWHC performed data collection and statistical analysis. DS supervised statistical analysis and wrote the manuscript. KMCC read and approved the final manuscript.

## Competing interests
The authors declare that they have no competing interests.

## References
1. Arbit E, Pannullo S. Lumbar stenosis: a clinical review. Clin Orthop Relat Res. 2001;384:137–43.
2. Cheung JP, Samartzis D, Shigematsu H, Cheung KM. Defining clinically relevant values for developmental spinal stenosis: a large-scale magnetic resonance imaging study. Spine (Phila Pa 1976). 2014;39:1067–76.
3. Djurasovic M, Glassman SD, Carreon LY, Dimar 2nd JR. Contemporary management of symptomatic lumbar spinal stenosis. Orthop Clin North Am. 2010;41:183–91.
4. Singh K, Samartzis D, Biyani A, An HS. Lumbar spinal stenosis. J Am Acad Orthop Surg. 2008;16:171–6.
5. Verbiest H. Pathomorphologic aspects of developmental lumbar stenosis. Orthop Clin North Am. 1975;6:177–96.
6. Kirkaldy-Willis WH, Wedge JH, Yong-Hing K, Reilly J. Pathology and pathogenesis of lumbar spondylosis and stenosis. Spine (Phila Pa 1976). 1978;3:319–28.
7. Verbiest H. Further experiences on the pathological influence of a developmental narrowness of the bony lumbar vertebral canal. J Bone Joint Surg Br. 1955;37-B:576–83.
8. Verbiest H. Fallacies of the present definition, nomenclature, and classification of the stenoses of the lumbar vertebral canal. Spine. 1976;1:217–25.

9. Athiviraham A, Yen D, Scott C, Soboleski D. Clinical correlation of radiological spinal stenosis after standardization for vertebral body size. Clin Radiol. 2007;62:776–80.

10. Bolender NF, Schonstrom NS, Spengler DM. Role of computed tomography and myelography in the diagnosis of central spinal stenosis. J Bone Joint Surg Am. 1985;67:240–6.

11. Chatha DS, Schweitzer ME. MRI criteria of developmental lumbar spinal stenosis revisited. Bull NYU Hosp Jt Dis. 2011;69:303–7.

12. Cheung KM, Ruan D, Chan FL, Fang D. Computed tomographic osteometry of Asian lumbar pedicles. Spine (Phila Pa 1976). 1994;19:1495–8.

13. Fang D, Cheung KM, Ruan D, Chan FL. Computed tomographic osteometry of the Asian lumbar spine. J Spinal Disord. 1994;7:307–16.

14. Hamanishi C, Matukura N, Fujita M, Tomihara M, Tanaka S. Cross-sectional area of the stenotic lumbar dural tube measured from the transverse views of magnetic resonance imaging. J Spinal Disord. 1994;7:388–93.

15. Inui Y, Doita M, Ouchi K, Tsukuda M, Fujita N, Kurosaka M. Clinical and radiologic features of lumbar spinal stenosis and disc herniation with neuropathic bladder. Spine (Phila Pa 1976). 2004;29:869–73.

16. Lee HM, Kim NH, Kim HJ, Chung IH. Morphometric study of the lumbar spinal canal in the Korean population. Spine (Phila Pa 1976). 1995;20: 1679–84.

17. Singh K, Samartzis D, Vaccaro AR, Nassr A, Andersson GB, Yoon ST, Phillips FM, Goldberg EJ, An HS. Congenital lumbar spinal stenosis: a prospective, control-matched, cohort radiographic analysis. Spine J. 2005;5:615–22.

18. Boden SD, Davis DO, Dina TS, Patronas NJ, Wiesel SW. Abnormal magnetic-resonance scans of the lumbar spine in asymptomatic subjects. A prospective investigation. J Bone Joint Surg Am. 1990;72:403–8.

19. Lee SU, Lee JI, Butts K, Carragee E, Fredericson M. Changes in posterior lumbar disk contour abnormality with flexion-extension movement in subjects with low back pain and degenerative disk disease. PMR. 2009;1: 541–6.

20. Herzog RJ, Guyer RD, Graham-Smith A, Simmons Jr ED. Magnetic resonance imaging. Use in patients with low back or radicular pain. Spine (Phila Pa 1976). 1995;20:1834–8.

21. Modic MT, Ross JS. Magnetic resonance imaging in the evaluation of low back pain. Orthop Clin North Am. 1991;22:283–301.

22. Edwards WC, Larocca SH. The developmental segmental sagittal diameter in combined cervical and lumbar spondylosis. Spine (Phila Pa 1976). 1985;10: 42–9.

23. Eisenstein S. Measurements of the lumbar spinal canal in 2 racial groups. Clin Orthop Relat Res. 1976;115:42–6.

24. Jones RA, Thomson JL. The narrow lumbar canal. A clinical and radiological review. J Bone Joint Surg Br. 1968;50:595–605.

25. Williams RM. The narrow lumbar spinal canal. Australas Radiol. 1975;19:356–60.

26. Kitab SA, Alsulaiman AM, Benzel EC. Anatomic radiological variations in developmental lumbar spinal stenosis: a prospective, control-matched comparative analysis. Spine J. 2014;14:808–15.

27. Samartzis D, Mok FP, Karppinen J, Fong DY, Luk KD, Cheung KM. Classification of Schmorl's nodes of the lumbar spine and association with disc degeneration: a large-scale population-based MRI study. Osteoarthr Cartil. 2016; S1063–4584(16)30059-0.

28. Takatalo J, Karppinen J, Taimela S, Niinimaki J, Laitinen J, Sequeiros RB, Samartzis D, Korpelainen R, Nayha S, Remes J, Tervonen O. Association of abdominal obesity with lumbar disc degeneration—a magnetic resonance imaging study. Plos One. 2013;8:e56244.

29. Cheung KM, Samartzis D, Karppinen J, Luk KD. Are "patterns" of lumbar disc degeneration associated with low back pain?: new insights based on skipped level disc pathology. Spine (Phila Pa 1976). 2012;37:E430–8.

30. Samartzis D, Karppinen J, Chan D, Luk KD, Cheung KM. The association of lumbar intervertebral disc degeneration on magnetic resonance imaging with body mass index in overweight and obese adults: a population-based study. Arthritis Rheum. 2012;64:1488–96.

31. Cheung JP, Shigematsu H, Cheung KM. Verification of measurements of lumbar spinal dimensions in T1- and T2-weighted magnetic resonance imaging sequences. Spine J. 2014;14:1476–83.

32. Landis JR, Koch GG. The measurement of observer agreement for categorical data. Biometrics. 1977;33:159–74.

33. Vangeneugden T, Laenen A, Geys H, Renard D, Molenberghs G. Applying concepts of generalizability theory on clinical trial data to investigate sources of variation and their impact on reliability. Biometrics. 2005;61: 295–304.

34. Epstein BS, Epstein JA, Jones MD. Lumbar spinal stenosis. Radiol Clin North Am. 1977;15:227–39.

35. Schonstrom NS, Bolender NF, Spengler DM. The pathomorphology of spinal stenosis as seen on CT scans of the lumbar spine. Spine (Phila Pa 1976). 1985;10:806–11.

36. Kahanovitz N, Rimoin DL, Sillence DO. The clinical spectrum of lumbar spine disease in achondroplasia. Spine (Phila Pa 1976). 1982;7:137–40.

37. Fortuna A, Ferrante L, Acqui M, Santoro A, Mastronardi L. Narrowing of thoraco-lumbar spinal canal in achondroplasia. J Neurosurg Sci. 1989;33: 185–96.

38. Schkrohowsky JG, Hoernschemeyer DG, Carson BS, Ain MC. Early presentation of spinal stenosis in achondroplasia. J Pediatr Orthop. 2007;27: 119–22.

39. Yu W, Lin Q, Zhou X, Shao H, Sun P. Reconsideration of the relevance of mild wedge or short vertebral height deformities across a broad age distribution. Osteoporos Int. 2014;25:2609–15.

# 17

# The effects of scoliosis and subsequent surgery on the shape of the torso

Adrian Gardner[1,2]* (iD), Fiona Berryman[1] and Paul Pynsent[2]

## Abstract

**Background:** Adolescent idiopathic scoliosis (AIS) causes asymmetry of the torso, and this is often the primary concern of patients. Surgery aims to minimise the visual asymmetry. It is not clear how scoliosis makes the torso asymmetric or how scoliosis surgery changes that asymmetry when compared to the distribution of asymmetries seen in a non-scoliotic group of normal controls.

**Methods:** Surface topography images were captured for a group with AIS both pre-operatively and post-operatively. Identifiable points were compared between the images to identify the effects of AIS on the shape of the torso by looking at the relative heights and distances from the midline of the shoulders, axillae and waist in a two-dimensional coronal view. This was then compared to a previously reported group of normal non-scoliotic children to analyse whether surgery recreated normality.

**Results:** There were 172 pairs of images with 164 females and 8 males, mean age at pre-operative scan of 13. 7 years. The normal group was 642 images (237 females and 405 males) from 116 males and 79 females, mean age of 12.5 years.
The curve patterns seen in the scoliotic group matched the patterns of a main thoracic curve ($n = 146$) and main thoracolumbar curve ($n = 26$). The asymmetries seen in both shoulders, axillae and waist were different between the two different types of curve. Across both groups, the shoulder asymmetry was less than that of the corresponding axillae. There was a statistically significant reduction in all asymmetries following surgery in the main thoracic group ($p < 0.001$). This was not seen in the main thoracolumbar group, thought to be due to the small sample size. In the main thoracic group, there were statistically significant differences in the asymmetries between the post-operative and normal groups in the shoulders and axillae ($p < 0.001$) but not the waist.

**Conclusions:** This paper demonstrates quantitatively the range of asymmetries seen in the AIS torso and the degree to which surgery alters them. Surgery does not recreate normality but does cause a statistically significant change in torso shape towards that seen in a non-scoliotic group.

**Keywords:** Scoliosis, Surface topography, Surgery, Shoulders, Axillae, Waist, Normal, ISIS2

## Background

Within the clinical presentation of adolescent idiopathic scoliosis (AIS), it is common for concern to be raised by both patients and parents around visible asymmetry of the back [1]. This relates to various features including a difference in the height of the shoulders and axillae, inequality of the waist creases and a prominence of one of the scapulae. One of the goals of surgery for AIS is the equalisation of these asymmetries, which translates into improvement in the patient's self-esteem and life satisfaction [2].

The results of scoliosis surgery are routinely reported as changes in the radiographic Cobb angle [3]. This is a measure of the spinal shape internal to the body rather than the external appearance. There is inherent difficulty in using radiographs as a way of measuring areas and shapes within the body comprised of soft tissue rather than bone. Serial radiography also comes with the price tag of a cumulative radiation dose to the body [4]. Surface topography has been developed as a non-radiation

---

* Correspondence: adriangardnerd@googlemail.com
[1]The Royal Orthopaedic NHS Foundation Trust, Bristol Road South, Northfield, Birmingham B31 2AP, UK
[2]Department of Anatomy, Institute of Clinical Science, University of Birmingham, Edgbaston, Birmingham B15 2TT, UK

method of documenting the three-dimensional shape of the back. The Integrated Shape Imaging System (ISIS) [5] is now in its second version (ISIS2) [6]. The system analyses a digital photograph of the child's back which has horizontal lines projected on to it. Fourier transform profilometry is used to create a surface for analysis. The output gives both quantitative and graphical information on the shape for the back in three-dimensions. The use of ISIS2 has been reported previously [6–8].

This paper documents the variability of the relative height of the shoulders, axillae and waist, and also the distance from the midline of the axillae and waist in a group of patients with AIS both pre-operatively and post-operatively. The post-operative values are then compared to previously established normative values for non-scoliotic children [9].

## Methods

Ethical and research governance approval has been obtained for both groups in this study from the NRES committee West Midlands—South Birmingham (11/H1207/10) and the NRES committee East Midlands—Northampton (15/EM/0283).

This analysis is a comparison of two groups. The first is a group of children with AIS who, as part of standard care, have surface topography (ISIS2) measured both before and after surgery as a paired set of images. The second is a group of non-scoliotic children who are part of a longitudinal data collection of surface shape measured using ISIS2 and has been reported on previously [9]. Torso parameters were identified in both groups which were then compared.

All of the scoliotic group had an MRI scan of the whole spine as part of their routine care. Children with neural axis anomalies or other abnormal findings have been excluded from this analysis. None of the study group has been treated in a brace as part of their care. For the majority of subjects, surgery was undertaken using modern posterior based pedicle screw techniques ($n = 98$). An anterior release was used in selected cases for a large stiff

curve ($n = 63$). Anterior-only surgery was used selectively for main thoracolumbar curve patterns in the absence of a large compensatory thoracic curve ($n = 11$).

All images in the study were acquired using ISIS2. The degree of spinal curvature in the coronal plane (a two-dimensional measure) was measured with the Lateral Asymmetry parameter from the automated ISIS2 analysis. In this study, a positive number indicated that the scoliosis was convex to the right, and a negative number indicated convex to the left. The ISIS2 images were analysed to find the two dimensional torso points that identify the position of the axillae, shoulders and waist. The axillae points were the most superior points of the posterior axillary folds. The shoulder points were at the superior edge of the torso along a vertical line from the axillae points [10]. The waist points identified were the 'minimal waist' [11], which corresponds to the narrowest waist and is the most suitable definition of the waist in a scoliotic population.

The positions of the points were then processed to create parameters comparing the two sides of the trunk against each other, Diff Height for a difference in vertical height and Diff Off for a difference in horizontal distance from the midline. This created the parameters Shoulder Diff Height (ShDiffHt), Axillary Diff Height (AxDiffHt) and Waist Diff Height (WaistDiffHt), Axillary Diff Off (AxDiffOff) and Waist Diff Off (WaistDiffOff) (see Table 1 and Fig. 1). Again, a positive number for the measured torso parameter indicated that the right side was higher than the left (DiffHt parameters) or further from the midline than the left (DiffOff parameters).

The data on the torso points are presented as data ellipses [12], as this clearly represents the bivariate nature of the data [13]. The layouts are displayed in the same way for each plot for the main thoracic (main thoracolumbar) curves. Pre-operative data are in green (dark green), post-operative data in blue (purple) and the non-scoliotic data in red (orange). The mean point is the solid dot in each colour. The ellipse is the 95% confidence interval about the mean in the respective colour.

**Table 1** A table of the torso parameter and their definitions as shown pictorially in Fig. 1 [9]

| Orientation | Torso parameter | Definition |
| --- | --- | --- |
| Vertical measurements | ShDiffHt | The difference in vertical height between the shoulder points |
| | AxDiffHt | The difference in vertical height between the axillary points |
| | WaistDiffHt | The difference in vertical height between the waist points |
| Horizontal measurements | axRoff | The horizontal distance from the midline to the right axillary point |
| | axLoff | The horizontal distance from the midline to the left axillary point |
| | waistRoff | The horizontal distance from the midline to the right waist point |
| | waistLoff | The horizontal distance from the midline to the left waist point |
| | AxDiffOff | The difference between axRoff and axLoff |
| | WaistDiffOff | The difference between waistRoff and waistLoff |

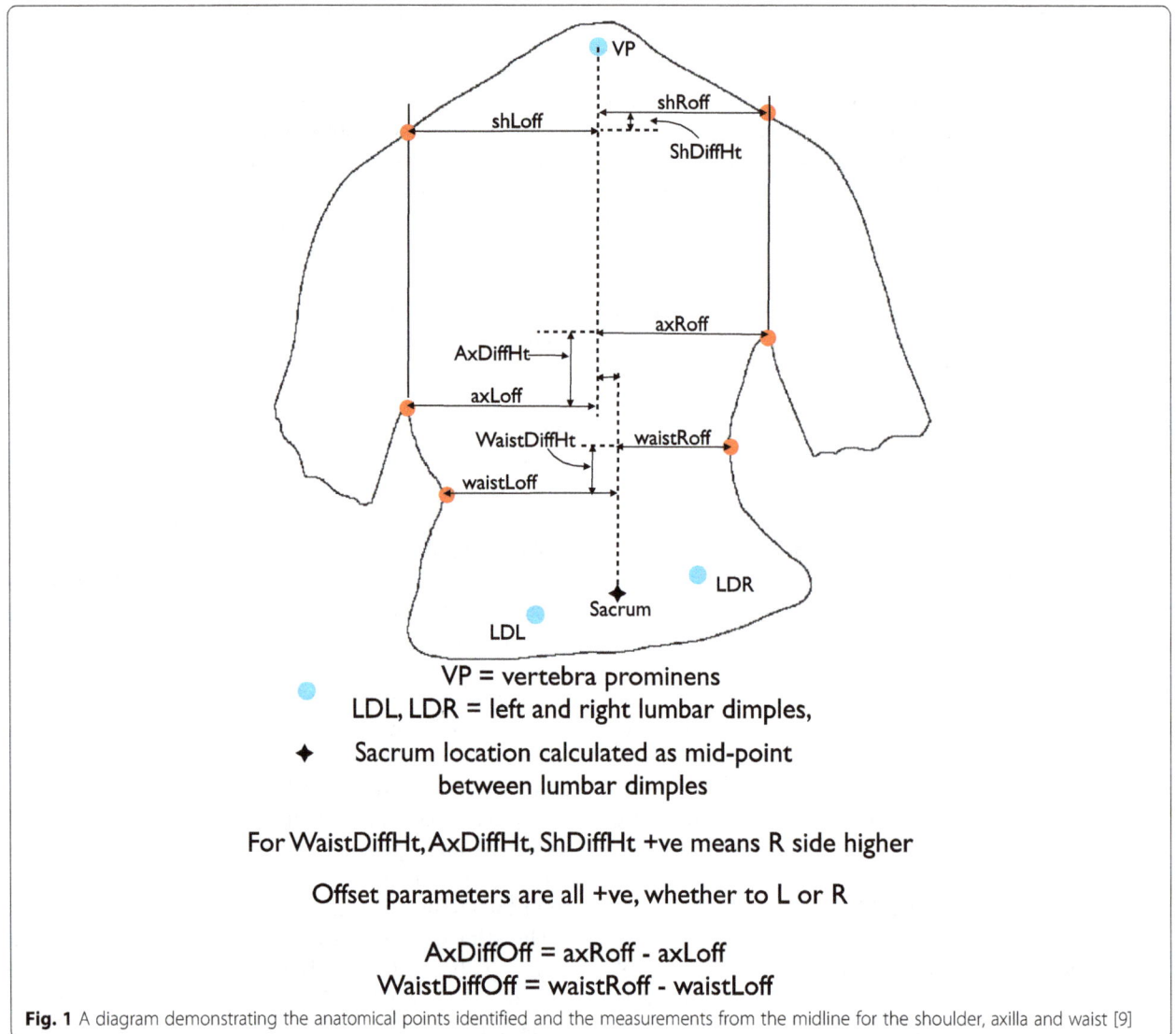

**Fig. 1** A diagram demonstrating the anatomical points identified and the measurements from the midline for the shoulder, axilla and waist [9]

In the $x$-axis, a positive number is a curve convex to the right. In the $y$-axis a positive number indicates that the right side is higher, or further from the midline, than the left. The box and whisker plots show the data spread of each individual parameter with the median value as the solid bar within the box, which represents the interquartile range. The whiskers from the box represent 1.5 times the interquartile range. Within the box, the dot is the mean value with the 95% confidence interval of the mean as the bars either side.

As there is a difference in the number of pre- and post-operative cases and that of the non-scoliotic group,

propensity matching was performed to confirm that this difference did not affect the results.

All analysis was carried out using R [14]. Comparisons of the data were performed with the $t$ test for parametric data and the Wilcoxon rank sum test for non-parametric data. Statistical significance was defined as $p < 0.05$.

## Results

The demographic information of both groups is shown in Table 2. In the non-scoliotic group, there have been serial measurements and images captured over 5 years of the same children, with subjects having between 1

**Table 2** The demographic information of both groups

|  | Males | Females | Mean age (years) | SD age (years) | Number of images for analysis |
|---|---|---|---|---|---|
| Non-scoliotic | 405 | 237 | 12.5 | 1.8 | 642 individual images |
| Scoliotic | 8 | 164 | 13.7 (at pre-operative scan) | 1.4 | 172 pairs of pre-operative and post-operative images |

and 5 images taken depending on the length of time they have been in the study. Thus, the number of individual images available for analysis is greater than the number of participants. This group consists of 116 males and 79 females. In the scoliotic group, each subject has a pre-operative and post-operative image giving 172 sets of paired data. Neither the time between the pre-operative image and surgery nor between surgery and the post-operative image was normally distributed. Surgery was a median of 346 days after the pre-operative image (IQR 320 days, range 1 to 1211 days). The median time from surgery to the post-operative image was 200 days (IQR 246 days, range 25–1321 days).

The ethnicity in each group was predominantly Caucasian with smaller numbers of participants with either an Afro-Caribbean or Indian heritage. In the scoliotic group, 11% of the total were not Caucasian. In the non-scoliotic group, 3% of the total were not Caucasian.

In the non-scoliotic group, a small curve in the spine in the coronal plane is seen in nearly all of the participants. The major curve was judged to be proximal thoracic (PT) in 21 subjects. There was no curve seen in eight subjects.

As described previously [9], patterns of curve were used to subdivide the data into a main thoracic group with compensatory thoracolumbar curve and a main thoracolumbar curve with compensatory thoracic curve [15]. In the scoliotic group, the largest subgroup had a main thoracic curve with a smaller number with a main thoracolumbar curve. There were no main PT curves. The numbers in each subdivision are shown in Table 3.

The data in the main thoracic curve group were normally distributed. The data in the main thoracolumbar curve group were not normally distributed. Figures 2, 3, 4, 5 and 6 show the data ellipses for the main thoracic curve with compensatory thoracolumbar curve (mean and 95% confidence interval ellipse) and Figs. 7, 8, 9, 10 and 11 show the data for main thoracolumbar curve with compensatory thoracic curve (median and 95% percentile ellipse). The individual data points for the non-scoliotic group are not presented as they obscure the data points of the pre-operative and post-operative groups.

Tables 4 and 5 show the mean (median) values for the parameters in the pre-operative and post-operative groups. The significance in the change from pre-operative to post-operative is also shown. Tables 6 and 7

**Table 3** The number in each subdivision of curve type in each group (PT- Proximal thoracic curve, NC- no curve)

| | Main thoracic | Main thoracolumbar | Others |
|---|---|---|---|
| Non-scoliotic | 387 | 227 | 28 (PT and NC) |
| Scoliotic | 146 | 26 | 0 |

compare the mean (median) values of the post-operative group to that of the non-scoliotic group.

The compensatory curves had no significant difference in effect (see Tables 4 and 5) on the anatomically distant points (for example the effect of the compensatory thoracolumbar curve on the shoulder or axillae points). The waist points and associated trunk imbalance in the main thoracic curve group are due to the effects of the thoracic curve rather than the smaller thoracolumbar curve. This point is further expanded in the 'Discussion' section.

Normalising the data for size of torso did not affect the distributions shown in the analysis. The effect of this analysis using a smaller group of non-scoliotic subjects after propensity matching was not appreciably different so the entire cohort of the non-scoliotic group was kept for the analysis.

## Discussion

AIS is a disorder affecting the adolescent spine and is known to come with a 'psychological burden'. There is a dislike of the asymmetry of the torso and overall body shape that presents with a spectrum of symptoms including mental health disorders [16, 17]. One of the aims of scoliosis surgery is to minimise the visible deformity, improving the symmetry of the torso as safely as possible. In a previous paper, using the same methodology as used here, Gardner et al. [9] have reported the range of normality based on two dimensional torso points in non-scoliotic children. This 'normal' group demonstrated that there is a degree of spinal curve in the coronal plane measurable in most children, with differences between the sides of the torso for the shoulder, axillae and waist points. That is, non-scoliotic children are not perfectly symmetrical in the coronal plane and tend to have some spinal curvature, although it is of low magnitude. The data from Gardner et al. [9] acts as a group of normative values to which the AIS group has been referenced.

The AIS group has a larger number of main thoracic curves with compensatory thoracolumbar curves than main thoracolumbar curves with compensatory thoracic curves. This is a similar distribution to that previously reported [15]. The main thoracic curves are mainly convex to the right and an increasing curve is associated with increasing difference between the right and left sides of the torso. The axillae are both more superior (AxDiffHt) and further from the midline (AxDiffOff) on the right in comparison to the left with an increasing scoliosis (Figs. 3 and 4). No effect of an increasing curve on ShDiffHt is seen (Fig. 2). This suggests that the shoulder girdle is compensating for an asymmetry of the underlying torso (demonstrated by the difference in position of the right and left axillae). The independence of

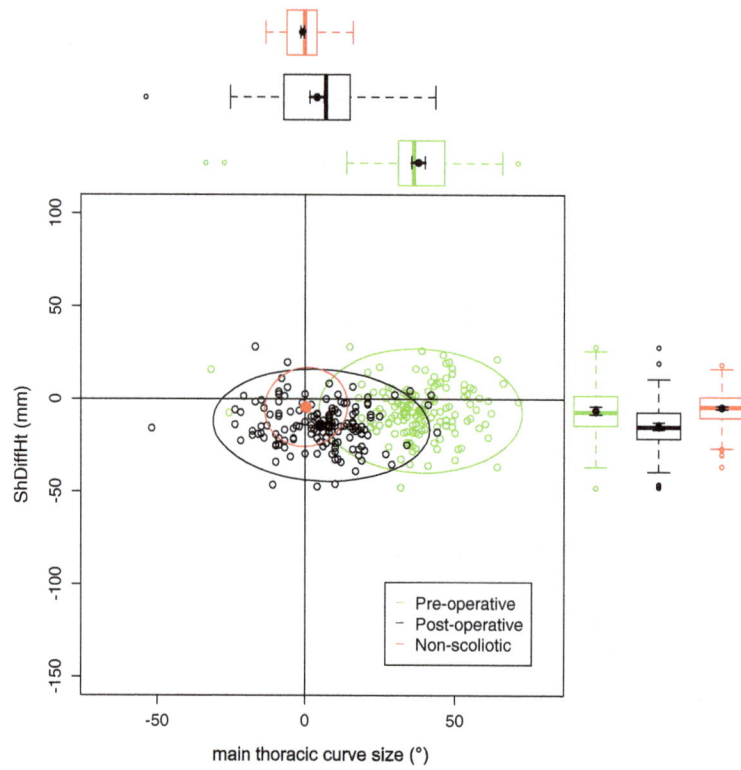

**Fig. 2** Data ellipses for the main thoracic curve pattern (main thoracic curve) showing ShDiffHt

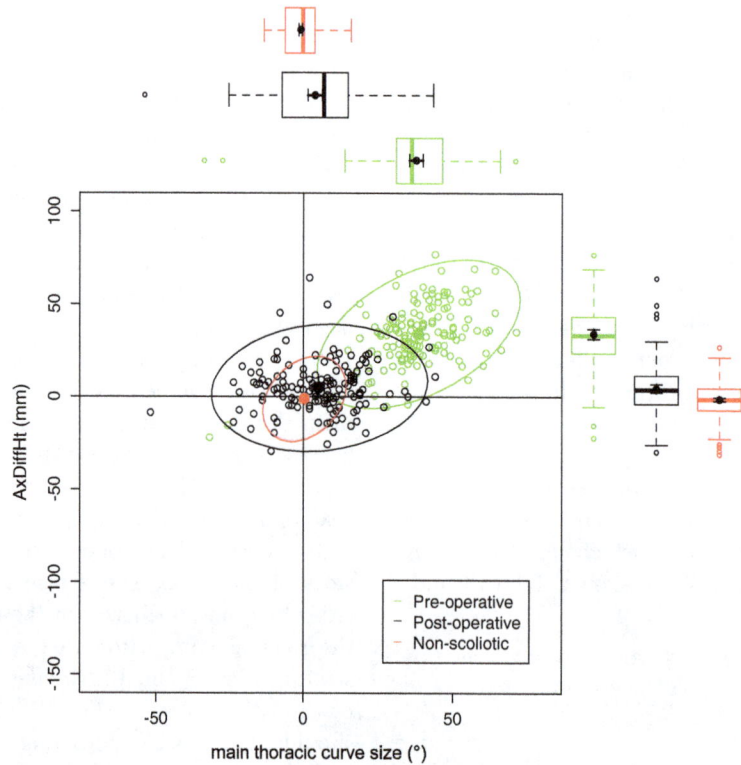

**Fig. 3** Data ellipses for the main thoracic curve pattern (main thoracic curve) showing AxDiffHt

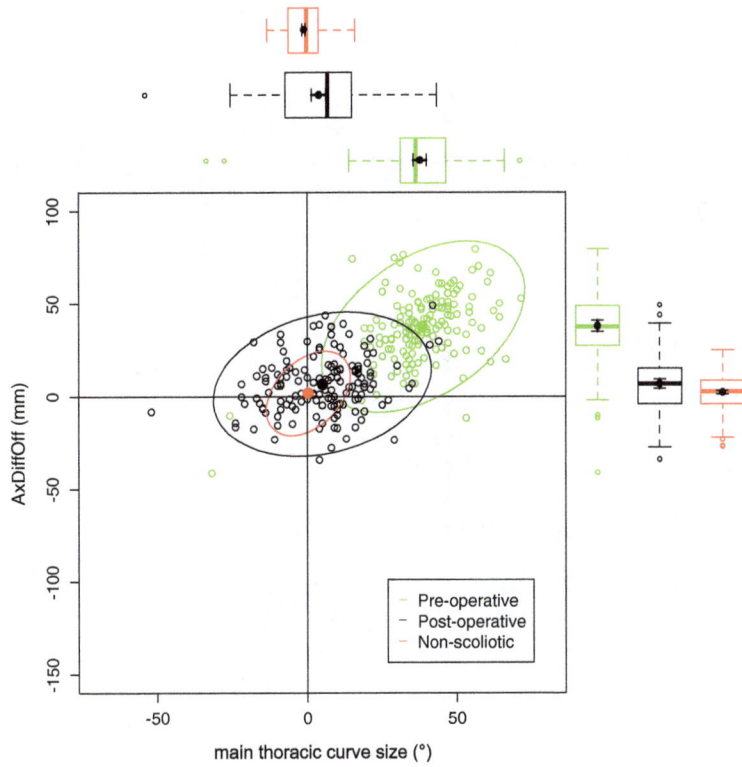

**Fig. 4** Data ellipses for the main thoracic curve pattern (main thoracic curve) showing AxDiffOff

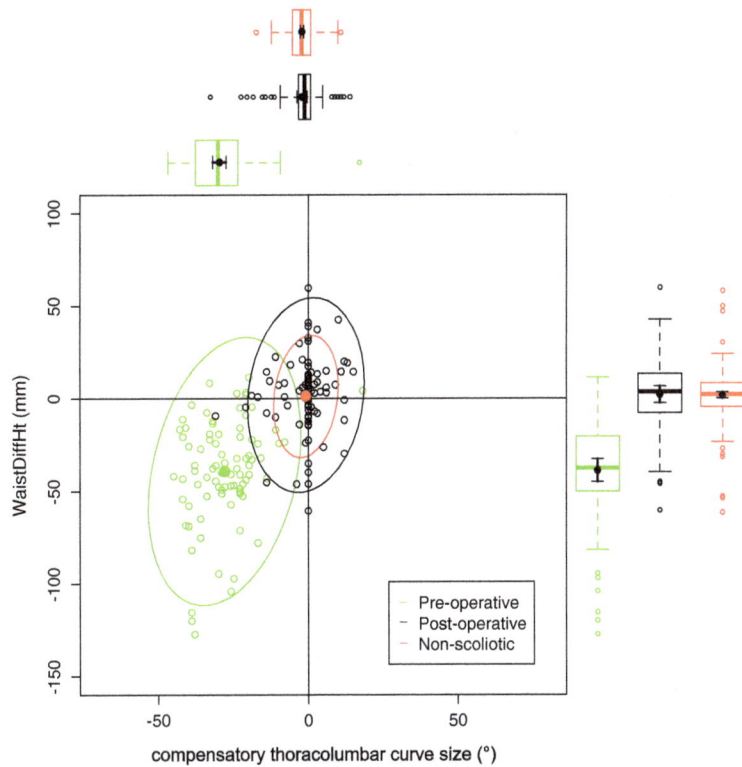

**Fig. 5** Data ellipses for the main thoracic curve pattern (compensatory thoracolumbar curve) showing WaistDiffHt

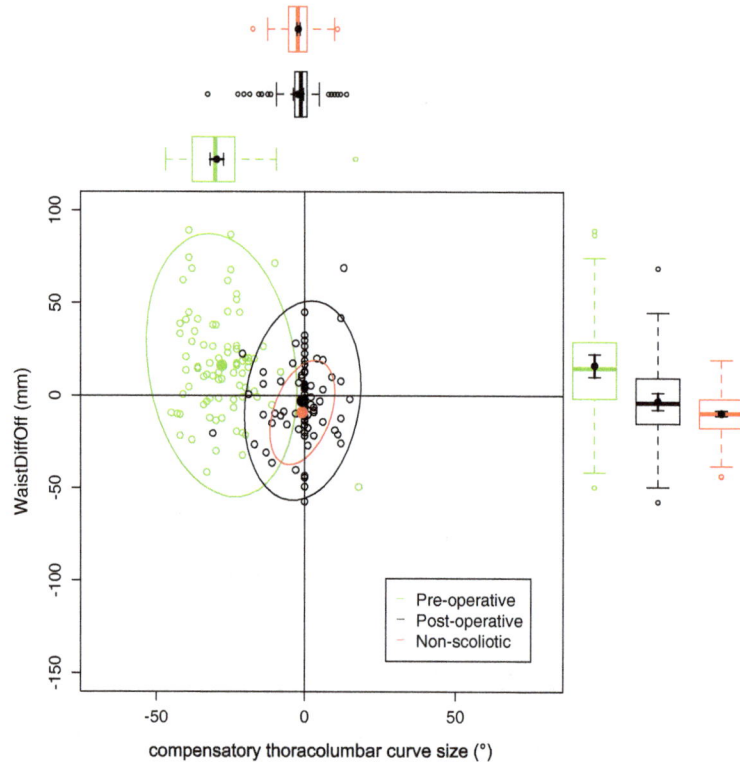

**Fig. 6** Data ellipses for the main thoracic curve pattern (compensatory thoracolumbar curve) showing WaistDiffOff

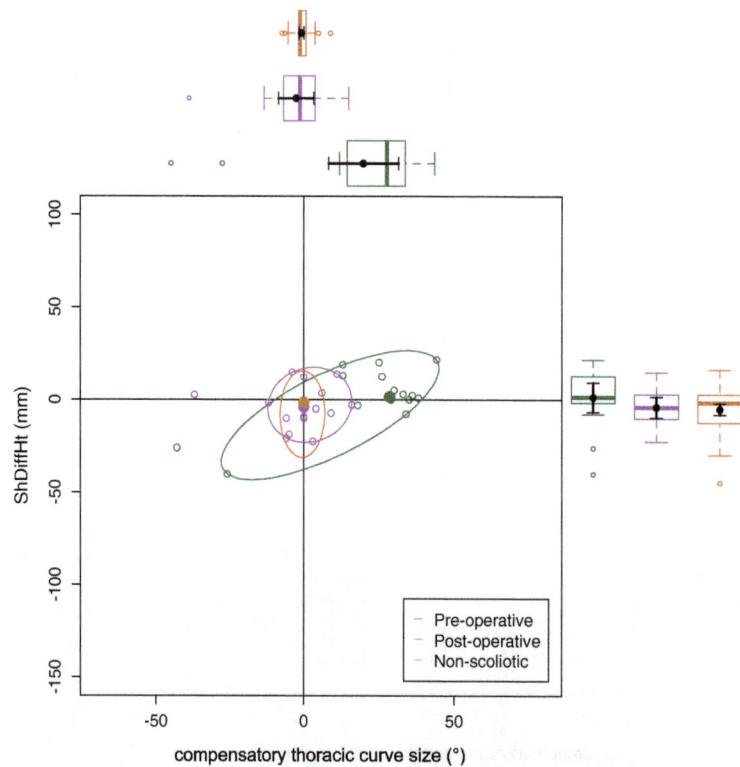

**Fig. 7** Data ellipses for the main thoracolumbar curve pattern (compensatory thoracic curve) showing ShDiffHt

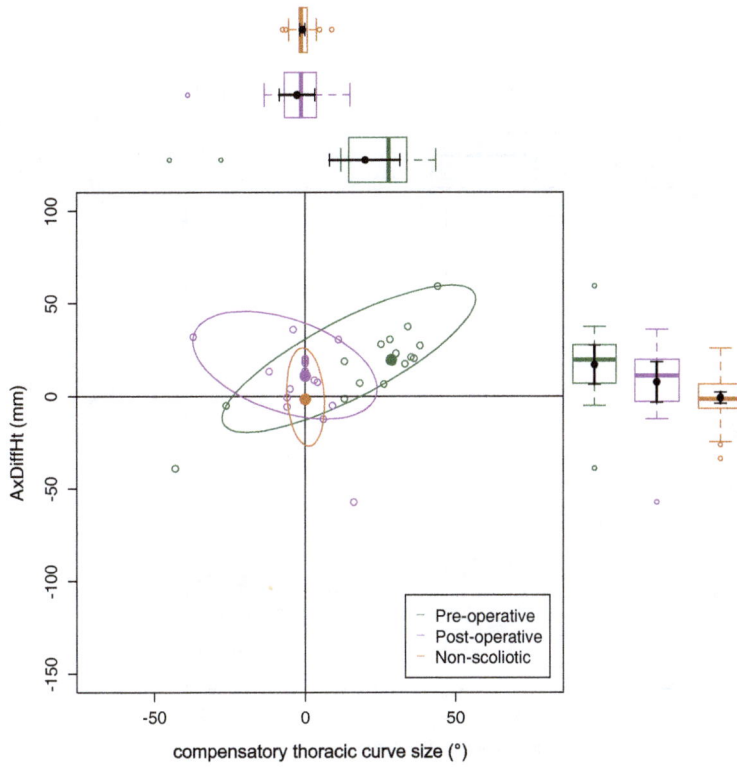

**Fig. 8** Data ellipses for the main thoracolumbar curve pattern (compensatory thoracic curve) showing AxDiffHt

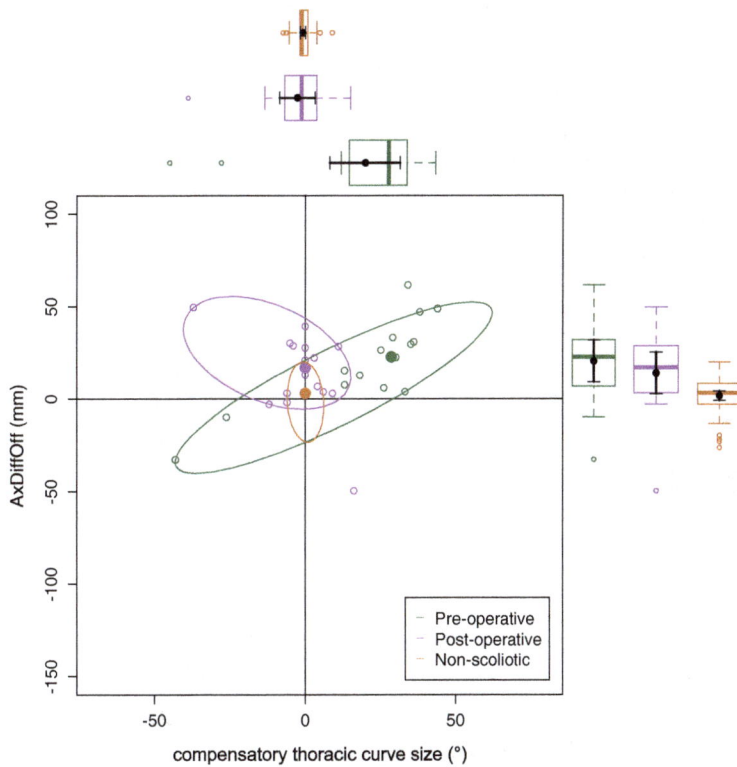

**Fig. 9** Data ellipses for the main thoracolumbar curve pattern (compensatory thoracic curve) showing AxDiffOff

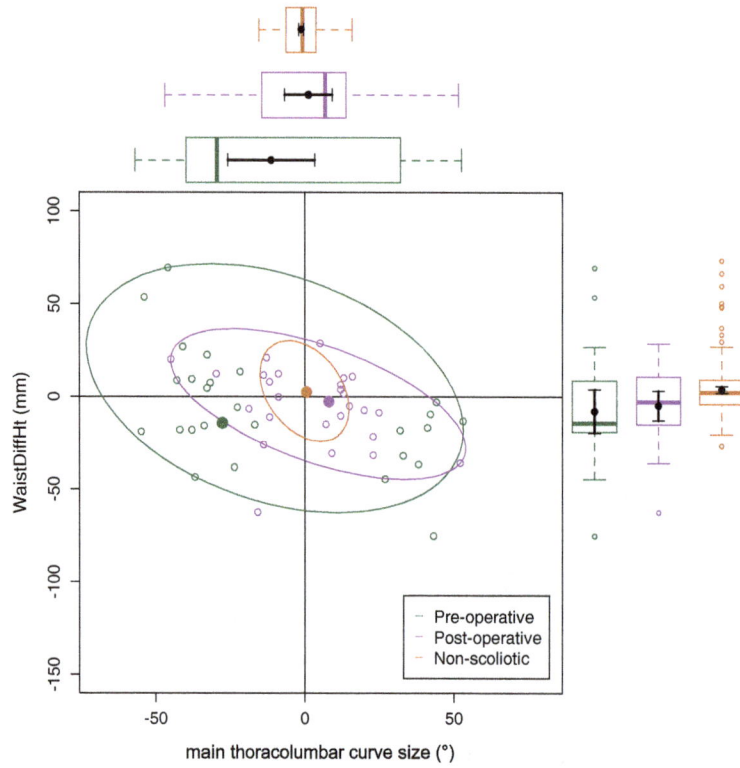

**Fig. 10** Data ellipses for the main thoracolumbar curve pattern (main thoracolumbar curve) showing WaistDiffHt

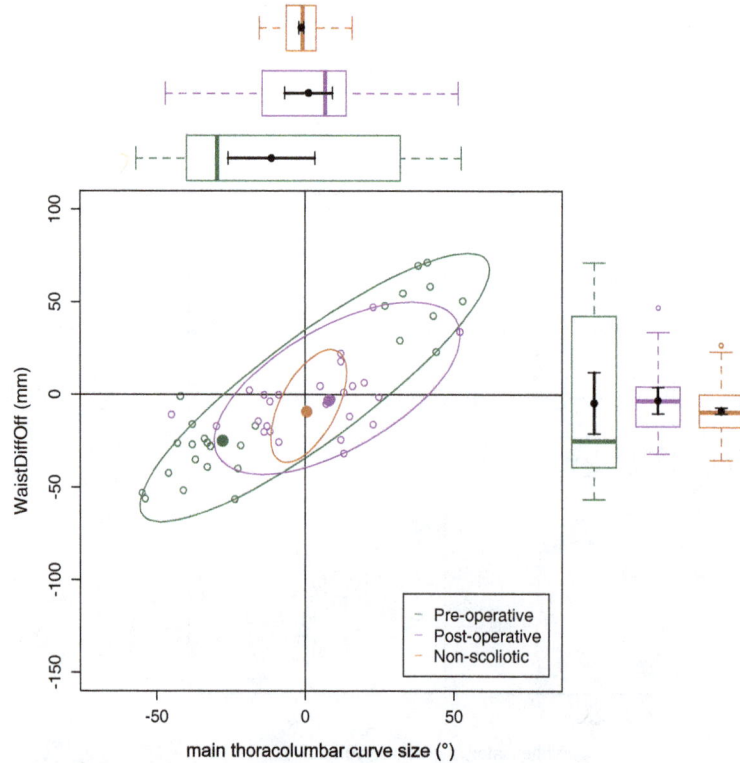

**Fig. 11** Data ellipses for the main thoracolumbar curve pattern (main thoracolumbar curve) showing WaistDiffOff

**Table 4** A table demonstrating the mean value (and standard deviation) of the parameters measured in the main thoracic pattern for the pre-operative and post-operative scoliotic group with the significance of the change also shown

| | Pre-operative | Post-operative | Significance |
|---|---|---|---|
| Curve size (°) | 38.5 (13.6) | 5.1 (14.6) | < 0.001 |
| ShDiffHt (mm) | −6.1 (13.5) | −14.3 (13.8) | < 0.001 |
| AxDiffHt (mm) | 34.1 (16.1) | 4.8 (13.8) | < 0.001 |
| WaistDiffHt (mm) | −38.8 (28.6) | 1.9 (20.8) | < 0.001 |
| AxDiffOff (mm) | 37.9 (18.5) | 6.6 (15.6) | < 0.001 |
| WaistDiffOff (mm) | 16.3 (28.2) | −2.9 (21.3) | < 0.001 |

**Table 6** A table showing the statistical analysis of the post-operative group for the main thoracic curve group compared to the non-scoliotic group

| | Post-operative scoliosis | Non-scoliotic | Significance of difference |
|---|---|---|---|
| ShDiffHt (mm) | −14.3 (13.8) | −4.3 (8.7) | < 0.001 |
| AxDiffHt (mm) | 4.8 (13.8) | −1.0 (9.4) | < 0.001 |
| WaistDiffHt (mm) | 1.9 (20.8) | 1.4 (13.2) | 0.838 |
| AxDiffOff (mm) | 6.6 (15.6) | 2.0 (9.2) | < 0.001 |
| WaistDiffOff (mm) | −2.9 (21.3) | −9.2 (11.1) | 0.013 |

Non-scoliotic data form Gardner et al. [9]

movement of the shoulder girdle relative to the torso may well explain why there is moderate to poor correlation of the intraoperative radiographic features of shoulder position to the post-operative shoulder position [18].

The waist is also increasingly asymmetric with an increasing compensatory thoracolumbar curve. As already stated, with an increasing curve, the axillary points become higher and further from the midline on the same side as the convexity of the curve. However, with the waist points, both DiffHt and DiffOff increase in magnitude but in differing directions to each other (Figs. 5 and 6). The reasons for this are unclear but may represent the difference between the relationship of the waist to the spine and the spine to the shoulder girdle. In thoracolumbar curves, the pelvis is the fixed base on which the spine deforms. In thoracic curves the shoulder girdle moves around the already deformed spine.

The effects of the compensatory curve (a thoracic curve on the waist points or a thoracolumbar curve on the axillae and shoulder points) are less clear, although the main thoracolumbar curve has only a small effect on the shoulder and axilla (Figs. 7, 8 and 9). The effect of the main thoracic curve on the waist is more marked

and reflects trunk asymmetry caused by a large thoracic curve (Figs. 5 and 6). The effects of the compensatory curve inferior to this thoracic curve are hidden in the effects of the thoracic curve. This is partly due to the mismatch of curve sizes between the main and compensatory curves, with the main curve exerting a relatively larger effect on the shape of the torso. In the main thoracolumbar curve group, a number had a small compensatory thoracic curve. In this circumstance, the overall curve pattern is known to present primarily with waist asymmetry [19]. This could explain the relationship of a thoracolumbar curve on the shoulder and axillae points suggesting that the small thoracic curve exerts a minimal effect.

The number of patients in the main thoracolumbar group is much smaller compared to the number in the main thoracic group. This is the likely reason for the skewed distribution of the data (Figs. 7, 8, 9, 10 and 11) and supports the decision to use non-parametric statistics to analyse this subgroup. With a greater sample size, it would be reasonable to expect a lessening of the effect of the outliers on the average value and a more uniform distribution allowing the use of the mean and 95% predictive confidence ellipse.

Surgical intervention leads to a statistically significant reduction in the size of the scoliosis in both coronal curve patterns (Tables 4 and 5). In the main thoracic group, this is accompanied by a reduction in the amount

**Table 5** A table demonstrating the median value (and values of quartile 1 and 3) of the parameters measured in the main thoracolumbar curve pattern for the pre-operative and post-operative scoliotic group with the significance of the change also shown

| | Pre-operative | Post-operative | Significance |
|---|---|---|---|
| Curve size (°) | −28.0 (−38.0 to 32.8) | 8.0 (−12.8 to 14.5) | 0.148 |
| ShDiffHt (mm) | 1.5 (−0.8 to 12.5) | −3.9 (−10.9 to 2.8) | 0.117 |
| AxDiffHt (mm) | 19.6 (6.9 to 27.4) | 10.9 (−1.9 to 19.4) | 0.044 |
| WaistDiffHt (mm) | −14.1 (−18.7 to 8.4) | −2.5 (−13.9 to 10.7) | 0.473 |
| AxDiffOff (mm) | 22.8 (7.1 to 31.4) | 17.0 (3.1 to 28.5) | 0.348 |
| WaistDiffOff (mm) | −24.9 (−37.9 to 39.4) | −3.0 (−16.7 to 4.1) | 0.727 |

**Table 7** A table showing the statistical analysis of the post-operative group for the main thoracolumbar curve group compared to the non-scoliotic group

| | post-operative scoliosis | non-scoliotic | significance of difference |
|---|---|---|---|
| ShDiffHt (mm) | −3.9 (−10.9 to 2.8) | −3.9 (8.5) | 0.844 |
| AxDiffHt (mm) | 10.9 (−1.9 to 19.4) | −2.2 (9.8) | 0.004 |
| WaistDiffHt (mm) | −2.5 (13.9 to 10.7) | 2.6 (14.0) | 0.136 |
| AxDiffOff (mm) | 17.0 (3.1 to 28.5) | 1.0 (8.4) | < 0.001 |
| WaistDiffOff (mm) | −3.0 (−16.7 to 4.1) | −9.1 (13.1) | 0.215 |

Non-scoliotic data form Gardner et al. [9]

of asymmetry in the torso at the axillae and waist in both DiffOff and DiffHt (Figs. 3, 4, 5 and 6), and this is statistically significant for all parameters. Interestingly, there is a statistically significant increase in the difference between the left and right sides in ShDiffHt (Fig. 2) with the mean value suggesting that the left is more superior than the right following surgery, a worsening of shoulder height asymmetry, for reasons unknown. The difficulties in achieving balanced shoulders in the post-operative patient remain a challenge [20]. It has been shown that the effect of unbalanced shoulders can reduce over time through other compensatory mechanisms [21]. Reviewing the torso as a whole, surgery is successful in reducing the size of the curve and equalising the shape of the posterior torso.

In the main thoracic group, the ellipses show that surgery improves the torso asymmetry towards that seen in the non-scoliotic group (Figs. 2, 3, 4, 5 and 6). There is still a statistically significant difference in the means for shoulder and axillae points between the post-operative group and the non-scoliotic group (Table 6). However, there is no significant difference in waist position between the post-operative and non-scoliotic groups. The change that occurs following scoliosis surgery is towards the range of asymmetries seen in the non-scoliotic group, although surgery does not completely recreate normality. It is worth noting that in all of the parameters, although the average values are similar, the spread of the data is more dispersed in the post-operative group compared to the non-scoliotic group. Whilst scoliosis surgery changes body shape towards a non-scoliotic population, there is still a difference seen. The answer to the question 'does scoliosis surgery recreate normality?' has to be no, but surgery provides a statistically significant change towards a normal shape.

The methodology for the torso points used here is scalar and linear rather than angular as used by Matamalas et al. [22, 23]. The criticism of a non-angular measurement is that it is vulnerable to bias related to differing size between subjects that is not seen in an angular measurement. When all of data presented here was normalised using back length for ShDiffHt, AxDiffHt and WaistDiffHt, axillary width for AxDiffOff or waist width for WaistDiffOff, there were no differences seen in the analysis results and normalisation did not add to the conclusions drawn. Angular measures can be difficult to convert to useful, measurable information in a clinical practice. Linear measures are easy to understand and reproduce and thus are preferred here.

It is noted that the results quoted here represent the position of the torso at the point in time that the post-operative image was taken. With continued growth and then subsequent changes through the ageing process, it is possible that over time, the position described here would change. It would be a valid study to revisit this scoliotic group at 5 years post-surgery to document how the torso has changed over the intervening period.

## Conclusion

This work demonstrates the metrics of trunk asymmetry in a scoliotic group and the effects of scoliosis surgery in reducing these asymmetries. Current surgical techniques do not make the spine straight in the coronal plane, nor do they equalise all asymmetries in the trunk. Surgery can make a statistically significant difference to body shape and when compared to a non-scoliotic group does reduce the size of the torso asymmetries towards the shape of the non-scoliotic torso. Future directions for this work will compare this change in body shape with patient-derived measures of their own deformity, such as the Spinal Appearance Questionnaire [24], to examine what the patients feel about their outcomes from surgery, which previously have been noted to be different from what the surgeon feels has been the outcome [25].

### Acknowledgements

We would like to acknowledge Professor Joanne Wilton of the Department of Anatomy, Institute of Clinical Science, University of Birmingham for her continued support and the Birmingham Orthopaedic Charity for funding this work.

### Funding

This work was funded by the Birmingham Orthopaedic Charity and forms part of a PhD at the University of Birmingham which is separately part funded by the Royal Orthopaedic Hospital NHS Foundation Trust.

### Authors' contributions

AG carried out the analysis and wrote the paper. FB collected the data and guided the analysis of the data. PP conceived the idea and provided statistical and technical support. All three authors have given final approval for the work to be published and agree to be accountable for all aspects of the work.

### Competing interests

The authors declare that they have no competing interests.

### References

1. Misterska E, Glowacki M, Harasymczuk J. Assessment of spinal appearance in female patients with adolescent idiopathic scoliosis treated operatively. Med Sci Moni. 2011;17:CR404–10.
2. Zhang J, He D, Gao J, Yu X, Sun H, Chen Z, et al. Changes in life satisfaction and self-esteem in patients with adolescent idiopathic scoliosis with and without surgical intervention. Spine. 2011;36:741–5.
3. Cobb J. Outline for the study of scoliosis. AAOS Instructional Course Lectures. 1948;5:261–75.
4. Law M, Ma W, Lau D, Chan E, Yip L, Lam W. Cumulative radiation exposure and associated cancer risk estimates for scoliosis patients: impact of repetitive full spine radiography. Eur J Radiol. 2016;85:625–8.
5. Turner-Smith A, Harris J, Houghton G, Jefferson R. A method for analysis of back shape in scoliosis. J Biomech. 1988;21:497–509.

6.    Berryman F, Pynsent P, Fairbank J, Disney S. A new system for measuring three-dimensional back shape in scoliosis. Eur Spine J. 2008;17:663–72.

7.    Berryman F, Pynsent P, Fairbank J. Thoracic kyphosis measurements with ISIS2. Stud Health Technol and Inform. 2008;140:68–71.

8.    Berryman F, Pynsent P, Fairbank J. Variability in Lateral Asymmetry measurements with ISIS2. J Bone Joint Surg Br. 2008;90(SUPP III):479.

9.    Gardner A, Berryman F, Pynsent P. What is the variability in shoulder, axilla and waist position in a group of adolescents? J Anat. 2017;231:221–8.

10.   Akel I, Pekmezci M, Hayran M, Genc Y, Kocak O, Derman O, et al. Evaluation of shoulder balance in the normal adolescent population and its correlation with radiological parameters. Eur Spine J. 2008;17:348–54.

11.   Mason C, Katzmarzyk P. Effect of the site of measurement of the waist circumference on the prevalence of the metabolic syndrome. Am J Cardiol. 2016;103:1716–20.

12.   Fox J, Weisberg S. An R Companion to Applied Regression. 2nd ed. New York: Sage Publications Inc; 2011.

13.   Friendly M, Monette G, Fox J. Elliptical insights: understanding statistical methods through elliptical geometry. Stat Sci. 2013;28:1–39.

14.   R Core Team R: A language and environment for statistical computing. R Foundation for Statistical Computing, 2016. Vienna, Austria [Online]. Available: http://www.R-project.org/.

15.   Lenke L, Betz R, Harms J, Bridwell K, Clements D, Lowe T, et al. Adolescent idiopathic scoliosis: a new classification to determine the extent of spinal arthrodesis. J Bone Joint Surg Am. 2001;83:1169–81.

16.   Payne W, Oligvie J, Resnick M, Kane R, Transfeldt E, Blum R. Does scoliosis have a psychological impact and does gender make a difference? Spine. 1997;22:1380–4.

17.   Smith F, Latchford G, Hall R, Millner P, Dickson R. Indications of disordered eating behaviour in adolescent patients with idiopathic scoliosis. J Bone Joint Surg Br. 2002;84:392–4.

18.   Sharma S, Anderson T, Wu C, Sun H, Wang Y, Hansen E, et al. How well do radiological assessments of truncal and shoulder balance correlate with cosmetic assessment indices in Lenke 1C adolescent idiopathic scoliosis? Clin Spine Surg. 2016;29:341–51.

19.   Qiu Y, Xu-sheng Q, Ma W, Wang B, Yu Y, Zhu Z, et al. How well do radiological measurements correlate with cosmetic indices in adolescent idiopathic scoliosis with Lenke 5, 6 curve types? Spine. 2010;35:E882–8.

20.   Amir D, Yaszay B, Bartley C, Bastrom T, Newton P. Does leveling the upper thoracic spine have any impact on postoperative clinical shoulder balance in Lenke 1 and 2 patients? Spine. 2016;41:1122–7.

21.   Matsumoto M, Watanabe K, Kawakami N, Tsuji T, Uno K, Suzuki T, et al. Postoperative shoulder imbalance in Lenke type 1A adolescent idiopathic scoliosis and related factors. BMC Musculoskelet Disord. 2014;15:366.

22.   Matamalas A, Bago J, D'Agata E, Pellise F. Reliability and validity study of measurements on digital photography to evaluate shoulder balance in idiopathic scoliosis. Scoliosis. 2014;9:23.

23.   Matamalas A, Bago J, D'Agata E, Pellise F. Validity and reliability of photographic measures to evaluate waistline asymmetry in idiopathic scoliosis. Eur Spine J. 2016;25:3170–9.

24.   Sanders J, Harrast J, Kuklo T, Polly D, Bridwell K, Diab M, et al. The Spinal Appearance Questionnaire: results of reliability, validity and responsiveness testing in patient with idiopathic scoliosis. Spine. 2007;32:2719–22.

25.   Buchanan R, Birch J, Morton A, Browne R. Do you see what I see? Looking at scoliosis surgical outcomes through orthopedists' eyes. Spine. 2003;28:2700–5.

# 18

# Systematic re-evaluation of intraoperative motor-evoked potential suppression in scoliosis surgery

Yew Long Lo[1,2*], Yam Eng Tan[3], Sitaram Raman[3], Adeline Teo[3], Yang Fang Dan[3] and Chang Ming Guo[3]

## Abstract

**Background:** Motor- (MEP) and somatosensory-evoked potentials (SSEP) are susceptible to the effects of intraoperative environmental factors.

**Methods:** Over a 5-year period, 250 patients with adolescent idiopathic scoliosis (AIS) who underwent corrective surgery with IOM were retrospectively analyzed for MEP suppression (MEPS).

**Results:** Our results show that four distinct groups of MEPS were encountered over the study period. All 12 patients did not sustain any neurological deficits postoperatively. However, comparison of groups 1 and 2 suggests that neither the duration of anesthesia nor speed of surgical or anesthetic intervention were associated with recovery to a level beyond the criteria for MEPS. For group 3, spontaneous MEPS recovery despite the lack of surgical intervention suggests that anesthetic intervention may play a role in this process. However, spontaneous MEPS recovery was also seen in group 4, suggesting that in certain circumstances, both surgical and anesthetic intervention was not required. In addition, neither the duration of time to the first surgical manoeuver nor the duration of surgical manoeuver to MEPS were related to recovery of MEPS. None of the patients had suppression of SSEPs intraoperatively.

**Conclusion:** This study suggests that in susceptible individuals, MEPS may rarely occur unpredictably, independent of surgical or anesthetic intervention. However, our findings favor anesthetic before surgical intervention as a proposed protocol. Early recognition of MEPS is important to prevent false positives in the course of IOM for spinal surgery.

**Keywords:** Intraoperative monitoring, Motor-evoked potential, Suppression, Amplitude, Scoliosis, Anesthesia

## Background

Motor-evoked potentials (MEPs) are routinely recorded during intraoperative monitoring (IOM) for spinal surgery to ensure integrity of the descending motor tracts. In addition, somatosensory-evoked potentials (SSEP) monitor the ascending dorsal column pathways of the posterior cord. Noteworthy, patients with scoliosis are neurologically intact in general, compared to those undergoing surgery for intramedullary or extramedullary spinal cord disorders.

MEPs and SSEPs are susceptible to the effects of intraoperative environmental factors. For MEPs, volatile anesthetic agents suppress excitability of the motor cortex, resulting in diminished amplitudes [1]. To mitigate the effects of inhalational anesthetics, total intravenous anesthesia (TIVA) has been shown to be effective [2].

SSEPs, in contrast, are less susceptible [3] to the dose-dependent effects of anesthetic agents compared to MEPs. However, blood pressure, anemia, and temperature appear to influence latency and amplitude of responses [4].

Hence, optimal conditions for IOM of spinal surgery include stable blood pressure and core temperature, avoidance of excessive blood loss, use of TIVA to maintain an adequate depth of anesthesia, as well as awareness of the effects of inhalational or neuromuscular blocking agents.

---

* Correspondence: lo.yew.long@singhealth.com.sg
[1]Department of Neurology, National Neuroscience Institute, Singapore General Hospital, Outram Road, Academia Level 4, Singapore 169608, Singapore
[2]Duke-NUS Medical School, Singapore, Singapore
Full list of author information is available at the end of the article

Gradual suppression of MEPs has been observed in patients under general anesthesia. MacDonald et al. [5] noted abrupt lower limb MEP loss during prolonged scoliosis surgery restored after instrumentation release without deficit and suggested increasing MEP stimulation parameters to offset this effect. Lyon et al. [6] described "anesthetic fade" by virtue of the rate of rise of stimulation voltage threshold proportional to anesthetic duration. The observed effect appears to be more pronounced in myelopathic than neurologically normal patients, but the underlying mechanism responsible remains unclear. In contrast, Holdefer et al. [7] reviewed MEP amplitudes of 50 patients receiving desflurane or propofol during spinal deformity surgery but found no evidence of reducing trend with time. This was corroborated by a separate study [8] which also found no significant MEP amplitude changes over 120 min during propofol anesthesia for spinal surgery. In all, there appears to be conflicting evidence for the occurrence of MEP amplitude reduction intraoperatively and if this phenomenon, if present, is related to anesthetic duration.

We attempt to re-examine these issues relating to motor-evoked potential suppression (MEPS) during IOM in the current study.

## Methods

The institution's ethics committee had previously approved the study protocols.

Over a 5-year period, 250 patients with adolescent idiopathic scoliosis (AIS) who underwent corrective surgery with IOM were retrospectively reviewed. All were previously determined by a neurologist to be without deficits. IOM recordings whereby MEP amplitude reductions beyond 50% of baseline value at maximum cortical stimulation of 400 V were defined as MEPS and identified for further analysis. Similarly, IOM recordings whereby SSEP amplitude reduction beyond 50% of baseline value identified for further analysis. The IOM protocol using TIVA and cortical stimulation methodology have been published previously [9, 10].

For induction of anesthesia, propofol at 1–2 mg/kg and fentanyl at 2 μg/kg was administered. A single administration of 0.8 mg/kg intravenous atracurium was used to facilitate endotracheal intubation. No further doses of neuromuscular blocking agents were used subsequently. Anesthesia was maintained using the regimen of 10 mg/kg propofol for the first 10 min, 8 mg/kg for the next 10 min, and 6 mg/kg for the subsequent length of operation. Fifty percent air in oxygen was administered. Remifentanil at a dose range of 0.03–0.1 μg/kg/min and morphine were titrated as required for pain relief. Electrocardiography, pulse oximetry, capnography, and direct radial artery pressures were monitored. A bispectral index (BIS) monitor was used in 6 of the patients. All patients were kept normothermic with a warming blanket, and normotensive anesthesia was maintained throughout the operation. Where the BIS monitor was used, the depth of anesthesia was kept to about 40 on the index. As 40 to 60 is considered the range for adequate depth of anesthesia, this was at the deeper end of the range.

After approximately 45 min post-induction, a train of four-twitch assessment was performed using a nerve stimulator (Fischer Paykel NS242, United Kingdom) on the median nerve at the wrist. Cortical stimulation was commenced only when the amplitude of the fourth twitch (abductor pollicis muscle) was visibly similar to the first, suggesting that the effects of neuromuscular blocking agents have subsided.

Cortical stimulation was delivered by 9-mm gold-plated disc electrodes at C3C4 (International 10-20 system) affixed with collodion. C3 was the active stimulating electrode position for left cortical stimulation, while C4 was for right cortical stimulation, correspondingly to a cross scalp stimulating configuration. A train of 5 square wave stimuli 0.5 ms in duration was delivered at 4 ms (250 Hz) interstimulus intervals. Stimulation output was increased in steps of 50 V until a morphologically reproducible MEP with the largest amplitude was elicited. The intensity was then increased and fixed at 10% above this threshold intensity to obtain a supramaximal MEP response recorded with 13-mm disposable subdermal needles (Technomed Europe, Beek, Netherlands) in the tibialis anterior (TA) bilaterally. Amplifier filter settings were set at 10 Hz and 2 kHz. Input impedance of stimulating and recording electrodes was maintained below 5 kΩ.

MEPs from the TA muscles were recorded bilaterally from the lower limbs by means of a Nicolet Endeavor CR IOM system (Natus Technology, USA). Peak to peak amplitudes and onset latency was measured for MEP responses in each limb, obtained from ipsilateral and contralateral cortical stimulation; ipsilateral MEPs refer to MEPs recorded from the TA on the same side as cortical stimulation. Ten consecutive supramaximal MEPs obtained before insertion of pedicle screws were averaged to obtain a final mean amplitude and latency as a baseline. The baseline sensitivity for signal acquisition was kept at 50 μV.

Surgical maneuver refers to screw placement or rod placement (Table 1).

Surgical intervention consisted of removal of pedicle screws, brackets, and rods, followed by a wake up test. The decision for wake up tests is left to the surgeon ultimately. No wake up tests were performed for cases 9 to 12 as it was felt that there was sufficient recovery of MEPs without surgical intervention.

Anesthetic intervention referred to the temporary reduction of TIVA and remifentanil to allow for the

**Table 1** Summary of MEPS events for 12 patients with AIS

| Patient | Age | Sex | Start anesthesia | Surgical maneuver | MEP suppression | Surgical intervention | Anesthetic intervention | MEP recovery | Stage of operation | Clinical outcome |
|---|---|---|---|---|---|---|---|---|---|---|
| Group 1 | | | | | | | | | | |
| 1 | 17 | F | 1319 | 1550 | 1609 | 1618 | 1622 | 1626 | Screw plac | N |
| 2 | 14 | F | 0850 | 0950 | 1001 | 1006 | 1204 | 1246 | Screw plac | N |
| 3 | 23 | M | 0959 | 1308 | 1346 | 1721 | 1730 | 1800 | Nil | N |
| 4 | 11 | F | 0845 | 1058 | 1101 | 1108 | 1150 | 1214 | Screw plac | N |
| Group 2 | | | | | | | | | | |
| 5 | 13 | F | 1334 | 1518 | 1534 | 1542 | 1647 | No | Screw plac | N |
| 6 | 21 | F | 1240 | 1416 | 1423 | 1426 | 1530 | No | Left rod plac | N |
| 7 | 29 | F | 0919 | 1131 | 1212 | 1258 | 1318 | No | Screw plc | N |
| 8 | 13 | F | 1411 | 1522 | 1535 | 1545 | 1600 | No | Left rod plac | N |
| Group 3 | | | | | | | | | | |
| 9 | 21 | M | 0908 | 1118 | 1133 | No | 1212 | 1329 | Screw plac | N |
| 10 | 11 | F | 1025 | 1041 | 1154 | No | 1317 | 1322 | Screw plac | N |
| 11 | 36 | F | 1428 | 1806 | 1811 | No | 1819 | 1849 | Screw plac | N |
| Group 4 | | | | | | | | | | |
| 12 | 31 | F | 0926 | 1004 | 1045 | No | No | 1112 | Screw plac | N |

*M* male, *F* female, *Plac* placement, *MEP* motor-evoked potential, *AIS* adolescent idiopathic scoliosis, *N* normal

reduction in the depth in anesthesia. In 6 cases where the BIS was used, the value rose to around 60 or more indicating a greater probability of deep sleep rather than anesthesia.

MEP amplitude recovery was defined as the recovery MEP amplitude to beyond 50% of baseline value or latency delay < 10% of baseline value.

SSEP amplitude recovery is similarly defined as the recovery cortical SSEP (P37) amplitude to beyond 50% of baseline value or latency delay < 10% of baseline value.

The following time intervals were noted for each case of possible MEPS:

1. Start of anesthesia to MEPS
2. MEPS to surgical intervention
3. MEPS to anesthetic intervention
4. Start of anesthesia to surgical maneuver
5. Surgical maneuver to MEPS

An anesthetist not involved in the management of each case reviewed intraoperative data to ensure that no confounding factors for MEPS, including vital signs, anesthetic protocol, and interventions, were present.

The Kruskal-Wallis and Mann-Whitney $U$ tests were used to compare interval between groups. A $p$ value < 0.05 denoted statistical significance.

## Results

A total of 12 AIS patients (2 men; mean age 20 (range 11 to 36)) were included in the final analysis. All were clinically well with no transient or permanent neurological deficits after surgical correction.

Based on 250 patients analyzed in this cohort, the estimated frequency of MEPS is 4.8%.

We identified four groups of cases fulfilling MEPS criteria:

1. MEPS with anesthetic and surgical intervention, followed by MEP amplitude recovery
2. MEPS with anesthetic and surgical intervention, without MEP amplitude recovery
3. MEPS with anesthetic but no surgical intervention, followed by MEP amplitude recovery
4. MEPs without anesthetic and surgical intervention, followed by MEP amplitude recovery

Wake up tests performed for cases 1 to 8 all normal.

In group 3, intraoperative visual monitoring devices such as the O Arm (Medtronic, plc, Colorado, USA) were utilized to provide additional information to the surgical team.

There were no significant differences in time interval 1 between groups 1, 2, and 3 (Kruskal-Wallis test, $H = 0.712$, $p > 0.05$). For time interval 2, comparison between groups 1 and 2 did not reveal statistical significance (Mann-Whitney $U$ test, $Z = 0.104$, $p > 0.05$). In addition, no statistical difference between groups 1, 2, and 3 was found for time interval 3 (Kruskal-Wallis test, $H = 4.348$, $p > 0.05$), 4 (Kruskal-Wallis test, $H = 0.875$, $p > 0.05$), and 5 (Kruskal-Wallis test, $H = 1.095$, $p > 0.05$).

Of the 12 cases, all 8 cases with MEP recovery were associated with screw placement. Conversely 2 of 4 cases without MEP recovery (group 2) were associated with rod placement.

The MEP changes of control muscle groups in the upper extremities (first dorsal interossei) did not exceed amplitude reductions beyond 50% of baseline value at maximum cortical stimulation of 400 V.

No intraoperative SSEP changes were detected for all patients.

Tables 1 and 2 summarize clinical data of the 12 cases analyzed.

## Discussion

Our results show that four distinct groups pf MEPS were encountered over the study period. All 12 patients did not sustain any neurological deficits postoperatively. However, comparing groups 1 and 2 suggest that neither the duration of anesthesia nor speed of surgical or anesthetic intervention were associated with recovery to a level beyond the criteria for MEPS. For group 3, spontaneous MEPS recovery despite the lack of surgical intervention suggests that anesthetic intervention may play a role in this process. However, spontaneous MEPS recovery was also seen in group 4, suggesting that in certain circumstances, both surgical and anesthetic interventions were not required. In addition, comparing groups 1, 2, and 3 suggests that neither the duration of time to the first surgical maneuver nor the duration of surgical manoeuver to MEPS were related to recovery of MEPS.

However, it appears that rod placement (group 2) (Table 1) is associated with more closely with failure of MEP recovery. As the numbers involved are small, it would be difficult to make broad conclusions based purely on these observations.

Overall, this study suggests that in susceptible individuals, MEPS may rarely occur unpredictably, independent of surgical or anesthetic intervention, although the observations made were not on an intentional interference basis. The eventual clinical outcomes were, most importantly, favorable. However, anesthetic intervention was performed in 11 of 12 cases and surgical intervention in 8 of 12 cases. Of note, case 4 in group 1 and cases 9, 10, and 11 in group 3 all had anesthetic intervention and MEP amplitude recovery under BIS monitoring. While the exact reasons remain unclear, the results overall favor anesthetic intervention over surgical intervention. In addition, over the study period, there were no identified cases fulfilling the criteria for significant SSEP changes, suggesting that this form of monitoring may be less vulnerable to interference by external factors intraoperatively. This was seen in contrast to previous reports [11, 12].

There is a lack of published information with regard to MEPS. One previous study [6] found the measured voltage threshold needed to produce an MEP of 50 µV to be greater at the end of surgery than at baseline. The rate of rise of this threshold was also greater in relation to operating duration and presence of myelopathy. However, direct comparison to our findings may not be valid in view of differences in stimulating and recording parameters, as well as inclusion of neurologically abnormal patients.

To our knowledge, no further published studies have attempted to address MEPS during IOM systematically in a similar manner.

What can we conclude on the physiological basis of MEPS? Several mechanisms have been proposed previously regarding the effect of anesthetic agents on MEPs. These include actions on synaptic transmission, prolongation of axonal refractory period, depressing spinal motor neuron excitability, and facilitation of GABA-mediated inhibitory interneuron actions [13–15]. Our findings are based on elimination of confounding intraoperative factors of blood loss, hypotension, hypothermia, and a standardized anesthetic intervention strategy in neurologically normal patients. In spite, the results do not suggest a duration-dependent suppression of cortical excitability for MEPS. Rather, individual factors predisposing to desynchronization of descending volleys summating at spinal interneurons or motor neurons may play a role, but this remains to be further explored.

Hence, we prefer the term MEPS over "anesthetic fade" in view of uncertainty over the purported physiological

**Table 2** Summary of time intervals for 12 patients with AIS

| Interval | 1 | 2 | 3 | 4 | 5 |
|---|---|---|---|---|---|
| Group 1 | | | | | |
| 1 | 170 | 9 | 13 | 189 | 19 |
| 2 | 71 | 5 | 123 | 60 | 11 |
| 3 | 225 | 218 | 224 | 188 | 54 |
| 4 | 136 | 7 | 49 | 133 | 3 |
| Group 2 | | | | | |
| 1 | 120 | 8 | 73 | 104 | 16 |
| 2 | 160 | 3 | 67 | 96 | 7 |
| 3 | 173 | 46 | 66 | 131 | 41 |
| 4 | 84 | 10 | 25 | 70 | 13 |
| Group 3 | | | | | |
| 1 | 145 | | 184 | 130 | 15 |
| 2 | 89 | | 172 | 16 | 13 |
| 3 | 99 | | 261 | 218 | 5 |
| Group 4 | | | | | |
| 1 | 79 | | | 38 | 41 |

All values shown are in minutes

mechanisms, as well as lack of evidence of dose or duration anesthesia plays in AIS patients.

As current studies are limited by small patient numbers, collation of experiences among multiple IOM centers utilizing similar protocols may shed more light on MEPS. Anesthetic depth measurements such as the bispectral index and electroencephalograhy can be incorporated to reduce additional confounders. Monitoring MEPs obtained from an extra muscle group in the lower limb may help mitigate the possibility of recording MEPs with diminished amplitude as a result factor not directly related to neurophysiological dysfunction.

Figure 1 is a flow diagram of a suggested protocol when MEPS is encountered, highlighting the use of anesthetic before surgical intervention based on findings of the current study. Early recognition is important to prevent false positives in the course of IOM for spinal surgery.

Conversely, a recent study examining 62,038 spine surgeries of all categories retrospectively had determined that false negatives occur at a rate of 0.04% [16]. It would appear that if MEPS occurring at 4.8% contributes to false positives, then the only patient in group 4 could be considered as a "true" false positive, rendering the

overall rate to be 0.4%. Our study, however, consisted of only neurologically normal AIS patients instead of all patients undergoing spinal operations.

For IOM using MEPs overall, it is recommended that interpretation should take into consideration limitations, confounding factors, and the MEP warning criteria be tailored to the type of surgery, as well as the technique and experience of the monitoring team [17]. To date, disappearance of the recorded MEP signals is the main warning criterion yet proposed for spinal cord monitoring. This is based on variability that challenges other criteria, high sensitivity to central motor disturbances, the likelihood that pathophysiology will affect many corticospinal axons because the tract is very small in the spinal cord, and the rapid failure of ischemic lower motor neurons [18–20].

## Conclusions

This study suggests that in susceptible individuals, MEPS may rarely occur unpredictably, independent of surgical or anesthetic intervention. However, our findings favor anesthetic before surgical intervention as a proposed protocol. Early recognition of MEPS is important to prevent false positives in the course of IOM for spinal surgery.

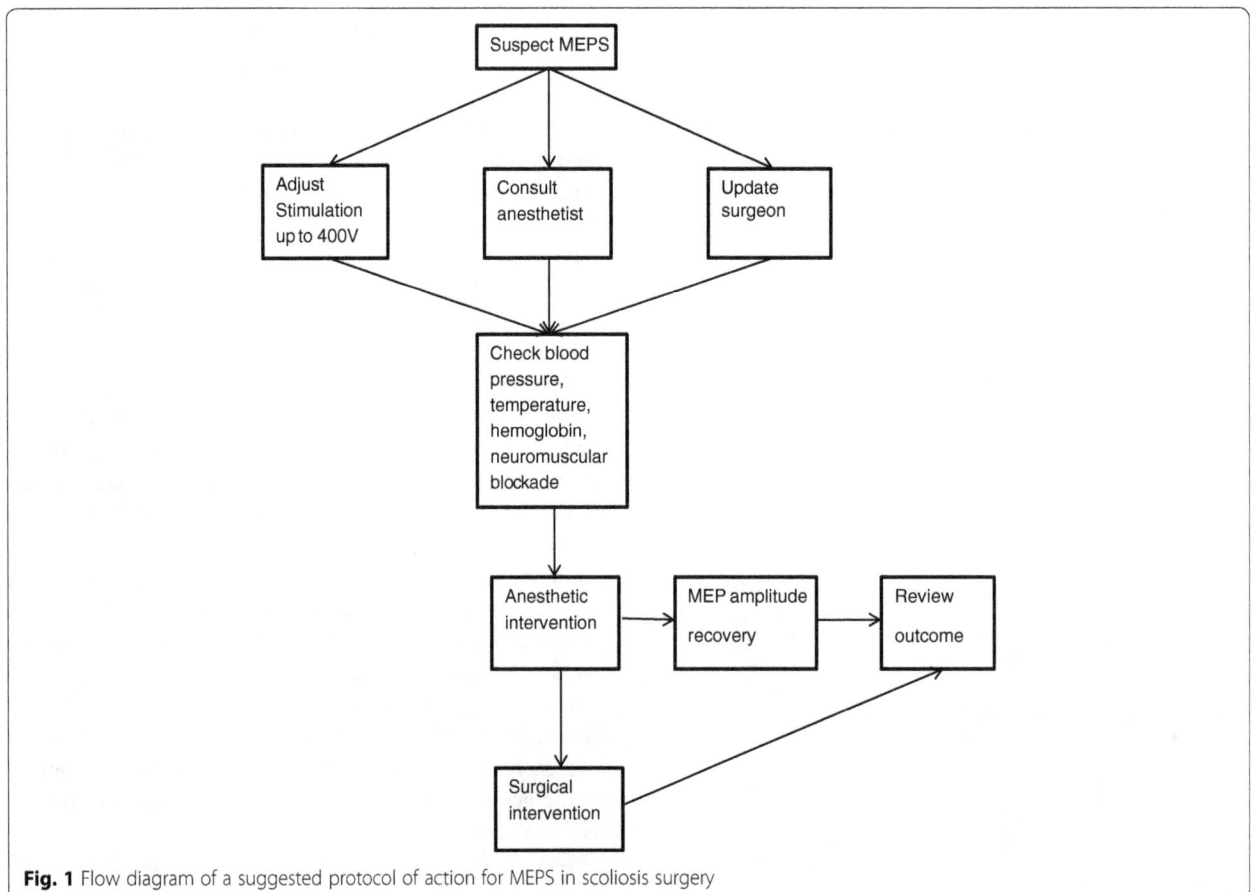

**Fig. 1** Flow diagram of a suggested protocol of action for MEPS in scoliosis surgery

## Abbreviations
BIS: Bispectral index; IOM: Intraoperative monitoring; MEP: Motor-evoked potential; MEPS: Motor-evoked potential suppression; SEP: Somatosensory-evoked potential; TA: Tibialis anterior; TIVA: Total intravenous anesthesia

## Authors' contributions
YLL wrote the paper and conceptualized the study. YET and AT analyzed the data. SR contributed to the data collection and paper writing. YFD monitored and collected the data. GCM operated and conceptualized the study. All authors have read and approved the manuscript.

## Competing interests
The authors declare that they have no competing interests.

## Author details
[1]Department of Neurology, National Neuroscience Institute, Singapore General Hospital, Outram Road, Academia Level 4, Singapore 169608, Singapore. [2]Duke-NUS Medical School, Singapore, Singapore. [3]Singapore General Hospital, Singapore, Singapore.

## References
1. Calancie B, Klose KJ, Baier S, et al. Isoflurane-induced attenuation of motor evoked potentials caused by electrical motor cortex stimulation during surgery. J Neurosurg. 1991;74:897–904.
2. Liu EH, Wong HK, Chia CP, Lim HJ, Chen ZY, Lee TL. Effects of isoflurane and propofol on cortical somatosensory evoked potentials during comparable depth of anesthesia as guided by bispectral index. Br J Anaesth. 2005;94(2):193–7.
3. Freye E, Hartung E, Schenk GK. Somatosensory-evoked potentials during block of surgical stimulation with propofol. Br J Anaesth. 1989;63:357–9.
4. Nuwer M. Spinal cord monitoring. In: Evoked potential monitoring in the operating room. New York: Raven Press; 1986. p. 49–101.
5. MacDonald DB, Al Zayed Z, Khoudeir I, Stigsby B. Monitoring scoliosis surgery with combined multiple pulse transcranial electric motor and cortical somatosensory-evoked potentials from the lower and upper extremities. Spine (Phila Pa 1976). 2003;28:194–203.
6. Lyon R, Feiner J, Lieberman JA. Progressive suppression of motor evoked potentials during general anesthesia: the phenomenon of "anesthetic fade". J Neurosurg Anesthesiol. 2005;17:13–9.
7. Holdefer RN, Anderson C, Furman M, Sangare Y, Slimp JC. A comparison of the effects of desflurane versus propofol on transcranial motor-evoked potentials in pediatric patients. Childs Nerv Syst. 2014;30:2103–8.
8. Liu HY, Zeng HY, Cheng H, Wang MR, Qiao H, Han RQ. Comparison of the effects of etomidate and propofol combined with remifentanil and guided by comparable BIS on transcranial electrical motor-evoked potentials during spinal surgery. J Neurosurg Anesthesiol. 2012;24:133–8.
9. Lo Y, Dan Y, Tan Y, Teo A, Tan S, Yue W, Guo C, Fook-Chong S. Clinical and physiological effects of transcranial electrical stimulation position on motor evoked potentials in scoliosis surgery. Scoliosis. 2010;23(5):3.
10. Lo YL, Dan YF, Tan YE, Nurjannah S, Tan SB, Tan CT, Raman S. Intraoperative motor-evoked potential monitoring in scoliosis surgery: comparison of desflurane/nitrous oxide with propofol total intravenous anesthetic regimens. J Neurosurg Anesthesiol. 2006;18(3):211–4.
11. Kalkman CJ, ten Brink SA, Been HD, Bovill JG. Variability of somatosensory cortical evoked potentials during spinal surgery. Effects of anesthetic technique and high-pass digital filtering. Spine (Phila Pa 1976). 1991;16:924–9.
12. Maurette P, Simeon F, Castagnera L, Esposito J, Macouillard G, Heraut LA. Propofol anaesthesia alters somatosensory evoked cortical potentials. Anaesthesia. 1988;43(S):44–5.
13. Woodforth IJ, Hicks RG, Crawford MR, Stephen JP, Burke D. Depression of I waves in corticospinal volleys by sevoflurane, thiopental, and propofol. Anesth Analg. 1999;89:1182–7.
14. Antkowiak B. Different actions of general anesthetics on the firing patterns of neocortical neurons mediated by the GABA(A) receptor. Anesthesiology. 1999;91:500–11.
15. Kakinohana M, Fuchigami T, Nakamura S, Kawabata T, Sugahara K. Propofol reduces spinal motor neuron excitability in humans. Anesth Analg. 2002;94:1586–8.
16. Tamkus AA, Rice KS, McCaffrey MT. Perils of intraoperative neurophysiological monitoring: analysis of "false-negative" results in spine surgeries. Spine J. 2018;18:276–84.
17. Macdonald DB, Skinner S, Shils J, Yingling C. American Society of Neurophysiological Monitoring. Intraoperative motor evoked potential monitoring—a position statement by the American Society of Neurophysiological Monitoring. Clin Neurophysiol. 2013;124:2291–316.
18. MacDonald DB, Janusz M. An approach to intraoperative neurophysiologic monitoring of thoracoabdominal aneurysm surgery. J Clin Neurophysiol. 2002;19:43–54.
19. Calancie B, Molano MR. Alarm criteria for motor-evoked potentials: what's wrong with the "presence-or-absence" approach? Spine. 2008;33:406–14.
20. Macdonald DB, Al Zayed Z, Al Saddigi A. Four-limb muscle motor evoked potential and optimized somatosensory evoked potential monitoring with decussation assessment: results in 206 thoracolumbar spine surgeries. Eur Spine J. 2007;16(Suppl 2):S171–87.

# 19

# Non-structural misalignments of body posture in the sagittal plane

Dariusz Czaprowski[1,2], Łukasz Stoliński[3,4,5], Marcin Tyrakowski[6], Mateusz Kozinoga[4,5]* [ID] and Tomasz Kotwicki[4]

## Abstract

**Background:** The physiological sagittal spinal curvature represents a typical feature of good body posture in the sagittal plane. The cervical and the lumbar spine are curved anteriorly (lordosis), while the thoracic segment is curved posteriorly (kyphosis). The pelvis is inclined anteriorly, and the lower limbs' joints remain in a neutral position. However, there are many deviations from the optimal body alignment.

The aim of this paper is to present the most common types of non-structural misalignments of the body posture in the sagittal plane.

**Main body of the abstract:** The most common types of non-structural misalignments of body posture in the sagittal plane are as follows: (1) lordotic, (2) kyphotic, (3) flat-back, and (4) sway-back postures. Each one may influence both the skeletal and the muscular system leading to the functional disturbance and an increased strain of the supporting structures. Usually, the disturbances localized within the muscles are analyzed in respect to their shortening or lengthening. However, according to suggestions presented in the literature, when the muscles responsible for maintaining good body posture (the so-called stabilizers) are not being stimulated to resist against gravity for an extended period of time, e.g., during prolonged sitting, their stabilizing function is disturbed by the hypoactivity reaction resulting in muscular weakness. The deficit of the locomotor system stability triggers a compensatory mechanism—the stabilizing function is overtaken by the so-called mobilizing muscles. However, as a side effect, such compensation leads to the increased activity of mobilizers (hyperactivity) and decreased flexibility, which may finally lead to the pathological chain of reaction within the musculoskeletal system.

**Conclusions:** There exist four principal types of non-structural body posture misalignments in the sagittal plane: lordotic posture, kyphotic posture, flat-back posture, and sway-back posture. Each of them can disturb the physiological loading of the musculoskeletal system in a specific way, which may lead to a functional disorder. When planning postural corrective exercises, not only the analysis of muscles in respect to their shortening and lengthening but also their hypoactivity and hyperactivity should be considered.

**Keywords:** Body posture, Corrective exercises, Faults of body posture, Lordotic posture, Kyphotic posture, Flat-back posture, Sway-back posture

## Background

### Human body posture

Human posture is commonly understood as the relationship between human body parts in the upright position. Particular body parts, such as the head and neck, the trunk, and the upper and lower limbs, are involved in the final body posture. A *good body posture* is considered (1) ergonomically advantageous while standing, (2) mechanically effective while moving, and (3) supportive for the normal function of internal organs. Body posture is described and considered in three reference planes: sagittal, coronal, and transversal [1, 2]. Kendall et al. proposed a definition of good human posture: "good posture is that state of muscular and skeletal balance which protects the supporting structures of the body against the injury or progressive deformity, irrespective of the attitude (erect, lying, squatting or stooping) in which these structures are working or resting. Under such

* Correspondence: kozinoga@ump.edu.pl
[4]Spine Disorders and Pediatric Orthopedics Department, University of Medical Sciences, 28 Czerwca 1956 135/147 Street, 61-545 Poznań, Poland
[5]Rehasport Clinic, Górecka 30, 60-201 Poznań, Poland
Full list of author information is available at the end of the article

conditions, the muscles will function most efficiently, and the optimum positions are afforded for the thoracic and abdominal organs" [3]. Such a comprehensive definition of body posture will not be used in this paper since the authors focused on the description of human posture in the upright standing position.

*Poor posture* is an imprecise term commonly used in the clinical practice to describe a relationship between various body parts which may be considered as faulty and which could stretch the spectrum from the non-perfect to pathological posture. It is postulated that poor posture can produce an increased strain on the supporting structures and less-efficient balance of the body over its base of support [3].

The most difficult task of describing *good body posture* concerns the sagittal plane alignment, while both the coronal and the transversal planes are usually considered symmetrical. In fact, the human being is symmetrical neither in the coronal nor in the transversal plane [3–5]. However, this simplification is used in this paper for the clear presentation of the sagittal plane alignment.

The *physiological sagittal spinal curvature* represents a typical feature of good body posture in the sagittal plane. The cervical and the lumbar spine are curved anteriorly (*lordosis*), while the thoracic segment is curved posteriorly (*kyphosis*). The head remains horizontal, which denotes that the eye level corresponds to the horizontal plane, while the chin is positioned just above the sternum. The pelvis is inclined anteriorly, and the lower limb joints remain in a neutral position [1–3].

The optimal body posture should represent the following alignment: the *head line*, beginning at the external auditory meatus (or at the mastoid process of the temporal bone), should run vertically through the acromion, the lumbar vertebral bodies, the promontory, then slightly posteriorly to the hip joint axis, slightly in front of the knee joint axis, and finish at the lateral malleolus or slightly in front of it. The course of this line in a good body posture overlaps the *base line* joining the center of gravity with the central point of the supporting area (Fig. 1) [4–7].

As presented above, the detailed description of a good body posture in the sagittal plane is not explicit. Moreover, characterizing the deviations from a good posture can be ambiguous. The aim of this paper is to present the most common types of non-structural misalignments of body posture in the sagittal plane.

## Non-structural versus structural misalignments of body posture

From a clinical point of view, the disturbances of human posture can be classified as non-structural or structural. The non-structural pathologies represent the main topic of this article and will be discussed in detail. The structural misalignments comprise specific clinical entities: idiopathic scoliosis, Scheuermann juvenile kyphosis, congenital vertebral malformation, sequels of spine osteomyelitis, spondylolisthesis, and other clinical entities that produce disorders of body posture, e.g., thoracic hyperkyphosis, flat back, and pelvis malposition. The said body posture disorders are known as "structural disorders," as this term indicates the presence of morphological abnormalities within the bones and soft tissues (fascia, muscles, ligaments, tendons). Additionally, structural misalignments reveal a more severe clinical problem as they are less flexible and less prone to correction compared to the non-structural disorders. They require specific diagnostic and therapeutic approach and are not discussed in this paper apart from the differential diagnosis issue.

The clinical appearance of children with non-structural versus structural (e.g., Scheuermann disease) disturbances of body posture may be similar (Fig. 2 versus Fig. 3). Two boys, aged 12 and 14 respectively, diagnosed with the kyphotic posture (increased thoracic kyphosis, protraction of the head and shoulders), are presented in Figs. 2 and 3. Figure 2 shows the kyphotic posture reasonable due to the non-structural pathology, namely the combination of an incorrect postural habit and muscles' hypo- and hyperactivity. Figure 3 presents the kyphotic posture due to the structural thoracic hyperkyphosis, which is a structural spinal deformity.

Differential diagnosis represents an important part of the evaluation of every child addressed for the so-called poor posture. Despite the modern imaging techniques, including digital whole-body radiography, computed tomography, or nuclear magnetic resonance, the basic clinical examination retains its value. For example, the functional testing allows assessing the flexibility of thoracic hyperkyphosis which reveals good in non-structural (Fig. 4a–c) versus poor in structural misalignment (Fig. 5a–c).

## Non-structural sagittal misalignments of body posture
### Principal types of sagittal postural misalignments
The most common types of non-structural misalignments of body posture in the sagittal plane in both children and adults are: (1) *lordotic posture*, (2) *kyphotic posture* which can sometimes coexist with the lordotic one as a *kyphotic-lordotic posture*, (3) *flat-back posture*, and (4) *sway-back posture* [4, 7, 8]. The biomechanical analysis of body alignment and the functional analysis of the muscles involved in each type of faulty posture reveal the muscle groups that remain the target for corrective management. Therefore, before the detailed description of particular types of faulty postures is given, the concept of functional muscle classification will be presented.

### Functional muscle classification by Bergmark and Richardson in the context of body posture
Bergmark [9] and Richardson et al. [10] reported on the functional specificity of skeletal muscles, expressed in a

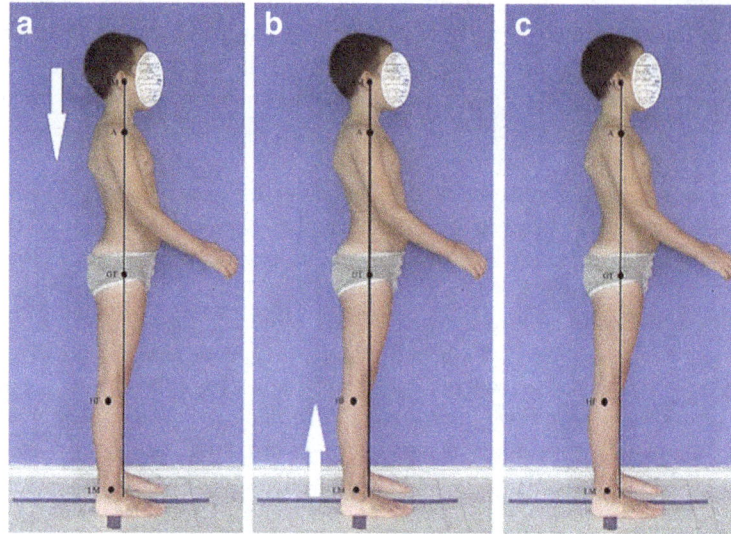

**Fig. 1** Good body posture in a 8-year-old boy—the head line (**a**) and the base line (**b**) overlaps each other (**c**). Note: AM—external auditory meatus; A—acromion; GT—greater trochanter; HF—head of fibula; LM—lateral malleolus

normal condition and response to stress. Many studies confirmed that individual skeletal muscles react differently to common events, such as injury of the associated joint, presence, or lack of gravitational load or specific patterns of use (e.g., ballistic exercises) [11–17], namely by *reflectory inhibition* or *reflectory excitation*. *Reflectory inhibition* results in muscle *hypoactivity* which may manifest clinically as *muscle weakness*. *Reflectory excitation* results in muscle *hyperactivity* which may manifest clinically as *reduced flexibility* [11–18]. Such reduced flexibility is usually reported on the clinical

examination as muscle shortening even though it does not involve the factual *shortening* of muscular fibers (contracture), which will be explained in the further part of the paper.

### Muscle groups maintaining good body posture

Bergmark [9] and Richardson et al. [10] proposed to classify the skeletal muscles into two groups: (1) *mono-articular*, also called local muscles or stabilizers, and (2) *multi-articular*, also called global or stabilizer/mobilizer muscles, depending on the subgroup (see

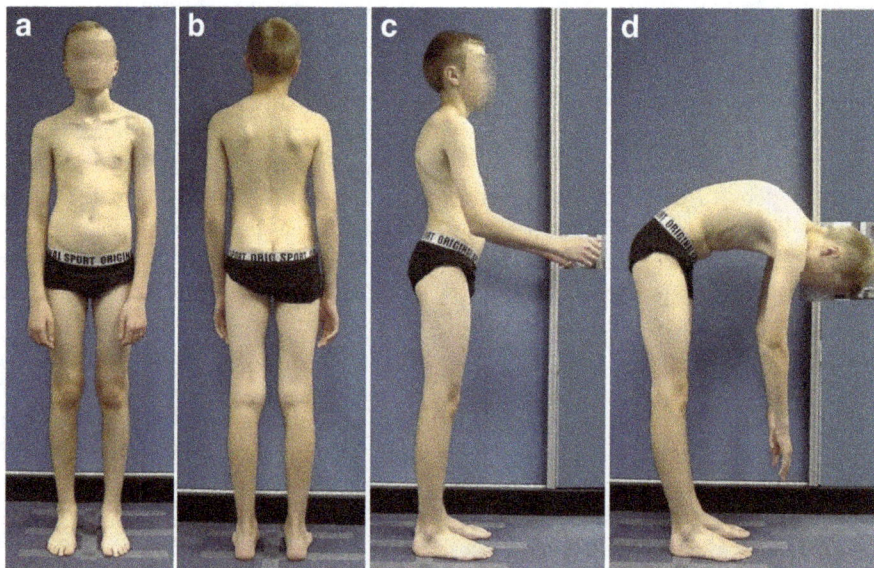

**Fig. 2** A 12-year-old boy with non-structural sagittal misalignment of body posture: postural thoracic hyperkyphosis. **a** Front view. **b** Back view. **c** Side view. **d** Forward bend view

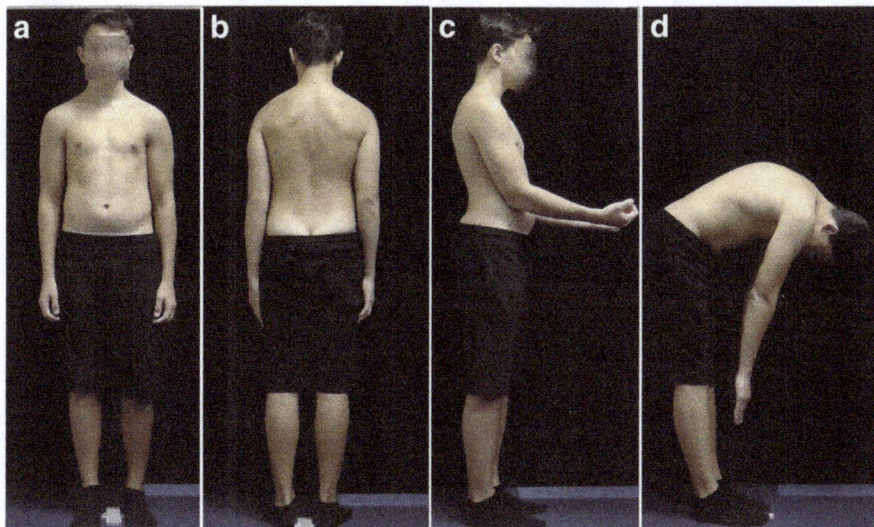

**Fig. 3** A 14-year-old boy with structural sagittal misalignment of body posture: structural thoracic hyperkyphosis. **a** Front view. **b** Back view. **c** Side view. **d** Forward bend view

below) [5, 9, 10]. According to the authors, the appropriate cooperation between these two muscle groups allows transferring the load from the thorax to the pelvis safely through the stabilized spinal segments and to minimize forces applied to the lumbar spine during functional activities [5, 6, 9, 10].

According to Bergmark [9] and Richardson et al. [10], the *local mono-articular* group comprises deep trunk muscles: multifidus, transversus abdominis, interspinalis, intertransversalis, semispinalis, posterior portion of the internal oblique, medial fibers of quadratus lumborum, the central portion of the erector spinae, diaphragm, and the muscles of the pelvic floor [9, 10]. These muscles are linked with joint stabilization, and they are capable of controlling the position of the joints or spinal segments. The stabilizers are responsible for preventing from

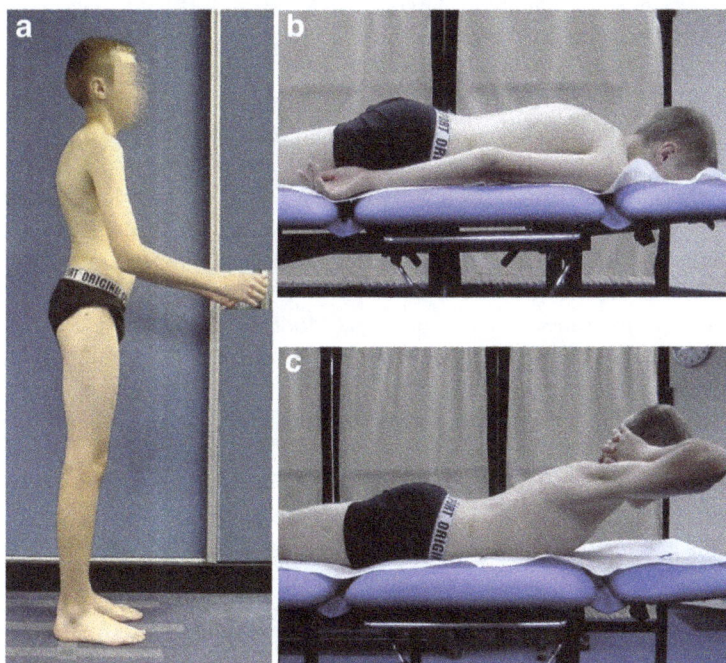

**Fig. 4** A 12-year-old boy with thoracic hyperkyphosis developing in habitual standing position. **a** Habitual standing position, lateral view. **b** Prone habitual lying position reveals thoracic hyperkyphosis. **c** Active trunk extension causes correction—flattening of thoracic hyperkyphosis

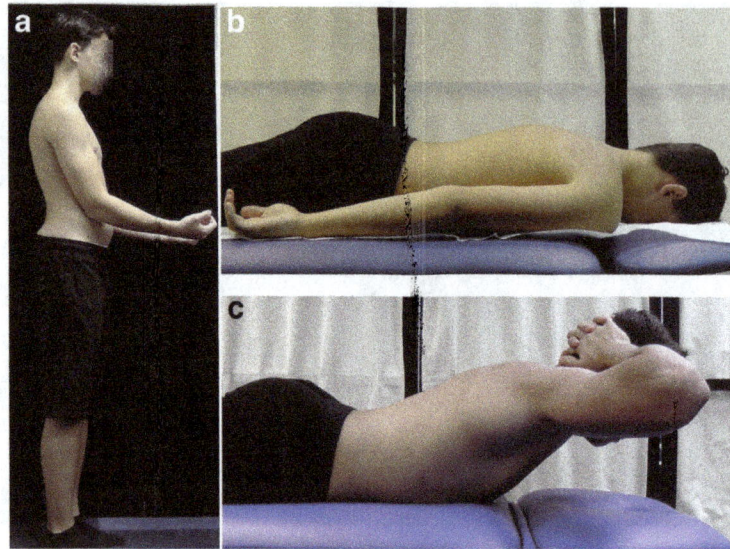

**Fig. 5** A 14-year-old boy with structural thoracic hyperkyphosis. **a** Habitual standing position, lateral view. **b** Lying prone position reveals maintaining thoracic hyperkyphosis. **c** Active trunk extension does not decrease the thoracic hyperkyphosis

local shifts of a particular spinal segment and provide segmental 3-D stability to maintain the global mechanical stability of the whole spine [2, 6, 8, 10, 19]. In response to stress, the local muscles are likely to undergo reflectory inhibition (hypoactivity). It may be caused by injury to the associated joint, ballistic repetitive exercises, or lack of use and lack of gravitational load [9–13, 15].

The *global multi-articular* muscles comprise large muscles which tend to be situated superficially in the trunk and the limbs. This muscle group provides the function of both stabilizing and force-generating moments in several joints at the same time. These muscles are considered phylogenetically the oldest [10, 11]. The global muscles are divided into two subgroups: the stabilizers and the mobilizers.

The *global stabilizers* comprise the antigravity muscles responsible for maintaining the erected posture. This group of muscles includes trapezius (middle and lower part), erector spinae (lumbar part), iliacus, gluteus maximus, gluteus medius, adductor magnus, and adductor brevis. These muscles are responsible for stabilizing the joint position while the joint movement is being performed [5, 6, 9–11].

The *mobilizers* comprise the muscles not related to antigravity postural action, e.g., erector spinae (thoracic part), rectus abdominis, external abdominal oblique, the anterior portion of internal abdominal oblique, the lateral portion of quadratus lumborum, psoas, hamstrings, tensor fasciae latae, rectus femoris, and adductor longus. These muscles are basically responsible for performing active movements in joints [5–11, 20].

## Muscle groups functioning in faulty body posture

Exposure of the human body to gravity forces, e.g., when standing or walking, is necessary to ensure proper activity of the skeletal muscles responsible for maintaining good body posture. When these muscles are not stimulated to resist gravity for an extended period, e.g., during prolonged sitting or lying, their stabilizing function is disturbed by the hypoactivity reaction resulting in muscular weakness and atrophy. The deficit of the locomotor system stability triggers a compensatory mechanism—the stabilizing function is overtaken by the mobilizing muscles. However, as a side effect, such compensation leads to mobilizers' increased activity (hyperactivity) and, subsequently, their decreased flexibility [7, 10, 11, 16, 18, 21, 22], which may finally lead to a pathological chain of reactions within the musculoskeletal system, as described below (Figs. 12, 13, 14 and 15).

## Lordotic posture
### Posture description

The lordotic posture represents a faulty posture that differs from the good one by the following: (1) increased lumbar lordosis and (2) increased pelvic anteversion (anterior tilt) (Fig. 6). Increased anterior tilt of the pelvis leads to increased flexion of hip joints. The knees can be in hyperextension and, due to this knee position, the plantar flexion of the feet occurs (Fig. 6) [3, 7, 8, 23].

In the lordotic posture the *head line* runs down posteriorly to lumbar vertebral bodies, passing near the intervertebral facet joints, which results in extensory overloading within the facets. The head line is also anterior to the knee joint axis, which leads to the

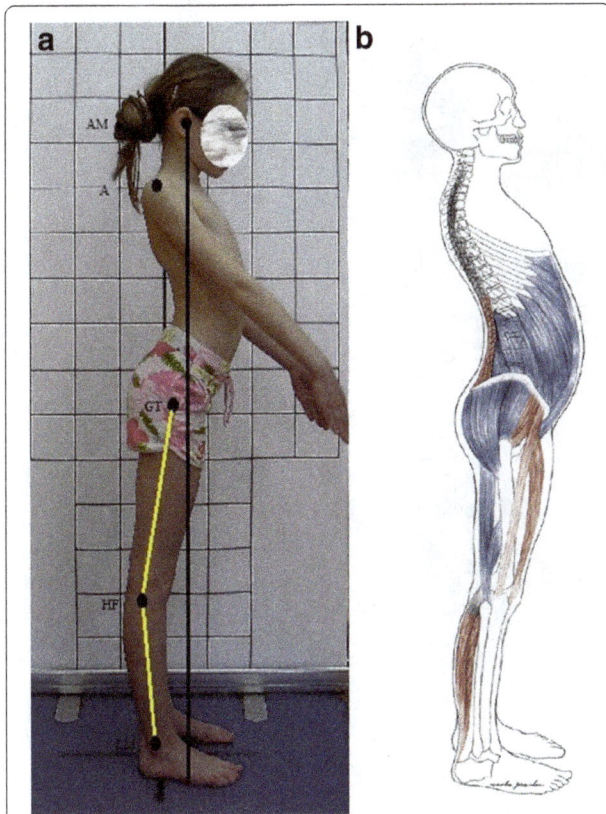

**Fig. 6** Lordotic posture in a 9-year-old girl. **a** Habitual standing, lateral view, note the hyperextension of the knees and plantar flexion of the feet. **b** Corresponding schematic representation of the shortened (red) and lengthened (blue) skeletal muscles. Note: AM—external auditory meatus; A—acromion; GT—greater trochanter; HF—head of fibula; LM—lateral malleolus

**Table 1** The position of body parts in the lordotic posture

| Part of the body | Position |
| --- | --- |
| Head | Neutral |
| Cervical spine | Normal curve = physiologically convex anteriorly (lordosis) |
| Thoracic spine | Normal curve = physiologically convex posteriorly (kyphosis) |
| Lumbar spine | Hyperextended (hyperlordosis) |
| Pelvis | Increased anterior tilt |
| Hip joints | Relatively flexed |
| Knee joints | Hyperextended |
| Ankle joints | Plantar flexed |

medial and the lateral portion. The medial portion of quadratus lumborum is responsible for spine stabilization and has a tendency to hypoactivity, while the lateral portion, related to trunk movements, has a tendency to hyperactivity (Fig. 6) [9, 10, 24].

The erector spinae is worthy of special attention as, according to both the literature and the biomechanical analysis of the standing posture, this muscle is likely to present shortening in the lumbar part of the spine [3]. However, the authors' experience reveals that this muscle is rarely shortened. We suspect that this phenomenon is a consequence of the lifestyle—spending the vast time in flexed sitting position [25, 26], so the lumbar part of erector spinae is constantly stretched. In turn, both standing and sitting position favors the shortening of hip flexors.

As a result of knee hyperextension and feet plantar flexion, the triceps surae may be shortened, including hypoactive soleus and hyperactive gastrocnemius (Table 2) [3, 9, 10].

overloading of the anterior knee compartment (Fig. 6). The *head line* may overlap the *base line*, or in the case of head protraction, it may run in front of it [3, 7, 8]. The description of the lordotic posture is given in Table 1.

*Functional state of muscles in the lordotic posture*
The abdominal muscles, gluteus maximus, posterior part of gluteus medius, and hamstrings are lengthened [3]. The stabilizers, mainly the gluteus maximus, are hypoactive. This, in turn, generates the hyperactivity of hamstrings that compensate the gluteus maximus in its function of stabilizing the pelvis and hip joints [10, 11].

The shortened muscles comprise quadratus lumborum as well as one-joint and two-joint hip flexors, namely the iliopsoas, rectus femoris, and tensor fasciae latae, respectively. However, from a clinical point of view, iliopsoas should be analyzed as two functionally independent muscles for the iliacus and the psoas, because each of them may be either hypo- (usually iliacus) or hyperactive (usually psoas). By the same token, quadratus lumborum comprises two functionally distinguished parts: the

**Kyphotic posture**
*Posture description*
The kyphotic posture represents a faulty posture that differs from the good one by the following: (1) increased thoracic kyphosis, (2) head protraction, (3) flattened or reversed lower cervical lordosis, (4) increased upper cervical lordosis, and (5) protraction of shoulders and scapulae (Fig. 7) [3, 7, 8].

In the kyphotic posture, the *head line* is shifted anteriorly to the thoracic spine, lumbar vertebral bodies, and hip and knee joint axis. The *base line* usually runs at the back of the head line (Fig. 7) [3, 7]. The description of the kyphotic posture is shown in Table 3.

*Functional state of muscle in the kyphotic posture*
In the kyphotic posture, the thoracic part of the erector spinae, rhomboids, serratus anterior, and the lower and middle parts of trapezius muscle are lengthened [3, 7].

The shortened muscles in the kyphotic posture are as follows: suboccipital, sternocleidomastoid, scaleni,

**Table 2** Functional characteristics of muscles in the lordotic posture

| Muscle | Lengthened | Shortened | Hypoactive | Hyperactive |
|---|---|---|---|---|
| Rectus abdominis | + | | | + |
| Abdominal internal oblique (anterior part) | + | | | + |
| Abdominal internal oblique (posterior part) | + | | + | |
| Abdominal external oblique | + | | | + |
| Gluteus maximus | + | | + | |
| Gluteus medius (posterior part) | + | | + | |
| Hamstrings | + | | | + |
| Erector spinae part lumbar (in sitting) | + | | + | |
| Erector spinae part lumbar (in standing) | | + | + | |
| Quadratus lumborum (medial part) | | + | + | |
| Quadratus lumborum (lateral part) | | + | | + |
| Iliacus | | + | + | |
| Psoas | | + | | + |
| Two-joint hip flexors | | + | | + |
| Gastrocnemius | | + | | + |
| Soleus | | + | + | |

Note: the symbol "+" means that the muscle meets a certain criteria

pectoralis major, pectoralis minor, and latissimus dorsi [3, 7]. Nevertheless, the latissimus dorsi may be shortened only in its part located close to the muscle insertion at the shoulder girdle (the crest of the lesser tubercle of the humerus) because of the shoulder protraction and internal rotation of the arms. On the other hand, the medial part of the latissimus dorsi may be lengthened due to increased thoracic kyphosis.

It is also worth taking a closer look at abdominal muscles. As a result of chest tilting, these muscles can be shortened, which has to be taken into consideration while selecting corrective exercises (Fig. 7) (Table 4).

**Kyphotic-lordotic posture**
In some individuals, the combination of the two aforementioned sagittal misalignments can be noted in the form of kyphotic-lordotic posture (Fig. 8) [3]. In this case, the influence of kyphotic and lordotic posture on the musculoskeletal system is combined [3, 7].

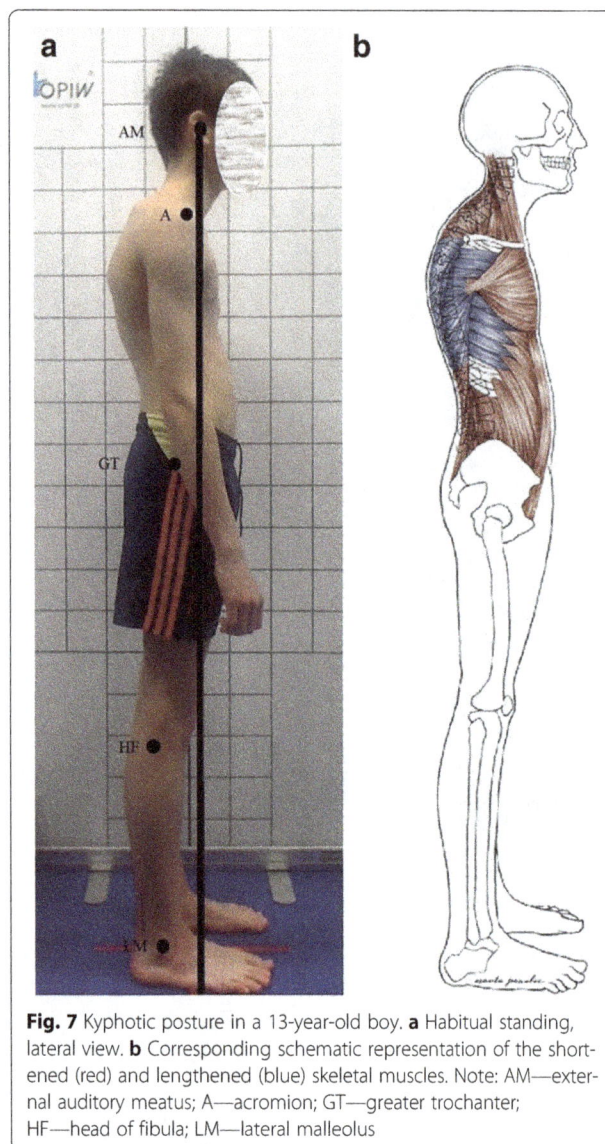

**Fig. 7** Kyphotic posture in a 13-year-old boy. **a** Habitual standing, lateral view. **b** Corresponding schematic representation of the shortened (red) and lengthened (blue) skeletal muscles. Note: AM—external auditory meatus; A—acromion; GT—greater trochanter; HF—head of fibula; LM—lateral malleolus

The authors would like to emphasize that difficulties in planning corrective exercises can occur in the kyphotic-lordotic posture. For instance, in lordotic posture, the abdominal muscles are lengthened and therefore should be shortened, while it is not recommended in the kyphotic posture. Although providing therapeutic schemata extends beyond the content of this paper, this example illustrates accurately the need for a nuanced physiotherapy: shortening the lower part of the abdominals (e.g., by moving upward their attachment to the pubic symphysis and iliac crest) while increasing the length of their upper part (Fig. 8).

**Flat-back posture**
*Posture description*
The flat-back posture represents a faulty posture that differs from the good one by the following: (1) flattened

**Table 3** The position of body parts in the kyphotic posture

| Part of the body | Position |
|---|---|
| Head | Protracted (moved forward) |
| Cervical spine | Upper part: extended (hyperlordosis)<br>Lower part: flexed (hypolordosis or kyphosis) |
| Scapulae | Abducted (moved laterally) |
| Shoulders | Protracted (moved forward) |
| Thoracic spine | Increased flexion (hyperkyphosis) |
| Chest | Tilted downward, sometimes flattened |
| Sternum | Tilted downward |
| Thoracic outlet | Increased obliquity |
| Lumbar spine | Neutral |
| Pelvis | Neutral |
| Hip joints | Neutral |
| Knee joints | Neutral |
| Ankle joints | Neutral |

**Table 4** Functional characteristics of muscles in the kyphotic posture

| Muscle | Lengthened | Shortened | Hypoactive | Hyperactive |
|---|---|---|---|---|
| Erector spinae (thoracic part) | + | | | + |
| Rhomboideus major and minor | + | | + | |
| Serratus anterior | + | | + | |
| Trapezius (middle and lower parts) | + | | + | |
| Latissimus dorsi (medial part) | + | | | + |
| Suboccipital | | + | | + |
| Sternocleidomastoid | | + | | + |
| Scaleni | | + | | + |
| Latissimus dorsi (area of insertion) | | + | | + |
| Trapezius (superior part) | | + | | + |
| Pectoralis minor and major | | + | | + |
| Rectus abdominis | | + | | + |
| Abdominal internal oblique (anterior part) | | + | | + |
| Abdominal internal oblique (posterior part) | | + | + | |
| Abdominal external oblique | | + | | + |

Note: the symbol "+" means that the muscle meets a certain criteria

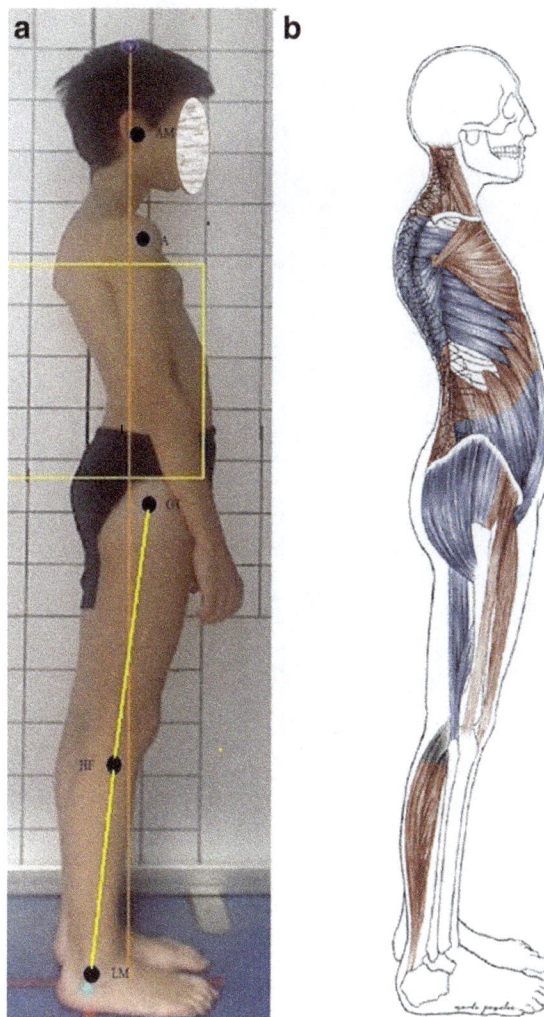

**Fig. 8** Kyphotic-lordotic posture in a 12-year-old boy. **a** Habitual standing, lateral view. **b** Corresponding schematic representation of the shortened (red) and lengthened (blue) skeletal muscles. Note: AM—external auditory meatus; A—acromion; GT—greater trochanter; HF—head of fibula; LM—lateral malleolus

lumbar lordosis and (2) flattened lower part of thoracic kyphosis. Moreover, increased kyphosis in the upper part of the thoracic region as well as kyphotisation of the cervico-thoracic junction may be present (Fig. 9). Pelvis remains in a neutral position or in a decreased anterior tilt [3, 7, 8, 27].

In the flat-back posture, the head line and the base line usually overlap and pass anteriorly to the lumbar vertebral bodies (leading to their flexion overload) and posterior to the hip joint axis (Fig. 9). The head may be moved anteriorly to the base line (Table 5) [3, 7].

### Functional state of muscles in the flat-back posture

The muscles which are usually lengthened in this posture include erector spinae (lumbar part), one-joint hip flexors (iliacus, psoas), and two-joint hip flexors (rectus

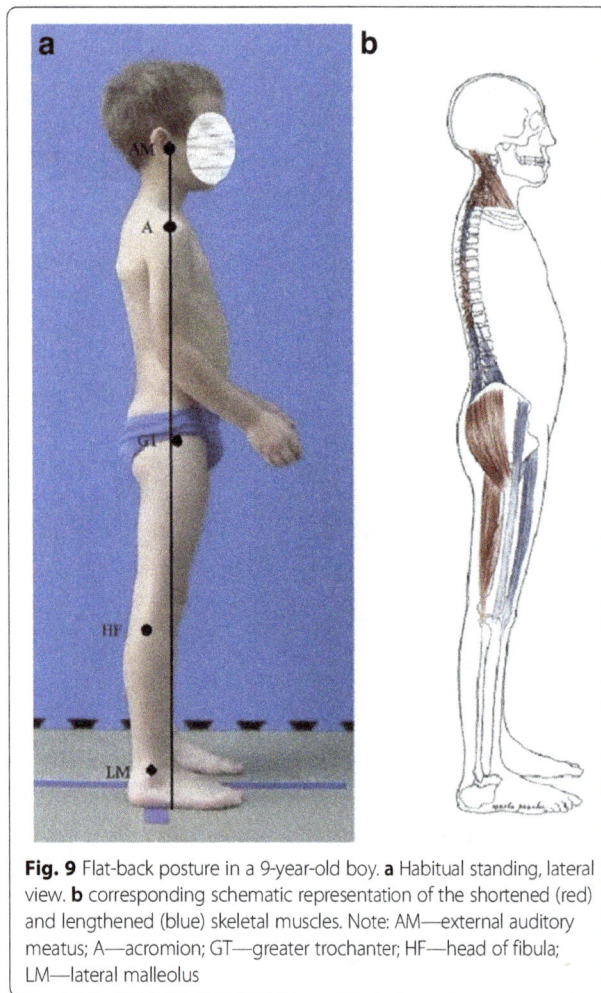

**Fig. 9** Flat-back posture in a 9-year-old boy. **a** Habitual standing, lateral view. **b** corresponding schematic representation of the shortened (red) and lengthened (blue) skeletal muscles. Note: AM—external auditory meatus; A—acromion; GT—greater trochanter; HF—head of fibula; LM—lateral malleolus

**Table 6** Functional characteristics of muscles in the flat-back posture

| Muscle | Lengthened | Shortened | Hypoactive | Hyperactive |
|---|---|---|---|---|
| Erector spinae part thoracic (upper part) | + | | | + |
| Erector spinae (lumbar part) | + | | + | |
| Iliacus | + | | + | |
| Psoas | + | | | + |
| Two-joint hip flexors | + | | | + |
| Suboccipital | | + | | + |
| Sternocleidomastoid | | + | | + |
| Scaleni | | + | | + |
| Erector spinae part thoracic (lower part) | | + | | + |
| Gluteus maximus | | + | + | |
| Hamstrings | | + | | + |

Note: the symbol "+" means that the muscle meets a certain criteria

### Sway-back posture
#### Posture description
The sway-back posture represents a faulty posture that differs from the good one by the following: (1) anterior pelvic shift, (2) thoracic kyphosis extended to the upper part of the lumbar spine (longer thoracic kyphosis is observed), (3) apparently shorter lumbar lordosis, (4) normal or slightly decreased anterior pelvic tilt (Fig. 10) [3, 7, 8, 27].

In the sway-back posture, the pelvis is in front of the head line, while the upper part of the trunk is usually moved posteriorly to this axis. The head line and the base line usually overlap each other suggesting the normal position of the head. However, the head is in a protraction because of the chest position that is in inclination in relation to the base and the head line [3, 7, 8]. The head line passes posteriorly to the lumbar vertebral bodies (resulting in their extension overload) and posteriorly to the hip joints axis (leading to overload of the hip joints) (Figs. 10 and 11, Table 7) [3, 5].

#### Functional state of muscles in the sway-back posture
Erector spinae in the upper thoracic and in the upper lumbar part, the muscles that stabilize the scapulae (serratus anterior, lower and middle part of trapezius and rhomboid muscles), abdominal muscles (their lower part), and one-joint (iliacus, psoas), and two-joint hip flexors (rectus femoris, tensor fascia latae) are lengthened [3, 7, 9, 10].

The shortened muscles are suboccipital, sternocleidomastoid, scaleni, chest muscles—pectoralis major and minor, erector spinae lumbar part (lower part), upper

femoris, tensor fasciae latae). Iliacus is usually hypoactive, while psoas is hyperactive. Two-joint hip flexors are hyperactive [3, 9, 10].

Gluteus maximus is shortened and hypoactive; hamstrings are also shortened yet hyperactive (Table 6, Fig. 9) [3, 9, 10].

**Table 5** The position of body parts in the flat-back posture

| Part of the body | Position |
|---|---|
| Head | Neutral or protracted (moved forward) |
| Cervical spine | Upper part: extended (hyperlordosis) Lower part: flexed (hypolordosis or kyphosis) |
| Thoracic spine | Upper part: increased flexion (hyperkyphosis) Lower part: straight (hypokyphosis) |
| Lumbar spine | Flexed (hypolordosis) |
| Pelvis | Neutral or decreased anterior tilt |
| Hip joints | Neutral or extended when decreased anterior tilt of pelvis occurs |
| Knee joints | Neutral |
| Ankle joints | Neutral |

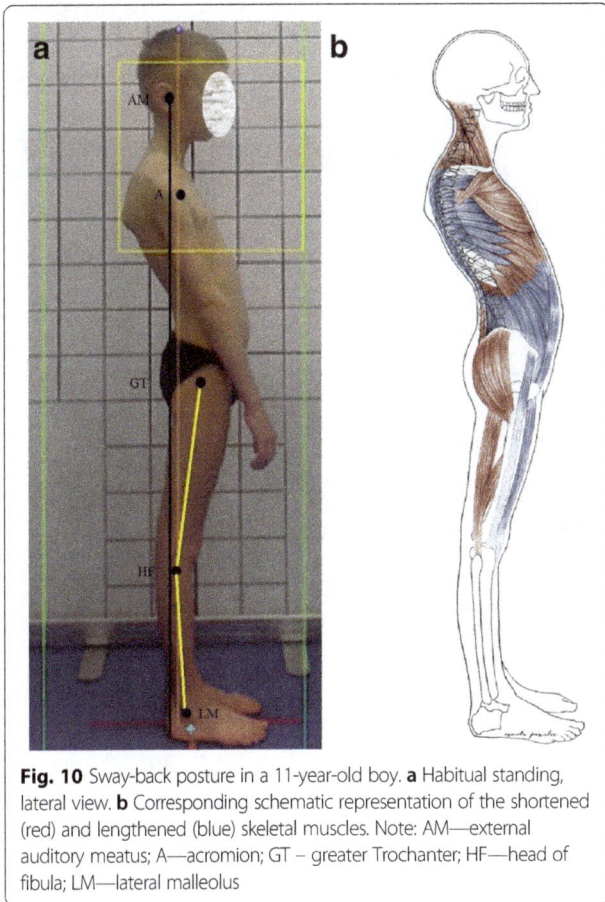

**Fig. 10** Sway-back posture in a 11-year-old boy. **a** Habitual standing, lateral view. **b** Corresponding schematic representation of the shortened (red) and lengthened (blue) skeletal muscles. Note: AM—external auditory meatus; A—acromion; GT – greater Trochanter; HF—head of fibula; LM—lateral malleolus

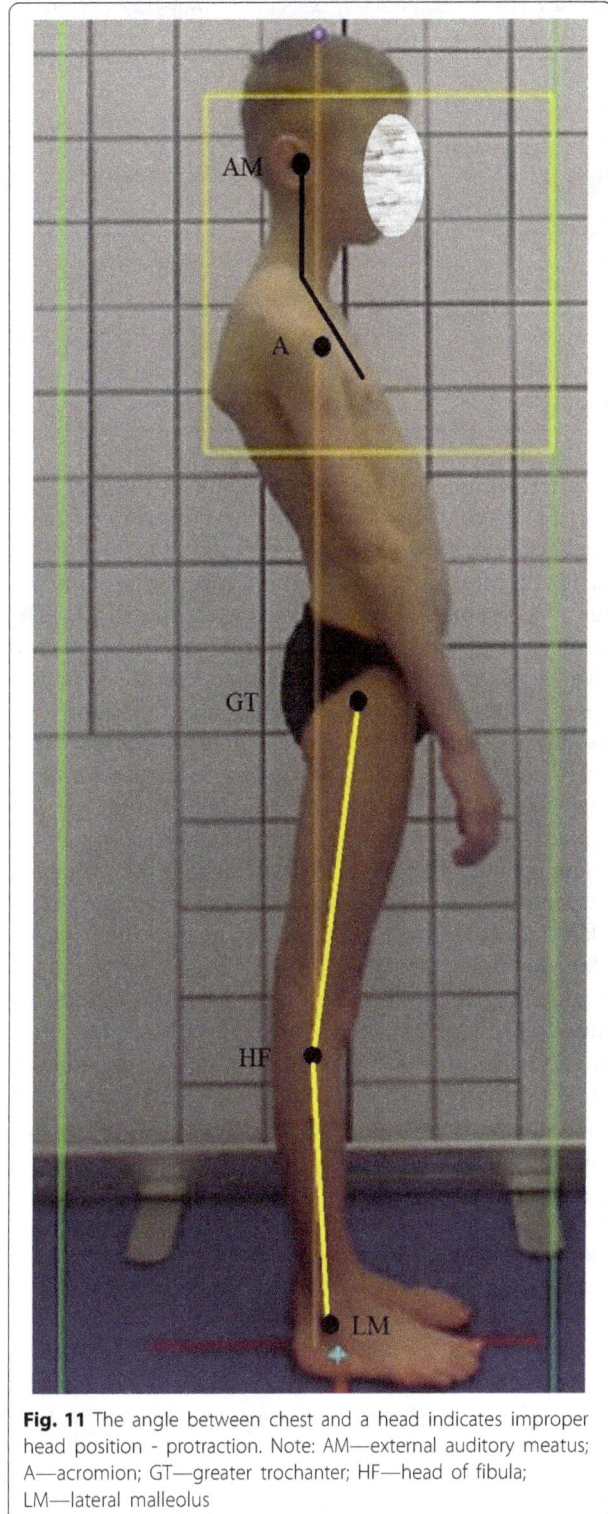

**Fig. 11** The angle between chest and a head indicates improper head position - protraction. Note: AM—external auditory meatus; A—acromion; GT—greater trochanter; HF—head of fibula; LM—lateral malleolus

fibers of abdominal muscles, gluteus maximus, and hamstrings. All these muscles demonstrate hyperactivity (except for the lower part of lumbar erector spinae, posterior part of internal oblique abdominal muscle, and gluteus maximus) (Table 8, Fig. 10) [3, 7, 9, 10].

## Discussion

The aim of the paper was to present the most common types of the sagittal, non-structural misalignments of the human body posture: namely the lordotic posture, kyphotic posture, flat-back posture, and sway-back posture. Each of them may influence both the skeletal and muscular systems leading to the functional disturbances, thus increasing the risk of back and peripheral joint pain or injuries [1–3, 5–8, 10, 19, 28, 29]. The paper was completed with the authors own experience in the diagnosis and treatment of body posture misalignments.

### Clinical relevance—considerations for the correction of non-structural misalignments of body posture

In a good body posture, balance should be maintained between the strength and the flexibility of the antagonistic muscles, for instance, between the hip flexors and the extensors or between the muscles of anterior and posterior part of the pectoral girdle [1–3, 6–10, 23].

According to the classification proposed by Kendall et al., muscles can be assessed in respect to their length and strength. Consequently, e.g., in lordotic

**Table 7** The position of body parts in the sway-back posture

| Part of the body | Position |
|---|---|
| Head | Protracted (moved forward) |
| Cervical spine | Upper part: extended (hyperlordosis)<br>Lower part: flexed (hypolordosis or kyphosis) |
| Thoracic spine | Upper part: increased flexion (hyperkyphosis)<br>Lower part: normal (kyphosis) |
| Lumbar spine | Upper part: flexion (kyphosis or hypolordosis)<br>Lower part: increased extension (hyperlordosis) |
| Pelvis | Shifted anteriorly, decreased anterior tilt |
| Hip joints | Extended due to decreased anterior tilt of pelvis |
| Knee joints | Neutral or hyperextended |
| Ankle joints | Neutral or plantar flexed |

**Table 8** Functional characteristics of muscles in the sway-back posture

| Muscle | Lengthened | Shortened | Hypoactive | Hyperactive |
|---|---|---|---|---|
| Trapezius (middle and lower part) | + | | + | |
| Serratus anterior | + | | + | |
| Rhomboideus major and minor | + | | + | |
| Erector spinae part thoracic (upper part) | + | | | + |
| Erector spinae lumbar part (upper part) | + | | + | |
| Rectus abdominis (lower fibers) | + | | | + |
| Abdominal internal oblique (anterior part, lower fibers) | + | | | + |
| Abdominal internal oblique (posterior part, lower fibers) | + | | + | |
| Abdominal external oblique (lower fibers) | + | | | + |
| Iliacus | + | | + | |
| Psoas | + | | | + |
| Two-joint hip flexors | + | | | + |
| Suboccipital | | + | | + |
| Sternocleidomastoid | | + | | + |
| Scaleni | | + | | + |
| Trapezius (superior part) | | + | | + |
| Pectoralis minor and major | | + | | + |
| Erector spinae lumbar part (lower part) | | + | + | |
| Rectus abdominis (upper fibers) | | + | | + |
| Abdominal internal oblique (anterior part, upper fibers) | | + | | + |
| Abdominal internal oblique (posterior part, upper fibers) | | + | + | |
| Abdominal external oblique (upper fibers) | | + | | + |
| Gluteus maximus | | + | + | |
| Hamstrings | | + | | + |

Note: the symbol "+" means that the muscle meets a certain criteria

posture, among others, the abdominal muscles, the gluteus maximus, the posterior part of gluteus medius, and hamstrings are lengthened. On the other hand, the erector spinae in the lumbar spine, quadratus lumborum, and hip flexors are shortened [3]. The authors suggested that the muscles which are excessive in length are usually weak and require strengthening, while these muscles that are too short are usually strong and maintain antagonistic muscles in a lengthened position [3]. According to our experience, this description of muscle function, based on the direct connection between the lengthening or shortening of muscles and their weakness or strength, respectively, is often taken into consideration while planning corrective exercises by many clinicians. A clinically important question remains: does the muscle lengthening mean that they prove weak, and does the muscle shortening correspond to their increased strength like in the classification proposed by Kendall et al.? The answer was attempted to be given with the detailed classification of muscles presented in the paper [9, 10].

**Muscle hyperactivity can be accompanied by muscle lengthening—the clinical example of hamstrings**

Figure 12 presents a boy whose anterior pelvic tilt is increased, which means that his hamstrings are probably lengthened and, according to Kendall et al., weak. It suggests that during corrective exercises these muscles should be strengthened. However, two functional tests performed by the boy (the long sitting test and the popliteal angle test) reveal interesting information [3, 7, 27]. Figure 13 presents the boy performing the maximal active knee extension while keeping the hip flexed at 90° (the popliteal angle test). The test indicates decreased hamstring flexibility. Accordingly, taking into consideration only the result of this test, the hamstrings would have to be stretched. Figure 14, in turn, shows a maximal trunk forward bending during the long-sitting test.

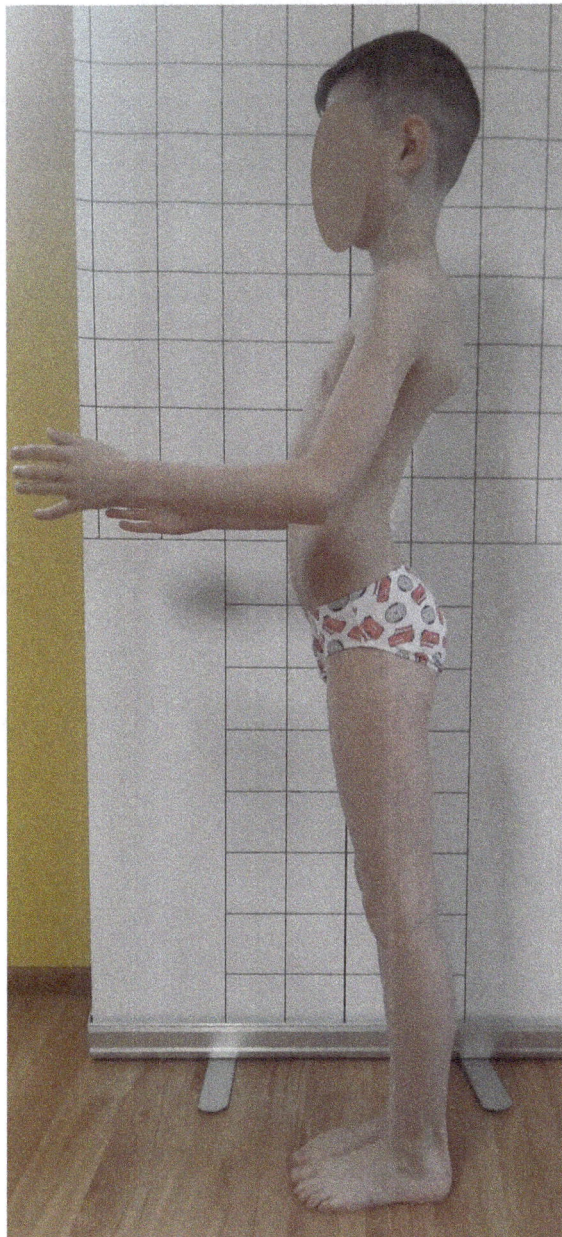

Fig. 12 A 10-year-old boy presenting a lordotic posture. Note the following elements: increased lumbar lordosis, increased anterior pelvic tilt

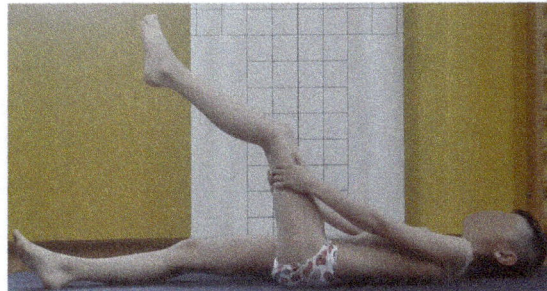

**Fig. 13** The maximal active knee extension keeping the hip flexed 90°—decreased flexibility of left hamstrings

with the use of the muscle classification proposed by Berg-mark and Richardson et al., which indicates that muscle lengthening may not be related to muscle weakness but can be analyzed in respect to its hyper- or hypoactivity [9, 10]. Taking into consideration the imbalance between the gluteus maximus muscle (hypoactive) and the hamstring muscles (hyperactive) (described detailed in the section "Lordotic posture"), the specific postural physiotherapy should not comprise hamstring exercises aimed at their strengthening (according to Kendall et al. [3]) or stretch-ing (according to functional tests results). The exercises should be focused rather on reducing their activity through regaining the activity of the stabilizers including, in this example, the gluteus maximus [7–10]. Further-more, the lengthened muscles should not be simply strengthened, but they should be shortened, so the exer-cises should be performed in the so-called internal (not full) range of motion [10].

In consequence, when planning the corrective exer-cises, it is important to verify not only the length of the muscles but also their function (hyper- or hypoac-tivity). It is also important to plan the exercises based on (1) the individual evaluation of the posture, especially when the characteristics of the posture does

The result of the test suggests the decreasing flexibility of hamstrings and trunk. However, the trunk flexion in sitting on the stool (knees flexed) indicates a good range of motion of the trunk, which confirms the limited flexi-bility of hamstrings (Fig. 15).

The abovementioned tests revealed the shortening of the hamstrings (Figs. 13 and 14). However, according to Fig. 12 and the description of the lordotic posture in the literature [3, 27], these muscles should be lengthened in this type of faulty posture. This question may be answered

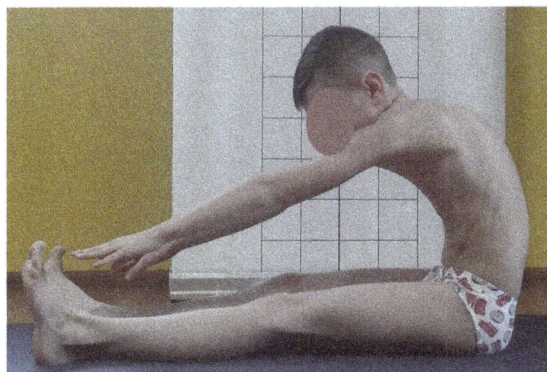

**Fig. 14** Trunk forward bend test—decreased flexibility of hamstrings and trunk

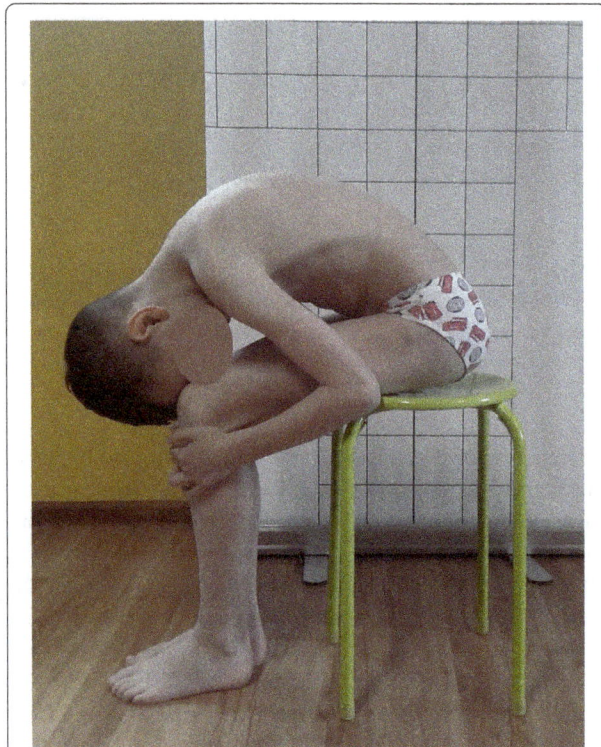

**Fig. 15** Normal trunk flexion in sitting position with knees flexed

not match any of the four types presented in the paper, and (2) the analysis of the posture in the usual position for a particular subject in which she/he spends most of the time during a day (e.g., sitting, position at work or while learning, position during learning or hobby).

### Limitations

The authors of this paper focused on the sagittal misalignments of the body posture and their relations with the muscular system. The paper is not discussing the relation of body posture with other factors: psychosocial, nutritional status, structural disorders, or fascial system. We did not discuss the important role of postural education to obtain the good results of corrective exercises.

Further studies are needed to verify a long-term influence of various types of non-structural sagittal misalignments of body posture on the disturbances in the muscular and skeletal system and the functional and structural status of the body.

### Conclusions

1. There exist four principal types of non-structural body posture misalignments in the sagittal plane: lordotic posture, kyphotic posture, flat-back posture, and sway-back posture. Each of them disturbs the

physiological loading of the musculoskeletal system, which may lead to functional disorders.

2. In individuals with sagittal misalignments of body posture, not only the evaluation of muscle length or strength should be performed, but also their primary function related to stabilization or mobilization in maintaining good body posture should be taken into consideration.

3. The correction of postural misalignments aimed at the restoration of a good sagittal alignment should start with detailed clinical examination followed by the application of specific corrective exercises directed to recover primary muscles' function.

**Acknowledgements**
Not applicable.

**Funding**
Not applicable.

**Authors' contributions**
DC performed the paper design, wrote and revised of the manuscript, and is the author of the figures. LS revised the manuscript and is the author of the figures. MT revised the manuscript. MK revised the manuscript and is the author of the figures. TK performed the paper design and wrote and revised of the manuscript. All authors read and approved the final manuscript.

**Competing interests**
The authors declare that they have no competing interests.

**Author details**
[1]Department of Physiotherapy, Józef Rusiecki University College in Olsztyn, Bydgoska 33, 10-243 Olsztyn, Poland. [2]Center of Body Posture, Bydgoska 33, 10-243 Olsztyn, Poland. [3]Spine Disorders Center, Rehasport Licensed Rehabilitation Center, Al. Niepodległości 4, 96-100 Skierniewice, Poland. [4]Spine Disorders and Pediatric Orthopedics Department, University of Medical Sciences, 28 Czerwca 1956 135/147 Street, 61-545 Poznań, Poland. [5]Rehasport Clinic, Górecka 30, 60-201 Poznań, Poland. [6]Department of Orthopaedics, Pediatric Orthopaedics and Traumatology, The Center of Postgraduate Medical Education in Warsaw, Konarskiego 13, 05-400 Otwock, Poland.

### References

1. Claus A, Hides JA, Moseley GL, Hodges PW. Different ways to balance the spine: subtle changes in sagittal spinal curves affect regional muscle activity. Spine. 2009;34(6):208–14.
2. O'Sullivan PB, Grahamslaw KM, Kendell M, et al. The effect of different standing and sitting postures on trunk muscle activity in a pain-free population. Spine (Phila Pa 1976). 2002;27:1238–44.
3. Kendall F, McCreary E, Provance PG, Rodgers M, Romani WA. Muscle testing and function with posture and pain. Baltimore: Lippincott Williams & Wilkins; 2005.
4. Janssen MM, Kouwenhoven JW, Schlösser TP, Viergever MA, Bartels LW, Castelein RM, Vincken KL. Analysis of preexistent vertebral rotation in the normal infantile, juvenile, and adolescent spine. Spine (Phila Pa 1976). 2011; 36(7):486–91.
5. Levangie PK, Norkin CC. Joint structure and function: a comprehensive analysis. F.A. Davis Company, 2005.

6.  McGill S. Low Back Disorders-3rd Edition with Web Resource: Evidence-Based Prevention and Rehabilitation. Human Kinetics; 3 edition, Champaign, USA; 2015.

7.  Sahrmann S. Diagnosis and treatment of movement impairment syndromes. St. Louis: Mosby; 2002.

8.  Comerford M, Mottram S. Kinetic control—e-book: the management of uncontrolled movement. Churchill Livingstone Australia; 2012.

9.  Bergmark A. Stability of the lumbar spine. A study in the mechanical engineering. Acta Orthop Scand Suppl. 1989;230:20–4.

10. Richardson CA, Hodges PW, Hides J. Therapeutic exercise for lumbopelvic stabilization: a motor control approach for the treatment and prevention of low back pain. 2nd ed. Edinburgh: Churchill Livingstone; 2004.

11. Richardson C. The muscle designation debate: the experts respond. J Bodyw Mov Ther. 2000;4(4):235–6.

12. Richardson C, Bullock MI. Changes in muscle activity during fast alternating flexion-extension movements of the knee. Scand J of Rehabil Med. 1986;18:51–8.

13. Appell HJ. Muscular atrophy following immobilization: a review. Sports Med. 1990;10:42.

14. Hides JA, Stokes MJ, Saide M, Jull GA, Cooper DH. Evidence of lumbar multifidus muscle wasting ipsilateral to symptoms in patients with acute/subacute low back pain. Spine. 1994;19:165–72.

15. Dilani Mendis M, Hides JA, Wilson SJ, Grimaldi A, Belavý DL, Stanton W, Felsenberg D, Rittweger J, Richardson C. Effect of prolonged bed rest on the anterior hip muscles. Gait Posture. 2009;30(4):533–7.

16. Hides JA, Belavý DL, Stanton W, Wilson SJ, Rittweger J, Felsenberg D, Richardson CA. Magnetic resonance imaging assessment of trunk muscles during prolonged bed rest. Spine (Phila Pa 1976). 2007;32(15):1687–92.

17. Hides JA, Lambrecht G, Stanton WR, Damann V. Changes in multifidus and abdominal muscle size in response to microgravity: possible implications for low back pain research. Eur Spine J. 2016 May;25(Suppl 1):175–82.

18. Hides JA, Belavý DL, Cassar L, Williams M, Wilson SJ, Richardson CA. Altered response of the anterolateral abdominal muscles to simulated weight-bearing in subjects with low back pain. Eur Spine J. 2009;18(3):410–8.

19. Reeve A, Dilley A. Effects of posture on the thickness of transversus abdominis in pain-free subjects. Man Ther. 2009;14(6):679–84.

20. Bogduk N, Twomey LT. Clinical anatomy of the lumbar spine. 2nd ed. London: Chruchill Livingstone; 1991.

21. Hides JA, Lambrecht G, Richardson CA, Stanton WR, Armbrecht G, Pruett C, Damann V, Felsenberg D, Belavý DL. The effects of rehabilitation on the muscles of the trunk following prolonged bed rest. Eur Spine J. 2011;20(5):808–18.

22. Belavý DL, Richardson CA, Wilson SJ, Rittweger J, Felsenberg D. Superficial lumbopelvic muscle overactivity and decreased cocontraction after 8 weeks of bed rest. Spine (Phila Pa 1976). 2007;32(1):232–9.

23. Lee DG. The Pelvic Girdle: An integration of clinical expertise and research. Churchill Livingstone; 4 edition USA; 2010.

24. Bullock-Saxton J, Murphy D, Norris C, Richardson C, Tunnel P. The muscle designation debate: the experts respond. J Bodyw Mov Ther. 2000;4(4):225–57.

25. Kędra A, Czaprowski D. Sedentary behaviours of 10-19-year-old students with and without spinal pain. Probl Hig Epidemiol. 2015;1(96):143–8.

26. Czaprowski D, Stoliński Ł, Szczygieł A, Kędra A. Sedentary behaviours of girls and boys aged 7-15. Polish Journal of Public Health. 2011;121(3):248–52.

27. Solberg G. Postural disorders & musculoskeletal dysfunction. Diagnosis, prevention and treatment. Philadelphia: Elsevier Churchill Livingstone; 2008.

28. Gajdosik RL, Albert CR, Mitman JJ. Influence of hamstring length on the standing position and flexion range of motion of the pelvic angle, lumbar angle, and thoracic angle. J Orthop Sports Phys Ther. 1994;20(4):213–9.

29. Fujitani R, Jiromaru T, Kida N, Nomura T. Effect of standing postural deviations on trunk and hip muscle activity. J Phys Ther Sci. 2017;29(7): 1212–5.

# 20

# Long-term outcome of posterior spinal fusion for the correction of adolescent idiopathic scoliosis

Hasan Ghandhari, Ebrahim Ameri, Farshad Nikouei, Milad Haji Agha Bozorgi[*], Shoeib Majdi and Mostafa Salehpour

## Abstract

**Background:** Adolescent idiopathic scoliosis (AIS) is the most common form of idiopathic scoliosis, and surgery is considered as one of the therapeutic options. However, it is associated with a variety of irreversible complications, in spite of the benefits it provides. Here, we evaluated the long-term outcome of posterior spinal fusion (PSF) of AIS to shed more light on the consequences of this surgery.

**Methods:** In a cross-sectional study, a total of 42 AIS patients who underwent PSF surgery were radiographically and clinically inspected for the potential post-operative complications. Radiographic assessments included the device failure, union status, and vertebral tilt below the site of fusion. Clinical outcomes were evaluated using the Oswestry disability index (ODI) and visual analogue scale (VAS).

**Results:** The mean age of the surgery was $14.4 \pm 5.1$ years. The mean follow-up of the patients was $5.6 \pm 3.2$ years. Complete union was observed in all patients, and no device failure was noticed. Pre- and post-operative vertebral tilt below the site of fusion were $11.12° \pm 7.92°$ and $6.21° \pm 5.73°$, respectively ($p < 0.001$). The mean post-operative ODI was $16.7 \pm 9.8$. The mean post-operative VAS was $2.1 \pm 0.7$. ODI value was positively correlated with follow-up periods ($p = 0.04$, $r = 0.471$). New degenerative disc disease (DDD) was observed in 6 out of 37 (16%) patients.

**Conclusion:** In spite of the efficacy and safety of PSF surgery of AIS, it might result in irreversible complications such as DDD. Moreover, the amount of post-operative disability might increase over the time and should be discussed with the patients.

**Keywords:** Adolescent idiopathic scoliosis, Posterior spinal fusion, Complications

## Background

Scoliosis is a spinal deformity which refers to deviation of the spine greater than 10° in the coronal plane. Idiopathic scoliosis is the most common type of scoliosis and spinal deformity as well. According to the age of onset, idiopathic scoliosis can be classified as infantile, juvenile, and adolescent [1, 2]. Adolescent idiopathic scoliosis (AIS) is the most common form of idiopathic scoliosis, occurring at the age of 10 years or greater [3].

The treatment options for AIS include observation, bracing, and surgery, and the general goal is to keep curves under 50° at maturity [2, 4]. Available surgical options for the treatment of idiopathic scoliosis include posterior spinal fusion (PSF), anterior spinal fusion (ASF), or a combination of both [5]. PSF remains as the gold standard for the treatment of thoracic and double major curves (most cases). ASF is indicated for thoracolumbar and lumbar cases having a normal sagittal profile. A combination of ASF and PSF could also be used for the management of large curves (> 75°) or stiff curves, young age, and to prevent crankshaft phenomenon [6–9]. The study of Geck et al. on the outcome of surgical management of adolescents with Lenke 5C curves revealed statistically significantly better curve correction, less loss of correction over time, and shorter hospitalization time when treated with a PSF compared with ASF for similar patient populations [10]. Superior

* Correspondence: mld_bozorgi86@yahoo.com
Bone and Joint Reconstruction Research Center, Shafa Orthopedic Hospital, Iran University of Medical Sciences, Tehran, Iran

outcome of PSF has been reported in other investigations as well [11].

Although the safety and efficacy of both techniques have been demonstrated [5], many patients and surgeons are concerned about the long-term outcome of an extensive fusion in terms of spinal function, the development of degenerative disc disease (DDD), and pain [12]. Weiss et al. reviewed the long-term risks of fusion spinal surgery with respect to the etiology of scoliosis to enable establishing a cost/benefit relation of this intervention. According to their study, average rate of complications was 44% in AIS, ranging from 10 to 78%. They concluded that long-term complications have not yet been fully evaluated and further studies are needed to address this concern adequately [13].

Here, we aimed at evaluating long-term effects of PSF in Iranian AIS patients. To the best of our knowledge, no similar investigation has been earlier performed in Iranian AIS population.

## Methods

In a cross-sectional study, AIS patients who underwent PSF surgery at our center during 2003–2015 were included. Exclusion criteria were (1) congenital, neuromuscular, or infantile scoliosis; (2) history of previous spinal surgery, i.e., discectomy; (3) presence of diseases which might affect the outcome such as rheumatoid arthritis and diabetes mellitus; (4) and unavailable imaging. Accordingly, from a total of 145 AIS patients who were treated with PSF, 52 were identified as eligible for this study. These patients were invited for the evaluation process; from them, 42 patients attended the evaluation session.

Plain standing spinal radiograph of C1–S1 in anteroposterior (AP) and lateral views, along with a lumbosacral MRI without contrast, was taken for radiographic assessments including the evaluation of device failure, union status of fusion site, and vertebral tilt below the site of fusion. Vertebral tilt was measured in both radiographs of before and after surgery using the superior end plate of the inferior disc at the fusion site. Clinical outcome was evaluated using the Oswestry disability index (ODI) and visual analogue scale (VAS), which in both a higher score was equivalent to an inferior outcome.

DDD classification was performed using the J. Khanna classification method. Based on this method, DDD was categorized into three classes. Accordingly, grade 1 was defined as a decrease in disc signal in T2 MRI. Grades 2 and 3 were defined as partial and complete disc collapse, respectively, in MRI imaging [14] (Fig. 1).

### Statistical analysis

Descriptive analysis was performed using mean and standard deviation (SD). $T$ test or analysis of variance (ANOVA) was used to compare the mean values between the groups. Pearson's or Spearman's correlation coefficient was used to evaluate the potential correlation between the variables. Data analysis was performed using SPSS for windows, version 16. A $p$ value of less than 0.05 was considered significant.

## Results

A total of 42 patients with the mean age of $20.5 \pm 6.8$ years, ranging from 16 to 25 years, were evaluated in this study. The mean age of surgery was $14.4 \pm 5.1$ years. The mean post-operative follow-up period of patient was $5.6 \pm 3.2$ years, ranging from 3 to 10 years. The most common level of fusion was L4 followed by L3 and L2. Screw or hook was used as the fusion device. The surgical and demographic characteristics of the patients have been summarized in Table 1.

Radiographic assessment of the patients confirmed a complete union in all cases. Furthermore, no device failure occurred in any patient of the study population. Mean vertebral tilt below the site of fusion before and after surgery were $11.12° \pm 7.92°$ and $6.21° \pm 5.73°$, respectively. This difference was statistically significant ($p < 0.001$).

The mean post-operative ODI was $16.7 \pm 9.8$. The mean post-operative VAS was $2.1 \pm 0.7$. No significant correlation was observed between the values of VAS and follow-up period ($p = 0.321$, $r = -0.157$). However, a significant positive correlation was seen between ODI values and follow-up periods ($p = 0.04$, $r = 0.471$), so that a higher ODI value was present in patients with longer follow-up after the surgery. Moreover, ODI values were significantly correlated with post-operative vertebral tilt ($p = 0.038$, $r = 0.389$). No significant association was observed between the fusion level and ODI or VAS ($p = 0.59$ and $p = 0.44$, respectively). The mean ODI and VAS were not significantly different when different devices were used ($p = 0.6$ and $p = 0.47$, respectively).

In total, DDD was present in 5 (15%) patients before the surgery, whereas the disc was normal in the remaining 37 (85%) patients. While at the evaluation session the disc was still normal in 31 (83.8%) out of these 37 patients, grade 1 and grade 2 DDD was developed in 5 (13.5%) and 1 (2.7%) patient, respectively. Most of DDDs (72%) occurred in the first 3–5 years after the surgery. DDD development was not associated with the age of the patients ($p = 0.12$). Occurrence of DDD was also not significantly associated with pre-operative or post-operative vertebral tilt ($p = 0.3$ and $p = 0.08$, respectively). No significant association was also observed between the clinical scores (VAS and ODI) and DDD occurrence ($p = 0.5$ and $p = 0.53$: respectively). Moreover, the level of fusion was not significantly associated with the occurrence of DDD ($p = 0.87$). The DDD occurrence was not associated with the choice of fusion device as well ($p = 0.14$).

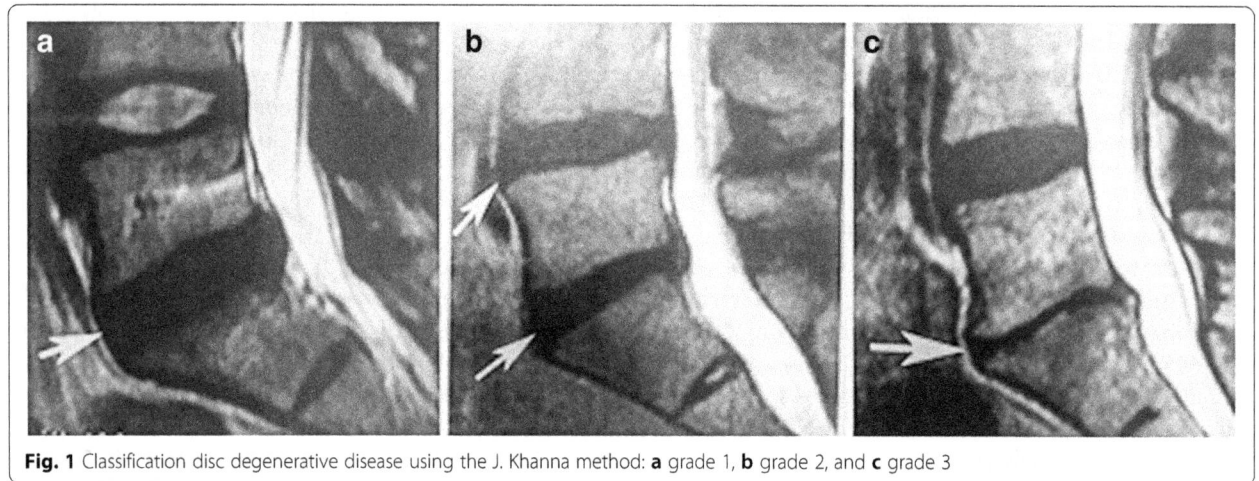

**Fig. 1** Classification disc degenerative disease using the J. Khanna method: **a** grade 1, **b** grade 2, and **c** grade 3

The results of surgery have been summarized in Table 2.

## Discussion

Corrective surgery of AIS can result in several benefits for the affected patients including improvements in esthetics, quality of life, disability, back pain, psychological well-being, and breathing function. It also can stop the progression of curve in adulthood, removing the need for further treatments in adulthood [15]. Based on the study of Ward et al., who compared the outcome of 190 non-operatively treated AIS subjects with 166 operatively treated patients, statistically significant differences in self-image, satisfaction, and total score were found in favor of the operative cohort [16].

On the other hand, AIS surgery still might result in a variety of complications whose long-term impact is poorly understood including neurological damage, loss of normal spinal function, strain on unfused vertebrae, curvature progression, decompensation and increased sagittal deformity, increased torso deformity, delayed paraparesis, and pseudarthrosis [13, 17]. Degenerative disc disease is also considered as one of the late complications of AIS both before and after the surgery, and its association with the severity of pain has been reported [18].

Thus, the surgeons must carefully weigh the potential for improvement against possible operative or post-operative complications. To this aim, further investigations are needed to shed more light on the long-term complications of AIS surgery and help the surgeon to choose the best therapeutic option.

Here, we evaluated the long-term outcome of PSF surgery in 42 AIS patients at a mean follow-up of 5.6 years. Radiographic markers of significant disc degeneration have been reported in nearly 7% of patients 10 years after surgery for AIS. However, the range of this rate varies between studies [19]. According to our study, new

**Table 1** The demographic and surgical characteristics of the patients

| Characteristic | Mean ± SD or number (%) |
| --- | --- |
| Age at the time of study (years) | 20.5 ± 6.8 |
| Age at the time of surgery (years) | 14.4 ± 5.1 |
| Post-operative follow-up (years) | 5.6 ± 3.2 |
| Gender | |
| • Male | 7 (15) |
| • Female | 35 (85) |
| Distal fusion level | |
| • L1 | 1 (2) |
| • L2 | 11 (25) |
| • L3 | 14 (33) |
| • L4 | 15 (35) |
| • L12 | 2 (5) |
| Fusion device | |
| • Screw | 27 (63) |
| • Hook | 15 (27) |

**Table 2** The outcome of the patients following the PSF surgery of AIS

| Patients' characteristics (n = 42) | Mean ± SD or number (%) |
| --- | --- |
| Pre-operative vertebral tilt | 11.12° ± 7.92° |
| Post-operative vertebral tilt | 6.21° ± 5.73° |
| Post-operative ODI | 16.7 ± 9.8 |
| Post-operative VAS | 2.1 ± 0.7 |
| New DDD | |
| • Grade 1 | 5 (13.5) |
| • Grade 2 | 1 (2.7) |

*PSF* posterior spinal fusion, *AIS* adolescent idiopathic scoliosis, *DDD* degenerative disc disease, *ODI* Oswestry disability index, *VAS* visual analogue scale

DDD was developed in 6 out of 37 (16%) patients with the preoperative normal discs.

Our study showed no association between the development of DDD and clinical findings (ODI and VAS). Similar results were reported in other investigations [20, 21].

While the DDD was more likely to present at the first post-operative 3–5 years in our patients, the clinical outcome was found to be associated with the time past the surgery, so that an inferior outcome was observed in patients with the longer follow-up period. In other words, the observed post-operative disability tended to increase over the time. The study of Upasani et al. also showed an increased pain at 5 years compared with 2 years after AIS surgical treatment [21]. Thus, we suggest surgeons to discuss this long-term complication with their patients prior to the surgery.

According to the study of Green et al., the lower level of fusion was associated with the higher rate and grade of disc degeneration after PSF surgery of AIS [22]. Similar results were reported by Luk et al. [23]. By contrast, Harding et al. found no correlation between disc degeneration and number of fused vertebrae [20]. Our results were in accordance with the results of Harding et al. [20].

Our results revealed a significant association between the preoperative vertebral tilt and post-operative ODI. This finding proposes that a pre-operative higher tilt distal to the site of fusion corresponds to a higher post-operative ODI and could be regarded as a prognostic marker of the surgery.

Our study has some weaknesses which should be pointed out. The small number of cases, caused by the high rate of loss of follow-up, could be regarded as the main weakness of this investigation. This limitation might have adversely affected the statistical power of the study. It also did not allow us to further analyze the data, such as to search an association between the grade of DDD and other variables. Thus, further studies with larger sample size are needed to confirm our results.

## Conclusion

In spite of the benefits it might bring to the affected patients, the surgery of AIS could result in a variety of irreversible complications, including the degenerative change of the discs. Thus, the surgeons must carefully weigh the potential benefits and complications of an AIS surgery prior to the procedure. Moreover, they should inform the patients that some of the observed improvements might reduce over the time.

## Abbreviations

AIS: Adolescent idiopathic scoliosis; ANOVA: Analysis of variance; AP: Anteroposterior; ASF: Anterior spinal fusion; DDD: Degenerative disc disease; MRI: Magnetic resonance imaging; ODI: Oswestry disability index; PSF: Posterior spinal fusion; SD: Standard deviation; VAS: Visual analogue scale

## Acknowledgements

The research team would like to thank Iran University of Medical Sciences for all the support and also all the participants and partners who played a role in the completion of this project.

## Funding

This study has been supported by Iran University of Medical Sciences.

## Authors' contributions

HG and EA supervised the project and edited the article critically. MS, MHAB, and SM did the project, filled the form, and prepared the first draft of the manuscript. FN analyzed and interpreted the data. All authors read and approved the final manuscript.

## References

1. Koop S. Infantile and juvenile idiopathic scoliosis. Orthop Clin North Am. 1988;19:331–7.
2. Janicki JA, Alman B. Scoliosis: review of diagnosis and treatment. Paediatr Child Health. 2007;12:771–6.
3. Burton MS. Diagnosis and treatment of adolescent idiopathic scoliosis. Pediatr Ann. 2013;42:e233–7.
4. Tari SHV, Mahabadi EA, Ghandehari H, Nikouei F, Javaheri R, Safdari F. Spinopelvic sagittal alignment in patients with adolescent idiopathic scoliosis. Shafa Orthop J. 2015;2(3):e739.
5. Wang Y, Fei Q, Qiu G, Lee CI, Shen J, Zhang J, Zhao H, Zhao Y, Wang H, Yuan S. Anterior spinal fusion versus posterior spinal fusion for moderate lumbar/thoracolumbar adolescent idiopathic scoliosis: a prospective study. Spine. 2008;33:2166–72.
6. Kotwicki T, Chowanska J, Kinel E, Czaprowski D, Tomaszewski M, Janusz P. Optimal management of idiopathic scoliosis in adolescence. Adolesc Health Med Ther. 2013;4:59.
7. Ghandhari H, Safari MB, Ameri E, Kheirabadi H, Tabrizi A. Correlation curve correction and spinal length gain in patients with adolescent idiopathic scoliosis. J Clin Diagn Res. 2017;11:RC01–4.
8. Lonner BS, Kondrachov D, Siddiqi F, Hayes V, Scharf C. Thoracoscopic spinal fusion compared with posterior spinal fusion for the treatment of thoracic adolescent idiopathic scoliosis. J Bone Join Surg. 2006;88:1022–34.
9. Viviani G, Raducan V, Bednar D, Grandwilewski W. Anterior and posterior spinal fusion: comparison of one-stage and two-stage procedures. Can J Surg. 1993;36:468–73.
10. Geck MJ, Rinella A, Hawthorne D, Macagno A, Koester L, Sides B, Bridwell K, Lenke L, Shufflebarger H. Comparison of surgical treatment in Lenke 5C adolescent idiopathic scoliosis: anterior dual rod versus posterior pedicle fixation surgery: a comparison of two practices. Spine. 2009;34:1942–51.
11. Huitema G, Willems PC, van Rhijn L, Kleijnen J, Shaffrey CI. Anterior versus posterior spinal correction and fusion for adolescent idiopathic scoliosis. Cochrane Libr. 2014. https://doi.org/10.1002/14651858.CD011280.
12. Bridwell KH, Shufflebarger HL, Lenke LG, Lowe TG, Betz RR, Bassett GS. Parents' and patients' preferences and concerns in idiopathic adolescent scoliosis: a cross-sectional preoperative analysis. Spine. 2000;25:2392–9.
13. Weiss H-R, Goodall D. Rate of complications in scoliosis surgery—a systematic review of the Pub Med literature. Scoliosis. 2008;3:9.
14. Khanna AJ. MRI for orthopaedic surgeons. New York: Thieme; 2010.
15. Negrini S, Grivas TB, Kotwicki T, Maruyama T, Rigo M, Weiss HR. Why do we treat adolescent idiopathic scoliosis? What we want to obtain and to avoid for our patients. SOSORT 2005 Consensus paper. Scoliosis. 2006;1:4.
16. Ward WT, Friel NA, Kenkre TS, Brooks MM, Londino JA, Roach JW. SRS-22r scores in nonoperated adolescent idiopathic scoliosis patients with curves greater than forty degrees. Spine. 2017;42:1233–40.

17. Hawes M. Impact of spine surgery on signs and symptoms of spinal deformity. Pediatr Rehab. 2006;9:318–39.

18. Buttermann GR, Mullin WJ. Pain and disability correlated with disc degeneration via magnetic resonance imaging in scoliosis patients. Euro Spine J. 2008;17:240–9.

19. Jones M, Badreddine I, Mehta J, Ede MN, Gardner A, Spilsbury J, Marks D. The rate of disc degeneration on MRI in preoperative adolescent idiopathic scoliosis. Spine J. 2017;17:S332.

20. Harding IJ, Charosky S, Vialle R, Chopin DH. Lumbar disc degeneration below a long arthrodesis (performed for scoliosis in adults) to L4 or L5. Euro Spine J. 2008;17:250–4.

21. Upasani VV, Caltoum C, Petcharaporn M, Bastrom TP, Pawelek JB, Betz RR, Clements DH, Lenke LG, Lowe TG, Newton PO. Adolescent idiopathic scoliosis patients report increased pain at five years compared with two years after surgical treatment. Spine. 2008;33:1107–12.

22. Green DW, Lawhorne TW III, Widmann RF, Kepler CK, Ahern C, Mintz DN, Rawlins BA, Burke SW, Boachie-Adjei O. Long-term magnetic resonance imaging follow-up demonstrates minimal transitional level lumbar disc degeneration after posterior spine fusion for adolescent idiopathic scoliosis. Spine. 2011;36:1948–54.

23. Luk K, Lee F, Leong J, Hsu L. The effect on the lumbosacral spine of long spinal fusion for idiopathic scoliosis. A minimum 10-year follow-up. Spine. 1987;12:996–1000.

# 21

# Effect of an elongation bending derotation brace on the infantile or juvenile scoliosis

John Thometz[1,2,5*], XueCheng Liu[1,2], Robert Rizza[3], Ian English[3] and Sergery Tarima[4]

## Abstract

**Background:** A wide variety of braces are commercially available designed for the adolescent idiopathic scoliosis (AIS), but very few braces for infantile scoliosis (IS) or juvenile scoliosis (JS). The goals of this study were: 1) to briefly introduce an elongation bending derotation brace (EBDB) in the treatment of IS or JS; 2) to investigate changes of Cobb angles in the AP view of X-ray between in and out of the EBDB at 0, 3, 6, 9, and 12 months; 3) to compare differences of Cobb angles (out of brace) in 3, 6, 9, and12 month with the baseline; 4) to investigate changes (out of brace) in JS and IS groups separately.

**Methods:** Thirty-eight patients with IS or JS were recruited retrospectively for this study. Spinal manipulation was performed using a stockinet. This was done simultaneously with a surface topography scan. The procedure was done in the operating room for IS, or in a clinical setting for JS. The brace was edited and fabricated using CAD/CAM method. Radiographs were recorded in and out of bracing approximately every 3 months from baseline to 12 months. A linear mixed effects model was used to compare in and out of bracing, and out of brace Cobb angle change over the 12 month period.

**Results:** Overall, 37.5% of curves are corrected and 37.5% stabilized after 12 months (Thoracic curves 48% correction, 19% stabilization; thoracolumbar curves 33% correction, 56% stabilization and lumbar curves 29% correction, 50% stabilization). The juvenile group had 25.7% correction and 42.9% stabilization, while the infantile group had 50% correction and 32.1% stabilization. There was a significant Cobb angle in-brace reduction in the thoracic (11°), thoracolumbar (12°), and lumbar (12°) ($p < 0.001$). There was no statistically significant change in out of brace Cobb angle from baseline to month 12 ($p > 0.05$). No patients required surgery within the 12 month span.

**Conclusions:** This study describes a new clinical protocol in the development of the EBDB. Short-term results show brace is effective in preventing IS or JS curve progression over a 12 month span.

**Keywords:** Early onset scoliosis, CAD/CAM, EBDB, Cobb angle

## Background

Approximately 70 years ago, Dr. Blount and Dr. Schmidt from our institution developed the Milwaukee brace to control curve progression for children with idiopathic scoliosis. Since then, a variety of other types of braces have been utilized clinically. The choices of bracing are prescribed based on the type of spinal deformity, and the extent of their success is due to bracing design and patient compliance [1–3]. For children with infantile

scoliosis (IS) or juvenile scoliosis (JS), the Milwaukee brace has been preferred over a thoraco-lumbar-sacral orthosis (TLSO). Bracing may lead to rib cage distortion and create a reduction in pulmonary function [4–6]. The design of the Milwaukee brace makes it preferable for the upper thoracic curvature [7].

Most universal designs, including the Milwaukee and most TLSO braces, follow a symmetric pattern. These usually apply a force to the apex of the curve through foam pads integrated to the bracing design by the orthotist. However, symmetric bracing do not provide the same in-brace correction as seen in asymmetric bracing, which is a common indication of long term out of bracing success [1, 8, 9]. Additionally, not all patients will

* Correspondence: jthometz@chw.org
[1]Department of Orthopedic Surgery, Children's Hospital of Wisconsin, Medical College of Wisconsin, Milwaukee, WI, USA
[2]Musculoskeletal Functional Assessment Center, Children's Hospital of Wisconsin, Medical College of Wisconsin, Milwaukee, WI, USA
Full list of author information is available at the end of the article

be able to tolerate a symmetric brace, since an asymmetric brace aims to provide a customized fit to improve wearability and comfort, and reduce brace weight [1, 10, 11]. One of the most popular asymmetric bracing includes the Chêneau brace, which aims to provide correction through a system of multipoint pressure zones [12, 13]. While these braces have proven to provide one of the highest in brace (IB) corrections, the indication for the use of these orthoses is to treat children with adolescent scoliosis [1]. Additionally, the Cheneau-Rigo brace includes a classification system with different types of braces, which allows the orthotists to design the brace.

Many clinicians perform serial casting on younger patients, since early-onset of scoliosis (EOS) patients are immature and have the largest potential for recovery through non-operative treatments [14]. It is common practice for bracing to be prescribed after casting to maintain the initial correction. Bracing is also prescribed to patients who are not able to tolerate casting [15]. Rather than serve as a corrective force, bracing will aim to halt curve progression, prevent respiratory dysfunctions, reduce pain, and enhance posture and cosmetic appearance [1, 15].

Overall, bracing studies are usually done on AIS populations. Although few are done on juvenile idiopathic scoliosis (JIS), or infantile idiopathic scoliosis (IIS), few studies have investigated the effects of bracing on the EOS population following a spinal manipulation procedure. To our knowledge, this will be the first study to investigate the effects of a computer aided design (CAD) and computer aided manufacturing (CAM) brace on patients with EOS. We will also introduce a new CAD/CAM bracing design, known as an elongation bending derotation brace (EBDB), which integrates the spinal manipulation procedure into its design. The purpose of this study was: 1) to briefly describe the preliminary results using the new EBDB in the treatment of IS or JS; 2) to investigate changes of Cobb angles in the AP view of X-ray between in and out of the EBDB bracing; 3) to compare differences of out of brace (OOB) Cobb angles in 3, 6, 9, and12 month with baseline; 4) to investigate OOB changes in JS and IS groups separately.

## Methods
### Study recruitment
Thirty-eight patients (22 males, 16 females; 17 IS, 21 JS) were recruited retrospectively for this study. 9 children were diagnosed with neuromuscular scoliosis, 1 congenital scoliosis, and 28 with IIS or JIS. This study was approved by IRB committee at Children's Hospital of Wisconsin. At the time of use of the EBDB, the average age was 6.2 years old (ranging from 4 months to 10 year-old). Criteria for inclusion includes: 1) All subjects are diagnosed with IS or JS (idiopathic, neuromuscular, or congenital); 2) Subjects must have not had any type of spinal surgery prior to bracing treatment; 3) Must be under 10 years old during the time of their first scan; 4) Must have had at least one follow up visit after their baseline scan before the 12 month mark.

Before their customized bracing treatment, 25 patients received some type of treatment (13 received TLSO bracing only, 8 received a series of casts only, 3 patients received casting and TLSO bracing, 1 patient received Physical therapy). 13 other patients received no prior treatment.

### Spinal manipulation, surface topography
In a clinic setting, the physicians determined the correction needed from the patients x-rays. The patient stood still in front of the physician with their arm held above their heads by the assistant. The physician used stockinet straps to provide translational and de-rotation force to correct the scoliosis curve. This allows for manipulation of the curve in the coronal and transverse plane, while also provide longitudinal traction by holding the upper limbs. While the patient was in the corrected position, a trained assistant used the handheld scanner (Polhemus FastSCAN Scorpion, Colchester, VT) to create a 3D scan of the patient's torso from the armpits down to the bilateral greater trochanter of the femur.

If the patient is unable to stand still in the clinic setting, the scanning was done in the OR while the patient was under general anesthesia. The patient was placed on a Spica casting table. Longitudinal traction was applied to the patient's arms and leg by assistants. A translational and de-rotation force was applied the scoliosis curve with stockinet straps to correct the curve in the coronal and transversal plane, with a mechanism was similar to the procedures mentioned above. The process differs in that the child is positioned with a much more dramatic bending movement used. The strap is similar.

### CAD, CAM and Fitting
Using a computerized aided design, the 3D shape of EBDB was created and sent to manufacturing. Afterwards, the patient returned to the clinic for a brace fitting. During fitting, the orthotist provided any necessary adjustments to the orthosis to make sure the orthosis fits properly. The costs of orthosis for children on the spica table with or without sedation are the same as TLSO, but additional charges are billed to children who needs to receive general anesthesia in OR. However, we have to remember that the brace is being used as an alternative to the cast for infantile scoliosis. Juvenile patients done in clinic have a similar charge for the brace.

## Radiographic analysis

All children were radiographically evaluated before their bracing treatment and in their brace during the day of fitting, which serves as our IB and OOB baselines. Follow up radiographic analyses were measured at approximately 3, 6, 9, or 12 months after the baseline scan, with missing measurements interpolated between the closest visits. Curve segments are classified to thoracic (T), thoracolumbar (TL), and lumbar (L) categories.

## Statistical analysis

We determined individual success of curve treatment based on the Scoliosis Research Society (SRS) criteria of spine correction for AIS, but followed up after approximately 12 months and used the criteria for EOS [16]. A $\geq 6°$ change or higher in Cobb angle indicates progression, $\leq -6°$change or lower indicates correction, while a range of changes between $\leq 5°$ or lower and $\geq -5°$ or higher indicates stabilization. Average Cobb angle change between IB and OOB were measured and compared after the data was standardized in terms of gender, age, bracing treatment time using a linear mixed effects model with random intercepts and fitted angles. This model was also used to test changes of Cobb angles for OOB from 0 to 12 months, and the interaction effects of age and gender on spinal curvature. Additionally, a Wilcoxon signed-rank test was applied to evaluate the effects of bracing at baseline for IS, JS, and combined groups. In a separate analysis, the IS and JS groups had their OOB Cobb angle changes compared separately. A $p$ value of less than 0.05 is considered significant.

## Results

The EBDB management protocols has been used in terms of children standing or supine position. In standing or supine position, children's spine was manipulated to correct the curvatures in three planes, then the corrected spine was scanned.

The starting Cobb angle was $38 \pm 14°$ (std) in the thoracic (ranging from 19° to 68°), $30 \pm 9.6°$ in the thoracolumbar (ranging from 19° to 42°), and $36 \pm 10.3°$ in the lumbar sections (ranging from 22° to 53°). No patients required surgery within the 12 month span. The findings for OOB Cobb angle changes are shown in Table 1. There were no significant differences of curves in terms of age and gender ($p > 0.05$).

When compared to the baseline radiographic measurements, the in-brace correction reduced the Cobb angle from 38° to 24.2° in the thoracic (36.3% reduction), 30° to 10.3° in the thoracolumbar (65.7% reduction), and 36° to 18.5° in the lumbar (48.3% reduction). The juvenile group had 23% correction, 47% stabilization, and 30% progression of curves. The infantile group had 50% correction, 32% stabilization, and 18% progression of

**Table 1** Cobb angle changes in children with out of brace over time (a Linear mixed effect model, $n = 36$, $P > 0.05$)

| Levels of Curve | Month | Cobb Angle (°) | Curve change (°) | % Change |
|---|---|---|---|---|
| Thoracic | 0 | 38.0 ± 14.0 | NA | NA |
| | 3 | 30.1 ± 19.7 | −5.6 | −15.6% |
| | 6 | 30.2 ± 21.5 | −5.5 | − 15.5% |
| | 9 | 31.5 ± 24.2 | −4.2 | −11.6% |
| | 12 | 29.4 ± 24.3 | −6.2 | −17.5% |
| Thoracolumbar | 0 | 30.0 ± 9.6 | NA | NA |
| | 3 | 25.2 ± 11.2 | 0.2 | 0.6% |
| | 6 | 24.8 ± 11.6 | −0.2 | −0.9% |
| | 9 | 24.3 ± 10.3 | −0.7 | −2.7% |
| | 12 | 23.9 ± 10.0 | −1.1 | −4.5% |
| Lumbar | 0 | 36.0 ± 10.3 | NA | NA |
| | 3 | 25.4 ± 14.3 | −3.5 | −12.2% |
| | 6 | 27.9 ± 14.5 | −1 | −3.5% |
| | 9 | 30.2 ± 14.2 | 1.3 | 4.5% |
| | 12 | 29.9 ± 14.2 | 1 | 3.6% |

curves. After the data was standardized in terms of age, gender, and time using a linear mixed effects model, significant in-brace changes were found in the T ($-11°$ reduction), TL ($-12°$ reduction), and L segment ($-12°$ reduction) ($P < 0.001$). Between juvenile and infantile scoliosis, overall, there was no significant difference in Cobb angle ($P > 0.05$). Changes between OOB and IB shows significant change for the IS, JS, and combined age groups ($P < 0.001$). There was no significant difference in Cobb angle changes over time ($p > 0.05$). Figures 1 and 2 show the Cobb angle changes in the thoracic region, and the OOB IS and JS groups, respectively. The curve improvement in one congenital scoliosis patient was in the compensatory curves.

## Discussion

The EBDB treatment showed to be effective in correcting nearly half of the thoracic curves and one third of the other curves. When combining all data curves, 75% of curves were corrected or stabilized and 25% of curves were progressed. The efficacy of our brace is further supported by finding no statistical significance of Cobb angle changes in relation to time in all three spinal segments.

Since children with EOS have ongoing spinal growth and development, EDF casting needs to be repeated every couple of months. This may be less cost effective and less patient friendly because visits are more frequent and may require casting to be done in the OR with the patient under general anesthesia. The brace technique does not need to repeat the casting process. Additionally, CAD/CAM modification holds a significantly

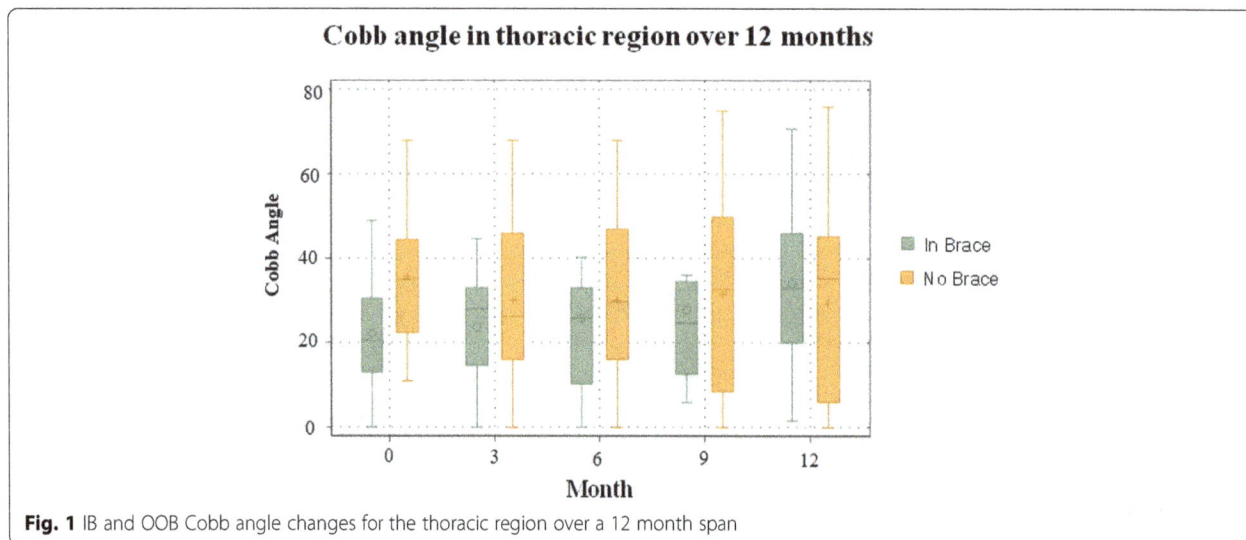

**Fig. 1** IB and OOB Cobb angle changes for the thoracic region over a 12 month span

reduced rectification time by 108 min (63.5% reduction) [7, 17]. However, we do bill the time of manipulation for scoliotic spine.

CAD/CAM can be done in different approaches, and has been shown to be equal to or improved over traditional methods. Wong et al. found a similar efficacy between TLSO fabrication through plaster molding compared to fabrication through CAD/CAM for IB reduction. They reported 41.9% in-brace reduction using CAD/CAM (– 12.8°) and 32.1% in-brace reduction using traditional approach (– 9.8°) [18]. Others integrated CAD/CAM with a finite element analysis (FEA) to fabricate bracing [11, 17]. Desbiens-Blais et al. did this using Boston brace guidelines, and found a similar efficacy to the traditional TLSO brace. They had an IB correction of 16° using their method vs. 11° with a TLSO for thoracic curves and 13° vs 16° for Thoracolumbar/Lumbar curves ($p > 0.05$) [17]. While these studies are

done on AIS patients, Sankar et al. found a better in-brace correction and increased comfort in a population of 10 scoliosis patients of various etiologies [19]. He used compared the CAD/CAM method to the traditional methods [19] Although their population is smaller and their patients' IB radiography was recorded 3 months after baseline, they found the highest percent in-brace correction of 51% in CAD/CAM and 44% in TLSO [19]. Our baseline in-brace corrections of 37.5% thoracic, 45.6% thoracolumbar, and 51.9% lumbar indicates the EBDB has a similar efficacy as compared to most CAD/CAM bracing studies.

This is a study utilizing a novel approach to create the CAD/CAM brace. This is clinical treatment protocol that will integrate the use of manipulation of the spine in its bracing design through either standing or supine position. Manipulation mechanisms will involve in the corrective forces by pulling the stockinet. Younger patients

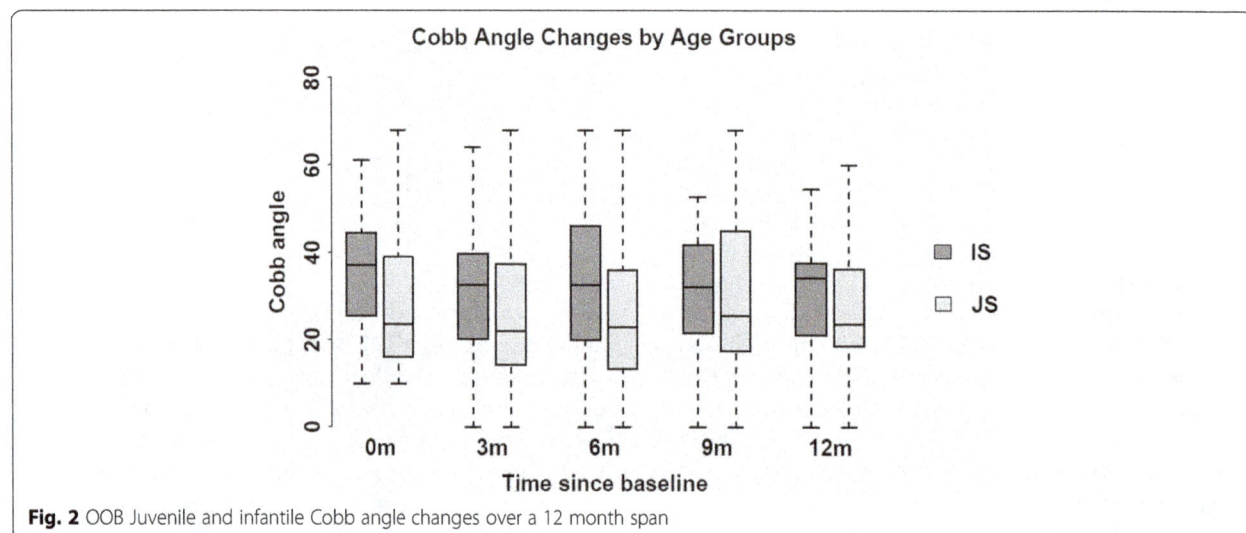

**Fig. 2** OOB Juvenile and infantile Cobb angle changes over a 12 month span

who are unable to stand still during spinal manipulation will be required to have these procedures in the OR, while older patients are done in the clinic. Thus the EBDB provides not only a CAD/CAM based asymmetric brace, but also adequate 3D correction of the spine deformity by manipulation.

There have been rare bracing studies on the IIS population. There is a case report of a 2 year-old with scoliosis due to Marfan's syndrome; there was a 12° IB correction and a 22° OOB reduction from baseline after approximately 2.5 years [20]. In our study, we found a comparable 11° (T), 12° (TL), and 12° (L) in-brace reduction ($P < 0.001$). Studies on younger populations usually investigate the effects of universal bracing designs on JIS populations. Their findings often have a wide variation due to differences in follow up timing, compliance, prescribed daily bracing wear, classification of curve change results, and study population [2, 4, 21–25]. Aulisa et al's prospective bracing study found that after a 24 month follow up using a Milwaukee, Lyon, or PSAB brace, OOB Cobb angle decreased from 29.6° to 16.9° (12.7° difference), and 77.8% of patients had spinal correction while 15.9% obtained stabilization [4]. However, another study only found an OOB change of 4° after 4 years using an Edinburgh brace, which is longer in duration compared to most bracing studies [21]. Tolo et al's study on JIS treatments found a 13% OOB Cobb angle reduction after 3 years of Milwaukee bracing treatment [22], but our results were only reported in one year follow-up and they were not comparable with studies with longer term follow-up. Overall, 48.3–56% of patients with naturally progressed JIS needed operation by the time they reach skeletal maturity, and 70% of all JIS curves progress over time [21, 22, 25, 26].

## Limitations

While our study has radiographic patient measurements every 3 months, missing measurements are interpolated using a linear regression analysis. Similar to most bracing studies, compliance can always be an issue in bracing studies. Our results with one year follow-up are preliminary and were not comparable with studies with longer follow-up. We would also like to extend the duration of our study to two years to validate the long term effect of the EBDB.

## Conclusions

The early onset of scoliosis can be treated with a custom fitted, asymmetric brace (EBDB) that integrates the 3D spinal manipulation correction into its design. It may provide users with a more patient friendly approach to treating EOS. This is especially helpful for patients who are not able to tolerate universal symmetric TLSO designs or repeated casting treatments.

## Abbreviations

CAD: Computer aided design; CAM: Computer aided manufacturing; EBDB: An elongation bending derotation brace (also previously named as Milwaukee Contoured Corrective CAD/CAM based brace, Mi3C™); EDF: Elongation-derotation-flexion; EOS: Early onset of scoliosis; FEA: Finite element analysis; IB: In brace; IIS: Infantile idiopathic scoliosis; IS: Infantile scoliosis; JIS: Juvenile idiopathic scoliosis; JS: Juvenile scoliosis; L: Lumbar; OOB: Out of brace; Std: Standard deviation; T: Thoracic; TL: Thoracolumbar; TLSO: Thoraco-lumbar-sacral orthosis

## Acknowledgements

We would like to thank J. Al-Ramahi, Biomedical Engineer, Musculoskeletal Functional Assessment Center, Children's Hospital of WI and Ziyang Yin, MS, Division of Biostatistics, Institute for Health and Society, MCW in the support of data collection and analysis.

## Authors' contributions

JT and XCL were two major contributors in developing study protocol, analyzing results, interpreting data, designing brace, and writing the manuscript. RR involved in the use of CAD for brace design. IE performed radiographic measurements for in and out of brace and evaluated patients information. ST provided statistical analysis for radiographic results. All authors read and approved the final manuscript.

## Competing interests

The authors declare that they have no competing interests.

## Author details

[1]Department of Orthopedic Surgery, Children's Hospital of Wisconsin, Medical College of Wisconsin, Milwaukee, WI, USA. [2]Musculoskeletal Functional Assessment Center, Children's Hospital of Wisconsin, Medical College of Wisconsin, Milwaukee, WI, USA. [3]Department of Mechanical Engineering, Milwaukee School of Engineering, Milwaukee, WI, USA. [4]Division of Biostatistics, Institution for Health & Society, Medical College of Wisconsin, Milwaukee, WI, USA. [5]Pediatric Orthopaedics, 9000 W. Wisconsin Ave., Suite 360, PO Box 1997, Milwaukee, WI 53201, USA.

## References

1.  SY N, et al. Bracing scoliosis-state of the art (mini-review). Curr Pediatr Rev. 2016;12:36–42.
2.  Aulisa AG, Giordano M, Falciglia F, Marzetti E, Poscia A, Guzzanti V. Correlation between compliance and brace treatment in juvenile and adolescent idiopathic scoliosis: SOSORT 2014 award winner. Scoliosis. 2014;9:6.
3.  Rahman T, et al. The association between brace compliance and outcome for patients with idiopathic scoliosis. J Pediatr Orthop. 2005;25:420–2.
4.  Akbarnia BA. Management themes in early onset scoliosis. J Bone Joint Surg Am. 2007;89(Suppl 1):42–54.
5.  Gillingham BL, Fan RA, Akbarnia BA. Early onset idiopathic scoliosis. J Am Acad Orthop Surg. 2006;14:101–12.
6.  Kahanovitz N, Levine DB, Lardone J. The part-time Milwaukee brace treatment of juvenile idiopathic scoliosis. Long-term follow-up. Clin Orthop Relat Res. 1982;167:145–51.
7.  Wong MS, et al. A work study of the CAD/CAM method and conventional manual method in the fabrication of spinal orthoses for patients with adolescent idiopathic scoliosis. Prosthetics Orthot Int. 2005;29:93–104.
8.  Emans JB, Kaelin A, Bancel P, Hall JE, Miller ME. The Boston bracing system for idiopathic scoliosis. Follow-up results in 295 patients. Spine. 1986;11:792–801.
9.  Landauer F, Wimmer C, Behensky H. Estimating the final outcome of brace treatment for idiopathic thoracic scoliosis at 6-month follow-up. Pediatr Rehabil. 2003;6:201–7.
10. Weiss H-R. "Brace technology" thematic series-the Gensingen brace™ in the treatment of scoliosis. Scoliosis. 2010;5:22.

11. Cobetto N, et al. Braces optimized with computer-assisted design and simulations are lighter, more comfortable, and more efficient than plaster-cast braces for the treatment of adolescent idiopathic scoliosis. Spine Deformity. 2014;2:276–84.

12. Kotwicki T, Cheneau J. Biomechanical action of a corrective brace on thoracic idiopathic scoliosis: Cheneau 2000 orthosis. Disabil Rehab Ass Technol. 2008;3:3.

13. Cheneau J. Scoliosis treating brace evaluation of our brace since 1970: an evaluation of the normalization of rotation, of rib static and of the wedge shaped vertebrae. Locomotor System. 2003;1:29–38.

14. Mehta MH. Growth as a corrective force in the early treatment of progressive infantile scoliosis. J Bone Joint Surg Br. 2005;87:1237–47.

15. Weinstein SL, et al. Effects of bracing in adolescents with idiopathic scoliosis. N Engl J Med. 2013;369:1512–21.

16. Richards BS, et al. Standardization of criteria for adolescent idiopathic scoliosis brace studies: SRS Committee on bracing and nonoperative management. Spine. 2005;30:2068–75.

17. Desbiens-Blais F, et al. New brace design combining CAD/CAM and biomechanical simulation for the treatment of adolescent idiopathic scoliosis. Clin Biomech. 2012;27(10):999–1005.

18. Wong MS, Cheng JCY, Lo KH. A comparison of treatment effectiveness between the CAD/CAM method and the manual method for managing adolescent idiopathic scoliosis. Prosthetics Orthot Int. 2005;29:105–11.

19. Sankar WN, et al. Scoliosis in-brace curve correction and patient preference of CAD/CAM versus plaster molded TLSOs. J Child Orthop. 2007;1:345–9.

20. Weiss H-R. Brace treatment in infantile/juvenile patients with progressive scoliosis is worthwhile. Stud Health Technol Inform. 2012;176:383–6.

21. Figueiredo UM, James JI. Juvenile idiopathic scoliosis. J Bone Joint Surg. 1981;63:61–6.

22. Tolo VT, Gillespie R. The characteristics of juvenile idiopathic scoliosis and results of its treatment. J Bone Joint Surg. 1978;60:181–8.

23. Coillard C, Circo AB, Rivard CH. SpineCor treatment for juvenile idiopathic scoliosis: SOSORT award 2010 winner. Scoliosis. 2010;5:25.

24. Jarvis J, Garbedian S, Swamy G. Juvenile idiopathic scoliosis: the effectiveness of part-time bracing. Spine. 2008;33:1074–8.

25. Charles YP, et al. Progression risk of idiopathic juvenile scoliosis during pubertal growth. Spine. 2006;31:1933–42.

26. Lenke LG, Dobbs MB. Management of juvenile idiopathic scoliosis. J Bone Joint Surg Am. 2007;89(Suppl 1):55–63.

# 22

# Two-dimensional digital photography for child body posture evaluation: standardized technique, reliable parameters and normative data for age 7-10 years

L. Stolinski[1,2,3*], M. Kozinoga[1,2], D. Czaprowski[4,5], M. Tyrakowski[6], P. Cerny[7,8,9], N. Suzuki[10] and T. Kotwicki[1]

**Abstract**

**Background:** Digital photogrammetry provides measurements of body angles or distances which allow for quantitative posture assessment with or without the use of external markers. It is becoming an increasingly popular tool for the assessment of the musculoskeletal system. The aim of this paper is to present a structured method for the analysis of posture and its changes using a standardized digital photography technique.

**Material and methods:** The purpose of the study was twofold. The first one comprised 91 children (44 girls and 47 boys) aged 7–10 (8.2 ± 1.0), i.e., students of primary school, and its aim was to develop the photographic method, choose the quantitative parameters, and determine the intraobserver reliability (repeatability) along with the interobserver reliability (reproducibility) measurements in sagittal plane using digital photography, as well as to compare the Rippstein plurimeter and digital photography measurements. The second one involved 7782 children (3804 girls, 3978 boys) aged 7–10 (8.4 ± 0.5), who underwent digital photography postural screening. The methods consisted in measuring and calculating selected parameters, establishing the normal ranges of photographic parameters, presenting percentile charts, as well as noticing common pitfalls and possible sources of errors in digital photography.

**Results:** A standardized procedure for the photographic evaluation of child body posture was presented. The photographic measurements revealed very good intra- and inter-rater reliability regarding the five sagittal parameters and good reliability performed against Rippstein plurimeter measurements. The parameters displayed insignificant variability over time. Normative data were calculated based on photographic assessment, while the percentile charts were provided to serve as reference values. The technical errors observed during photogrammetry are carefully discussed in this article.

**Conclusions:** Technical developments are allowed for the regular use of digital photogrammetry in body posture assessment. Specific child positioning (described above) enables us to avoid incidentally modified posture. Image registration is simple, quick, harmless, and cost-effective. The semi-automatic image analysis, together with the normal values and percentile charts, makes the technique reliable in terms of child's posture documentation and corrective therapy effects' monitoring.

**Keywords:** Standardization, Digital photography, Photogrammetry, Percentile charts, Normative data, Primary school children

* Correspondence: stolinskilukasz@op.pl
[1]Department of Spine Disorders and Pediatric Orthopedics, University of Medical Sciences, 28 Czerwca 1956r. no. 135/147, 61-545 Poznan, Poland
[2]Rehasport Clinic, Poznan, Poland
Full list of author information is available at the end of the article

## Background

### Human body posture

Body posture is defined as the alignment of body segments which is considered as an important health indicator [1]. Human body posture is also described as a motor habit accompanying daily activities [2]. Normal human posture is the characteristic of the vertical position which relies on spinal alignment and its position over the patient's head and pelvis [3, 4]. Human body posture undergoes large variability, which depends on age, sex, body growth, environmental factors, and psychophysical status of an individual [5–7]. The accurate description of human body posture represents a topic of interest for the scientists aiming to measure and to document the posture. For the clinicians, posture evaluation plays a role in the global health assessment. On the one hand, faulty posture may result from various disorders, while the posture itself may be even patognomic for certain diseases (ex. spondylolisthesis). On the other hand, incorrect body posture can have negative impact on the overall health, leading to pain or functional disorder, which means that it can affect the quality of life both in childhood and adulthood [8].

The quality of body posture results from individual settings of respective body parts, especially the spine [9] and pelvis [10] alignment in the sagittal plane. The gravity line is defined as the vertical line passing through the center of gravity in the entire body. For a standing subject, the reference posture is described by the relations between the gravity line and body segments [11]. Balanced arrangement of body parts provides the basis for the center of mass. Such arrangement of body parts enables the maintenance of horizontal gaze as well as effective muscle contraction and stretching without unnecessary loss of energy [12]. Diagnostic tools for measuring the sagittal spine curvatures and the pelvis alignment can be used to describe a correct posture while standing [13].

The multitude of methods and diagnostic tools makes it difficult to standardize the assessment of body posture. In addition, there is a lack of a clear range between the traditional and faulty posture—in particular, the number of quantitative posture parameters. Thus, the data on

the prevalence of faulty posture is very divergent and based on different diagnostic criteria [14].

The content of the paper fulfills the following objectives: (1) to standardize digital photography technique for posture assessment; (2) to determine the intra-observer reproducibility and the inter-observer reliability of photographic sagittal parameters: sacral slope (SS), lumbar lordosis (LL), thoracic kyphosis (TK), chest inclination (CI), and head protraction (HP); (3) to check the validity of photographic measurements against the Rippstein plurimeter measurements; (4) to analyze the variability of five sagittal photographic angles: SS, LL, TK, CI, HP, and two coronal parameters: Anterior Trunk Symmetry Index (ATSI) and Posterior Trunk Symmetry Index (POTSI) over time (1 week); (5) to present the normative values of sagittal photographic parameters based on photographic assessment of 7782 children aged 7–10; and (6) to discuss common pitfalls and sources of errors in digital photography used in posture evaluation.

## Methods

### Standardization of posture assessment with digital photography

The use of reliable tools and methods for clinical measurements is the first step towards evidence-based medicine [15] as the foundation of effective and safe clinical practice. Just like any tool, the photographic technique for posture evaluation should be checked and validated before use. Standardization required to assess body posture was performed as part of this study.

*Preparing a patient to photogrammetry*

**Marking anatomical body landmarks** In the procedure below, body posture is assessed without the use of external markers attached to the skin. Dots corresponding to the anatomical body landmarks are drawn on the skin with the use of a non-toxic color pencil. The following body landmarks are marked (Fig. 1):

– The center of the sternal notch

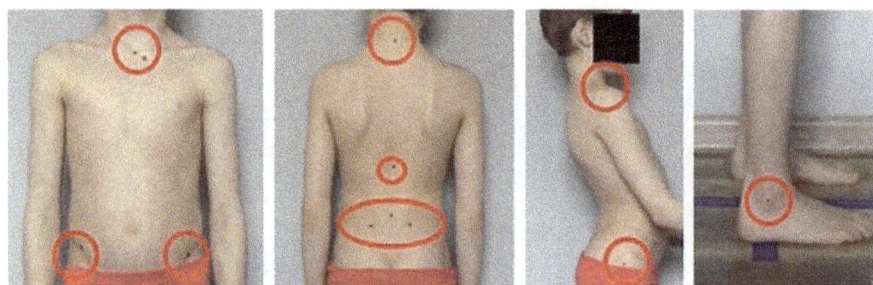

**Fig. 1** Anatomical points marked on the body

– Anterior superior iliac spine (ASIS)—right and left
– Posterior superior iliac spine (PSIS)—right and left
– Spinous process of C7
– The point between T12 and L1 spinous process
– The point between L5 and S1 spinous process
– The center of acromion—right and left
– The center of greater trochanter—right and left
– The center of external malleolus of the ankle joint

**Positioning the patient Positioning children during body posture evaluation** Standardized procedure for photographic body posture evaluation includes the photos presented in Fig. 2: spontaneous standing frontal posture (2a), sagittal profiles including photos of the left side (2b), left side actively corrected (2c), left side in forward bending (2d), spontaneous standing posture of the back (2e), right side (2f), right side actively corrected (2g), right side in forward bending (2h), as well as front (2i) and back forward bending (2j).

**Positioning children during scoliosis rib and lumbar prominence evaluation** In order to document the angle of trunk rotation at different trunk levels, one can take a sequence of photos (5–15) made during forward bending of a child (Fig. 3).

**Lower limb positioning in photographic examination** The undressed child (wearing the underwear and a narrow bra for girls) is barefoot with its knees extended and the feet hip-width apart. The feet are placed on longitudinal and crosswise lines marked on the ground so that their lateral malleoli are situated over the center of the crosswise line and the feet stay parallel to the longitudinal line (Fig. 4). Most of the upper part of the intergluteal cleft should be uncovered.

**Upper limb and head positioning in photographic examination** The hair is tied with the use of a hair clip to make the external auditory meatus and the upper body contours visible. Children are asked to look forward at eye level. For the front and back photos, the upper limbs are loosely hanging down. For the lateral photos, in order to uncover the contour of the back, the upper limbs are

slightly flexed in the gleno-humeral and the elbow joint at the angle of approx. 10°–20° and 20°–30° respectively. The gleno-humeral joint flexion is performed slowly to avoid any trunk movement, especially the backward trunk hyperextension (Fig. 5). For the front photos taken during forward bending, the upper limbs are kept together and directed forward to the ground as in Adam's test (Fig. 3). For lateral photos made during forward bending, the upper limbs are loosely hanging down (Fig. 2d, h).

*Photographic parameters for the frontal plane evaluation*
There are two main photographic parameters for the frontal plane trunk assessment and two for the lower limb assessment. The two trunk parameters are Anterior Trunk Symmetry Index and Posterior Trunk Symmetry Index.

Anterior Trunk Symmetry Index (ATSI)—the parameter is defined as the sum of six indices: three frontal plane asymmetry indices (sternal notch, axilla folds, and waist lines) and three frontal plane height difference indices (acromions, axilla folds, and waist lines). Frontal asymmetry index at sternal notch level (FAI-SN) is calculated by dividing the distance between the center of the sternal notch and the midline by the height of the trunk. The height of the trunk (e) is the vertical distance between the navel and the center of the sternal notch. Frontal asymmetry indexes at axilla level (FAI-A) and at trunk level (FAI-T) are calculated by dividing the difference in the distance between each trunk's edge and the midline ($c - d$, $a - b$) by the width of the trunk ($c + d$, $a + b$). Height indices of trunk asymmetry are calculated by dividing the difference in height at three levels of trunk: HDI-S for shoulders, HDI-A for axillas, and HDI-T for the trunk waistline by the trunk height measured from navel to the center of the sternal notch (e). The shoulder point is the point of intersection at shoulder level with a vertical line from each axilla. ATSI was introduced by Stolinski et al. in 2012 [16] (Fig. 6).

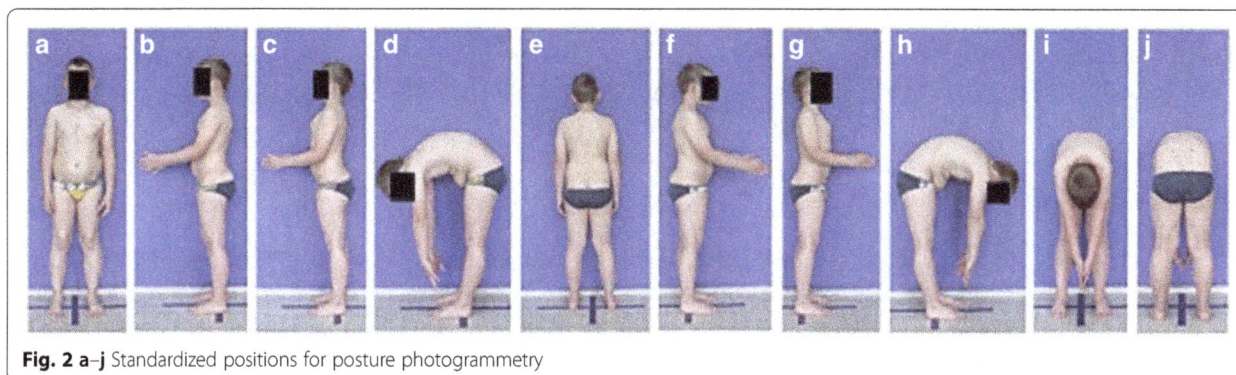

**Fig. 2 a–j** Standardized positions for posture photogrammetry

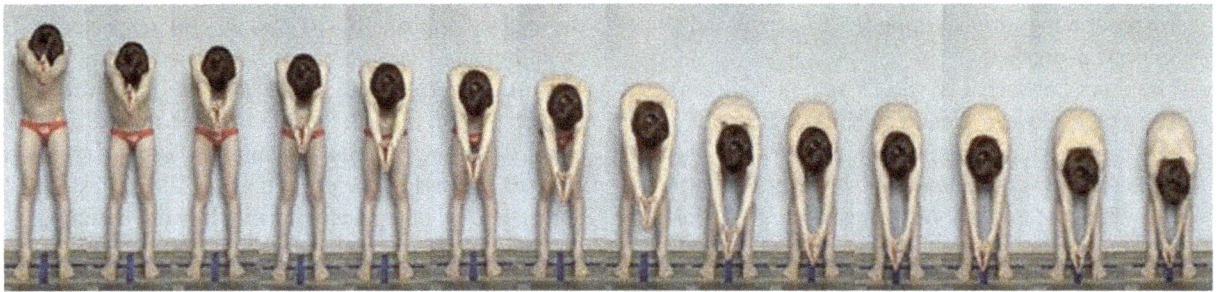

**Fig. 3** Photographic documentation of trunk rotation/trunk inclination deformity revealed during Adams' forward bending test (left to right—progressive forward bending)

$$ATSI = (FAI–SN + FAI–A + FAI–T )$$
$$+(HDI–S + HDI–A + HDI–T)$$

Posterior Trunk Symmetry Index (POTSI)—similarly to ATSI Index, the POTSI parameter is defined as the sum of six indices: three frontal plane asymmetry indices (C7, axilla folds, and waist lines) and three frontal plane height difference indices (acromions, axilla folds, and waist lines). Frontal asymmetry index at C7 level (FAI-C7) is calculated by dividing the distance between the C7 point and the midline by the height of the trunk. The height of the trunk (e) is the vertical distance between the C7 and the beginning of gluteal cleft. Frontal asymmetry indexes at axilla level (FAI-A) and trunk level (FAI-T) are calculated by dividing the difference in distance between each trunk's edge and the midline (c – d, a – b) by the width of the trunk (c + d, a + b). Height indices of trunk asymmetry are calculated by dividing the difference in the height at three levels of trunk: HDI-S for shoulders, HDI-A for axillas, and HDI-T for the trunk waistline by the trunk height (e). The shoulder point is the point of intersection at shoulder level with a vertical line from each axilla. POTSI was introduced by Suzuki et al. in 1999 [17, 18] (Fig. 7).

$$POTSI = (FAI-C7 + FAI-A + FAI-T )$$
$$+(HDI-S + HDI-A + HDI-T)$$

The two photographic postural parameters of lower limb frontal plane assessment are tibiofemoral angle and tibiocalcaneal angle.

Tibiofemoral angle (TFA)—the angle between the line drawn from the center of the ankle joint to the center of the knee joint and the line drawn from the center of the knee joint to ASIS of the same lower limb (Fig. 8a) [19, 20].

Tibiocalcaneal angle (TCA)—the angle between a line drawn between the center of the calcaneus and the Achilles tendon, and a second line drawn from the Achilles tendon to the mid-calf of the same lower limb (Fig. 8b) [21].

*Photographic parameters for the sagittal plane evaluation*
The following photographic parameters are assumed for the sagittal plane assessment:

Sacral slope angle (SS)—the angle between the vertical line and the line tangent to body contour at the sacral area (Fig. 9a) [22].
Lumbar lordosis angle (LL)—the angle between the line tangent to body contour at the level of T12-L1 spinous processes and the line tangent to body contour at the level of L5-S1 spinous processes (Fig. 9b) [23].
Thoracic kyphosis angle (TK)—the angle between the line tangent to body contour at the level of C7-Th1 spinous processes and the line tangent to body contour at the level of Th12–L1 spinous processes (Fig. 9c) [24].
Chest inclination angle (CI)—the angle between the horizontal line and the line connecting the C7 spinous process with the point at the anterior neck-anterior thorax junction (Fig. 9d) [25].
Head protraction angle (HP)—the angle between the horizontal line and the line connecting the C7 spinous process and the external auditory meatus (Fig. 9e) [26].

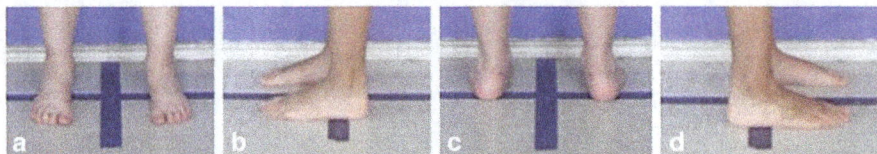

**Fig. 4** Feet positioning for posture photographic evaluation: **a** front view, **b** lateral left view, **c** back view, and **d** lateral right view

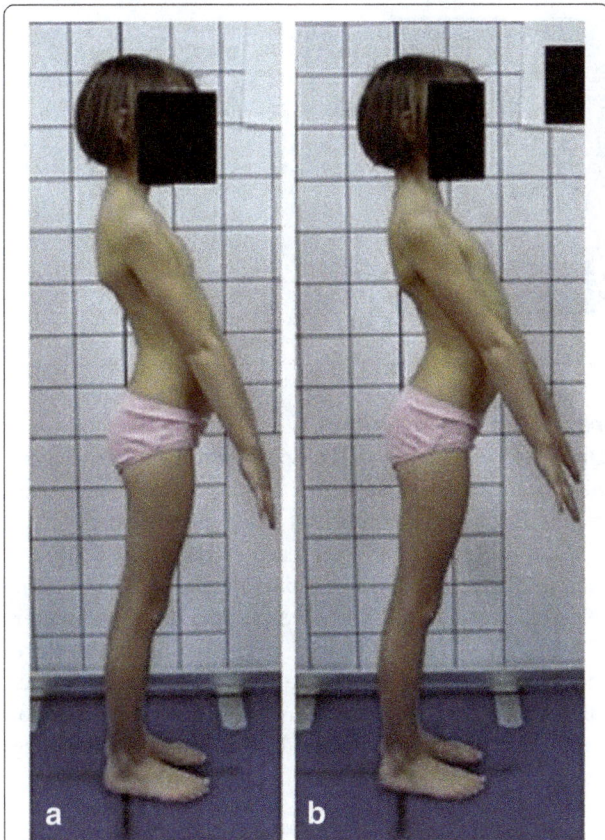

**Fig. 5** Child's posture taken for sagittal plane assessment: **a** spontaneous standing posture, **b** "actively corrected posture" in this child reveals backward trunk hyperextension which should be avoided; such image points out the importance of children education in what the correct human body posture consists of

Acromion-ankle angle (AA)—the angle between the vertical line drawn from the center of external malleolus of the ankle joint and the line drawn from the center of external malleolus of the ankle joint to the center of acromion (Fig. 10c).

Ear-ankle angle (EA)—the angle between the vertical line drawn from the center of external malleolus of the ankle joint and the line drawn from the center of external malleolus of the ankle joint to the external auditory meatus (Fig. 10d).

Enlarged photos of coronal and sagittal parameters are presented in Additional file 1: Appendix 1.

### Semi-automatic measurements of postural photographic parameters

All the abovementioned parameters can be measured manually, manually in ink, on a print or digitally on the monitor screen. To facilitate the measurement, a semi-automatic software named SCODIAC was created [28]. The software is available online and free to download [https://www.ortotika.cz/download/SetupSCODIAC_Full.zip]. The landmarks are manually placed on the screen. Afterwards, the software calculates the values of the required parameters. The initial version of software was checked against x-ray measurements [29]. The current version focused on digital photography images (Fig. 11). Placing the landmarks consists in moving small circles provided at the screen to the required anatomical points manually. The software calculations are automatic. The software explains all functions in a user-friendly way.

Sagittal pelvic tilt (SPT)—the angle between the horizontal line and the line joining the anterior and the posterior superior iliac spine (Fig. 10a) [27].

Trochanter-ankle angle (TA)—the angle between the vertical line drawn from the center of external malleolus of the ankle joint and the line drawn from the center of external malleolus of the ankle joint to the top of the greater trochanter (Fig. 10b).

### Validation of the photographic technique

We checked the reliability of the photographic technique above. Our objectives in this part of the study were (1) to determine the intra-observer reproducibility and the inter-observer reliability of the photographic sagittal parameters: sacral slope angle (SS), lumbar lordosis angle (LL), thoracic kyphosis angle (TK), chest inclination angle (CI), and head protraction angle (HP) (Fig. 9); and (2) to check the validity of photographic measurements

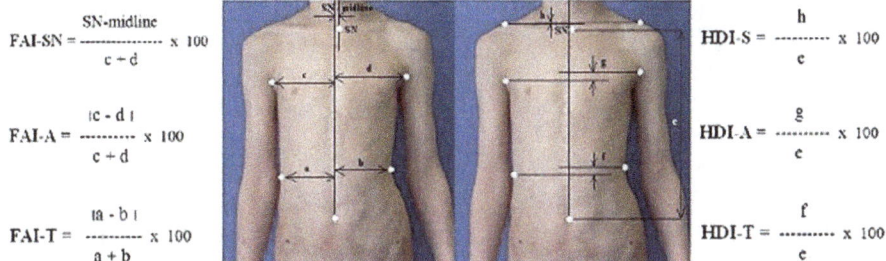

**Fig. 6** Diagram illustrating the measurements of ATSI Index

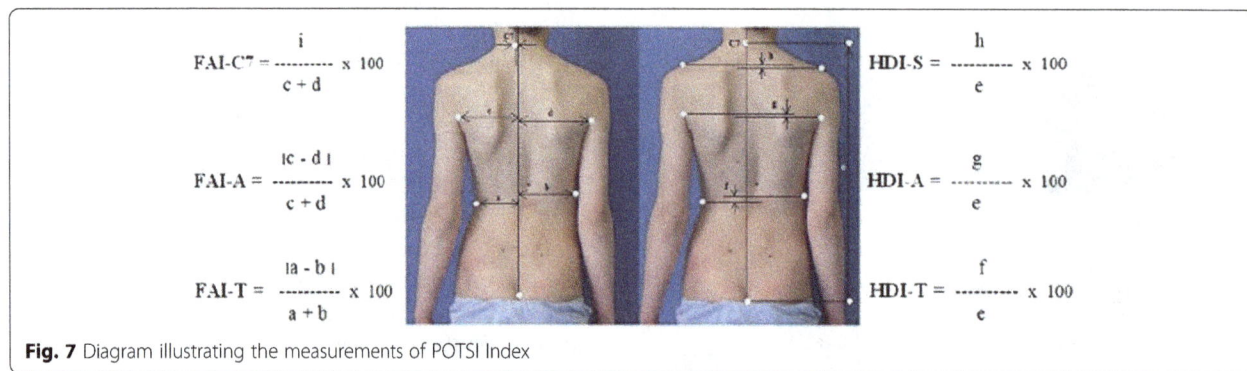

$$FAI\text{-}C7 = \frac{i}{c + d} \times 100$$

$$FAI\text{-}A = \frac{|c - d|}{c + d} \times 100$$

$$FAI\text{-}T = \frac{|a - b|}{a + b} \times 100$$

$$HDI\text{-}S = \frac{h}{e} \times 100$$

$$HDI\text{-}A = \frac{g}{e} \times 100$$

$$HDI\text{-}T = \frac{f}{e} \times 100$$

**Fig. 7** Diagram illustrating the measurements of POTSI Index

against the Rippstein plurimeter measurements by analyzing correlations between the corresponding angles.

The study group consisted of 91 healthy volunteers (44 girls and 47 boys) aged 7–10 (mean $8.2 \pm 1.0$ years). The exclusion criteria were history of any spine disorder, min. 7-degree ATR value, lower limbs discrepancy, and refusal to participate. Children were photographed in a relaxed (spontaneous, habitual) posture from the left (Fig. 2b) and right side (Fig. 2f). The study was performed in accordance with the 1964 Helsinki Declaration. All studies reported in this chapter were approved by the Institutional Review Board of Poznan University of Medical Sciences (No. 832/11, date 6/10/2011).

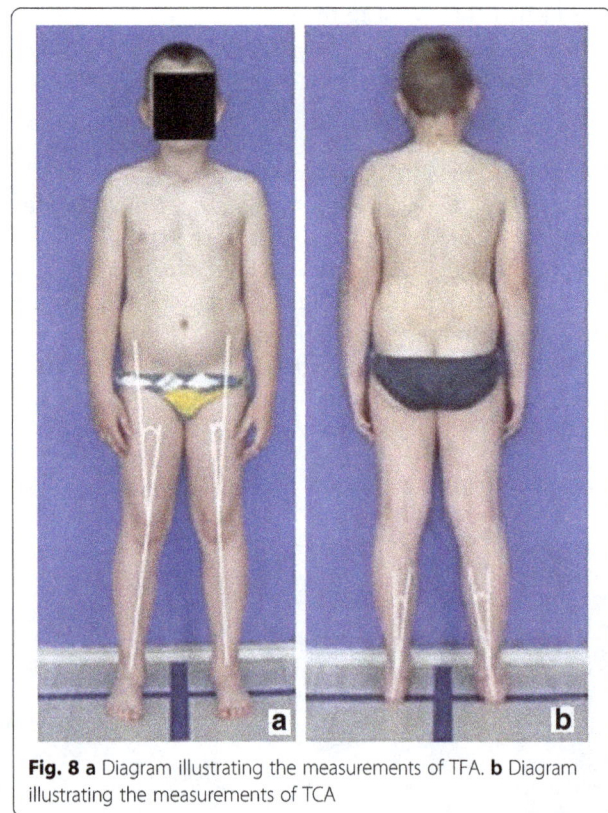

**Fig. 8 a** Diagram illustrating the measurements of TFA. **b** Diagram illustrating the measurements of TCA

### Intra-observer reproducibility

One observer (a physiotherapist with 10 years' experience) performed three series of photographic measurements. Each series comprised three measurements, with a 2-day interval between each series. The observer measured the photographic parameters of 30 randomly selected healthy children. Five photographic parameters (SS, LL, TK, CI, and HP) were measured using the aforementioned methodology. The intra-observer reproducibility was quantified by the use of intraclass correlation coefficient (ICC) and standard error for single measurement (SEM) [30].

### Inter-observer reliability

Three observers, physiotherapists with 10, 8, and 2 years' experience respectively, performed three series of photographic measurements. Each series included three measurements, with a 2-day interval between each series. The observer measured photographic parameters of 30 randomly selected healthy children. Five photographic parameters (SS, LL, TK, CI, and HP) were measured using the methodology described above. The inter-observer reliability was quantified by the use of intraclass correlation coefficient (ICC) and standard error for single measurement (SEM) [30].

### Validation of the photographic technique against Rippstein plurimeter

In order to determine the correlation of the photographic parameters versus Rippstein plurimeter measurements, three observers measured the sagittal curvatures (sacral slope, lumbar lordosis, and thoracic kyphosis) of 91 children three times with the use of the Rippstein plurimeter (Fig. 12) immediately after the children had the photos taken, one photo from the left side and one photo from the right side, according to standardized conditions described above. The values of the corresponding parameters (photographic thoracic kyphosis angle versus plurimeter thoracic kyphosis angle, etc.) were compared.

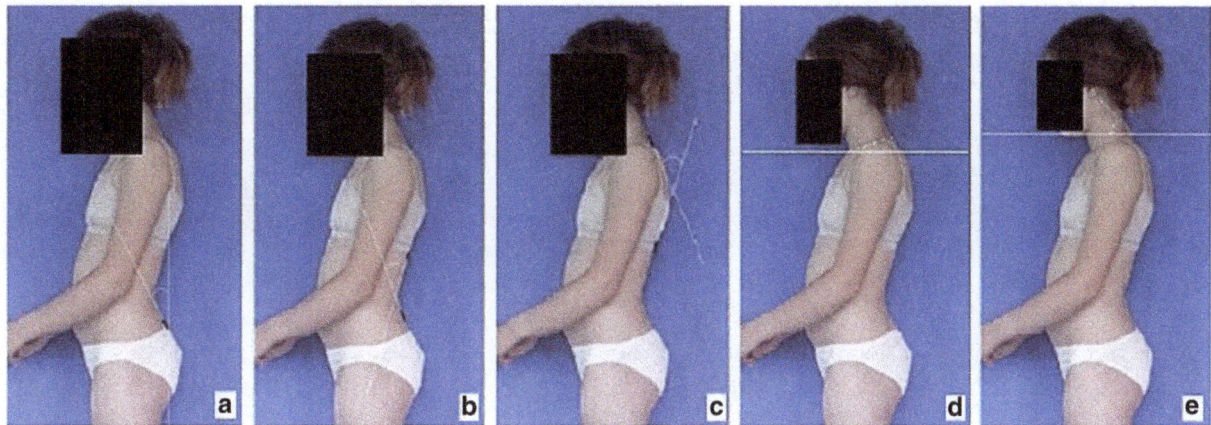

**Fig. 9 a** Diagram illustrating the measurements of SS. **b** Diagram illustrating the measurements of LL. **c** Diagram illustrating the measurements of TK. **d** Diagram illustrating the measurements of CI. **e** Diagram illustrating the measurements of HP

**Variability of photographic sagittal parameters over time**

The aim of the second part of the study was to analyze the variability over time (zero time, after 1 h, and after 1 week) of five 2D photographic angles: sacral slope (SS), lumbar lordosis (LL), thoracic kyphosis (TK), chest inclination (CI), and head protraction (HP).

The study group comprised 30 healthy volunteers (13 girls and 17 boys) aged 7–10 (mean $8.2 \pm 1.0$ years). The same exclusion criteria as in photographic technique validation XYZ were used. Children were photographed in a standardized relaxed (spontaneous, habitual) posture (Fig. 2b). At each of the three exposures, the digital photographs of the left profile of the body were taken three times one after another within 5 s. The exposure was made (1) at the time zero, (2) 1 h later, and (3) one week later.

In total, 270 photos were assessed. Five photographic parameters were calculated on each photo.

**Variability of photographic coronal parameters over time**

The aim of this part of the study was to analyze the variability in time (zero time, after one hour, after one week) of two coronal photographic parameters: ATSI (Anterior Trunk Symmetry Index) (Fig. 6) and POTSI (Posterior Trunk Symmetry Index) (Fig. 7) which serve to evaluate the symmetry of the trunk in coronal plane.

The study group comprised 30 healthy volunteers (13 girls and 17 boys) aged 7–10 (mean $8.1 \pm 1.1$ years). The same exclusion criteria as in photographic technique validation were used. Children were photographed in a standardized relaxed (spontaneous, habitual) posture in the coronal plane. Three digital photographs were taken within 5 s, including the front (Fig. 13) and back (Fig. 14)

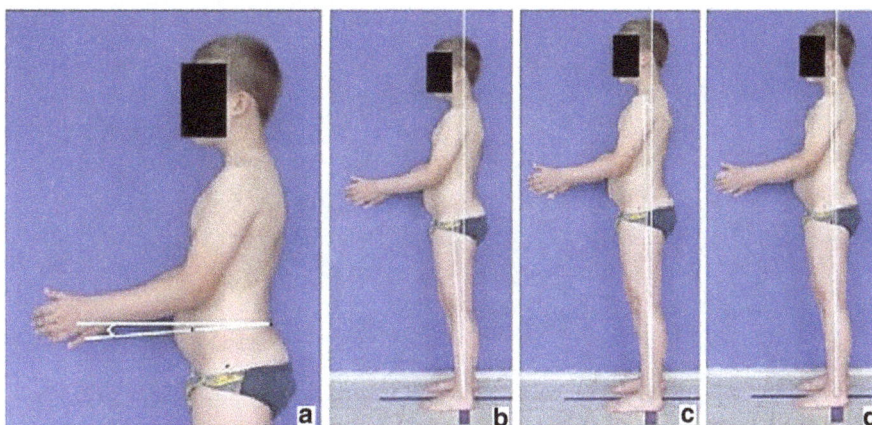

**Fig. 10 a** Diagram illustrating the measurements of SPT. **b** Diagram illustrating the measurements of TA. **c** Diagram illustrating the measurements of AA. **d** Diagram illustrating the measurements of EA

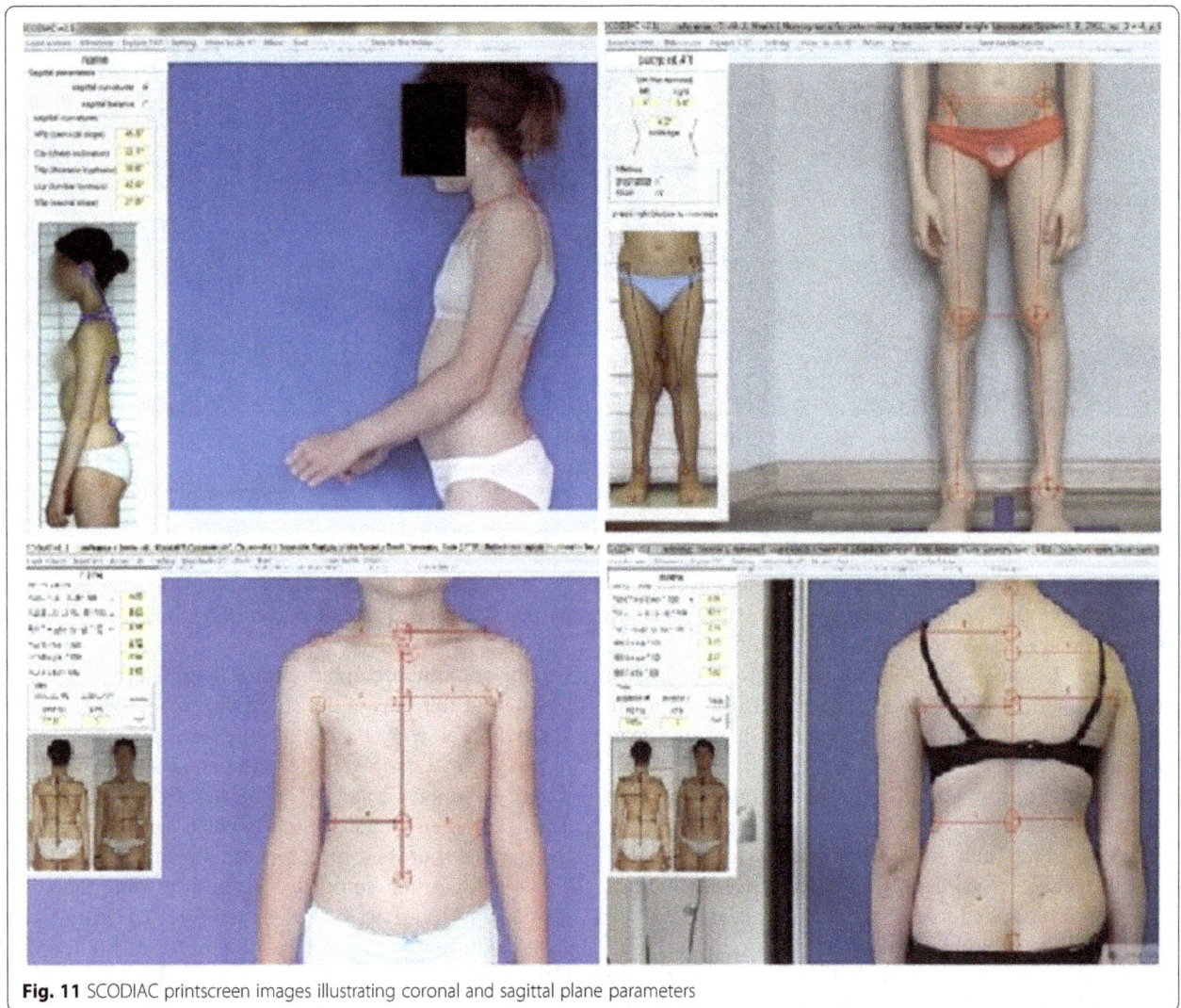

**Fig. 11** SCODIAC printscreen images illustrating coronal and sagittal plane parameters

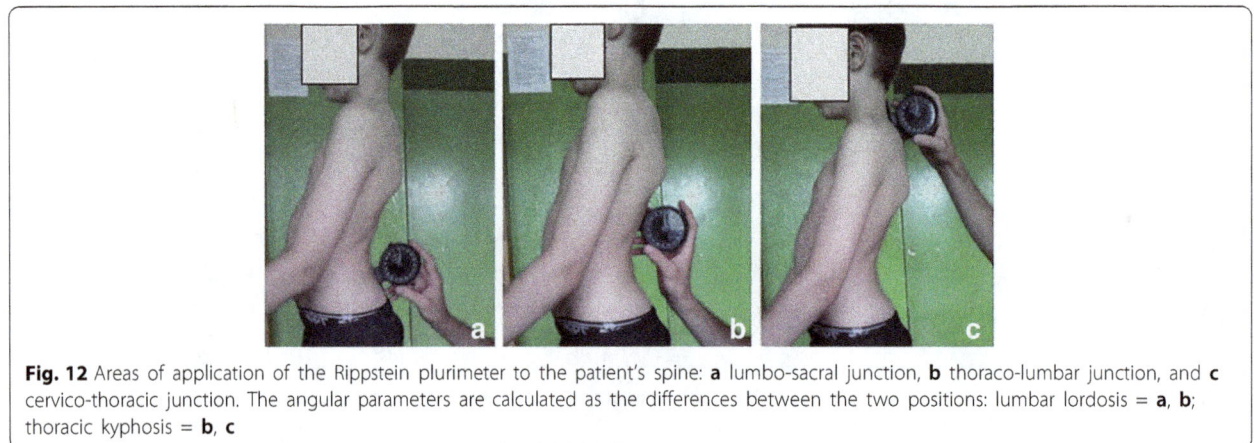

**Fig. 12** Areas of application of the Rippstein plurimeter to the patient's spine: **a** lumbo-sacral junction, **b** thoraco-lumbar junction, and **c** cervico-thoracic junction. The angular parameters are calculated as the differences between the two positions: lumbar lordosis = **a**, **b**; thoracic kyphosis = **b**, **c**

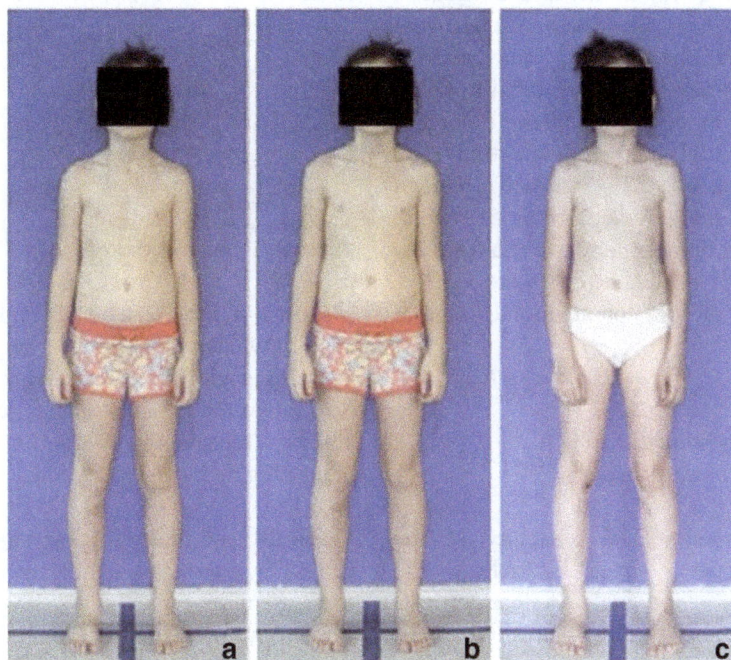

**Fig. 13** Positioning of the child during photographic documentation of front view: **a** zero time, **b** after 1 h, and **c** after 1 week

view. The same procedure was repeated after 1 h and after 1 week (540 photos were assessed).

## Normative values of sagittal photographic parameters in children aged 7–10

Normative values of sagittal photographic parameters were calculated based on photographic assessment of 7782 children of both sexes, aged 7–10. All photographs were taken respecting the abovementioned procedures.

### Statistical analysis

Statistical analyses were performed using Statistica 10 (StatSoft), Gretl and Microsoft Excel software. Statistical significance level was defined as $P < 0.05$. Reliability was determined with the intraclass correlation coefficient

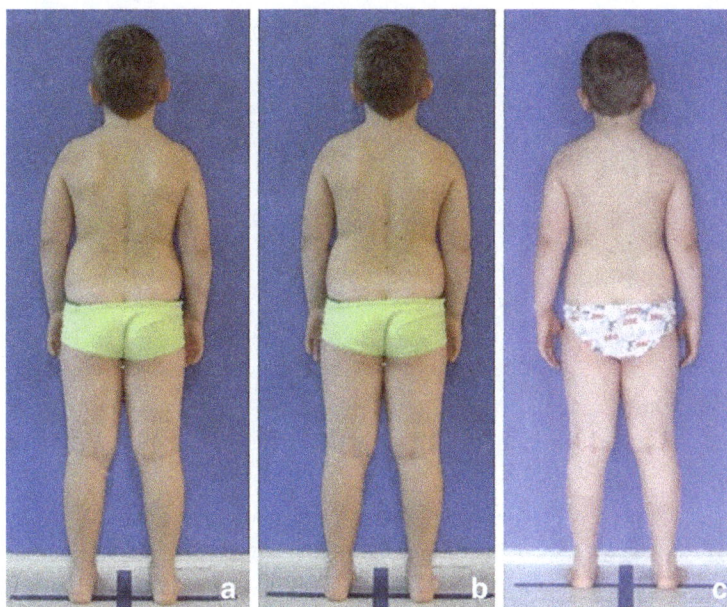

**Fig. 14** Positioning of the child during photographic documentation of back view: **a** zero time, **b** after 1 h, and **c** after 1 week

(ICC) by means of the two-way model and Cronbach's alpha. [30, 31]. The scale from Bland and Altman were used in the classification of the reliability values and relationship between plurimeter and photography [30]. ICC values smaller than or equal to 0.20 were considered poor, 0.21–0.40 fair, 0.41–0.60 moderate, 0.61–0.80 good, and 0.81–1 very good [32]. Standard error of measurement (SEM) was measured according to Shrout. [33]. Analysis of variance, homogeneity of variance, normality of distribution, and post hoc tests were used to examine the variation of five photographic sagittal parameters over time.

## Results
### Photogrammetry reliability studies
### *Validation of the photographic technique*

**Photographic measurements** The reliability of the photographic measurements is shown in Table 1. The ICC values for the sacral slope angle, lumbar lordosis angle, thoracic kyphosis angle, chest inclination angle, and head protraction angle revealed very good reliability, with the SEMs of the measurement ranging between 0.7 and 1.3.

**Photogrammetry versus plurimeter** The correlation of measurements using plurimeter and digital photography

**Table 2** Correlation of Rippstein plurimeter versus photographic measurements

| Variables | ICC | 95% | CI | SEM [°] | P value |
|---|---|---|---|---|---|
| Plurimeter SS—photo SS | 0.93 | 0.89 | 0.95 | 1.2 | 0.712 |
| Plurimeter LL—photo LL | 0.97 | 0.93 | 0.98 | 0.9 | 0.425 |
| Plurimeter TK—photo TK | 0.95 | 0.93 | 0.97 | 1.4 | 0.945 |

*ICC* intraclass correlation coefficient, *CI* confidence interval, *SEM* standard error of measurement
*Statistically significant difference (P < .05)

is shown in Table 2. The ICC values for the sacral slope angle (0.93), lumbar lordosis angle (0.97), and thoracic kyphosis angle (0.95) revealed very good reliability. All ICC values for the three angles reported very good interobserver repeatability, with the SEMs of the measurement ranging between 0.9 and 1.4.

**Variability of photographic sagittal parameters over time** There were no significant differences between the measurements ($p > 0.05$) at zero time, after 1 h, and after 1 week in any of the five sagittal photographic parameters. In the case of SS and CI, the 1 week measurement was different to the zero and the 1-h measurement, but the differences were not statistically significant (using analysis of variance and post hoc tests). The results of measurement of both parameters increased with time, so the largest difference was observed between the

**Table 1** Reliability of using photographic technique for measuring the sagittal trunk alignment

| Variables | Intraobserver reproducibility | | | | | Interobserver reliability | | | | |
|---|---|---|---|---|---|---|---|---|---|---|
| | ICC | 95% | CI | SEM [°] | P value | ICC | 95% | CI | SEM [°] | P value |
| Left side of the body | | | | | | | | | | |
| SS | 0.93 | 0.88 | 0.97 | 1.0 | 0.957 | 0.93 | 0.86 | 0.97 | 0.9 | 0.658 |
| LL | 0.97 | 0.95 | 0.99 | 1.0 | 0.975 | 0.97 | 0.95 | 0.99 | 1.0 | 0.987 |
| TK | 0.93 | 0.87 | 0.96 | 1.2 | 0.974 | 0.94 | 0.89 | 0.97 | 0.9 | 0.811 |
| CI | 0.96 | 0.92 | 0.98 | 0.7 | 0.953 | 0.92 | 0.83 | 0.96 | 0.9 | 0.540 |
| HP | 0.90 | 0.83 | 0.95 | 1.0 | 0.990 | 0.84 | 0.74 | 0.92 | 1.2 | 0.984 |
| Right side of the body | | | | | | | | | | |
| SS | 0.93 | 0.88 | 0.97 | 1.0 | 0.952 | 0.92 | 0.86 | 0.96 | 1.1 | 0.954 |
| LL | 0.96 | 0.93 | 0.98 | 1.2 | 0.936 | 0.96 | 0.92 | 0.98 | 1.1 | 0.852 |
| TK | 0.91 | 0.85 | 0.95 | 1.3 | 0.990 | 0.92 | 0.86 | 0.96 | 1.2 | 0.726 |
| CI | 0.93 | 0.87 | 0.96 | 0.9 | 0.931 | 0.88 | 0.79 | 0.94 | 1.1 | 0.689 |
| HP | 0.94 | 0.89 | 0.97 | 0.7 | 0.989 | 0.85 | 0.75 | 0.92 | 1.0 | 0.913 |
| Mean of the left and right side of the body | | | | | | | | | | |
| SS | 0.95 | 0.91 | 0.97 | 0.9 | 0.977 | 0.94 | 0.89 | 0.97 | 0.9 | 0.836 |
| LL | 0.97 | 0.95 | 0.98 | 1.0 | 0.952 | 0.98 | 0.95 | 0.99 | 0.9 | 0.936 |
| TK | 0.93 | 0.88 | 0.97 | 1.1 | 0.986 | 0.92 | 0.86 | 0.96 | 0.9 | 0.777 |
| CI | 0.96 | 0.92 | 0.98 | 0.7 | 0.950 | 0.92 | 0.84 | 0.96 | 0.9 | 0.622 |
| HP | 0.94 | 0.89 | 0.97 | 0.8 | 0.995 | 0.89 | 0.80 | 0.94 | 1.0 | 0.979 |

*ICC* intraclass correlation coefficient, *CI* confidence interval, *SEM* standard error of measurement
*Statistically significant difference (P < .05)

**Table 3** Variability of sagittal and frontal parameters over time

| Measurements | SS | | LL | | TK | | CI | | HP | | ATSI | | POTSI | |
|---|---|---|---|---|---|---|---|---|---|---|---|---|---|---|
| | Mean | SD | Mean | SD | Mean | SD | Mean | SD | Mean | SD | Mean | SD | Mean | SD |
| Zero time | 24.7 | 7.0 | 41.7 | 9.5 | 44.5 | 6.7 | 27.1 | 7.1 | 53.3 | 3.1 | 21.6 | 11.6 | 21.3 | 10.0 |
| After 1 h | 25.3 | 7.2 | 42.0 | 8.3 | 43.6 | 7.6 | 27.6 | 7.5 | 52.8 | 5.8 | 21.8 | 11.4 | 21.9 | 10.6 |
| After 1 week | 26.8 | 8.1 | 43.0 | 9.1 | 45.0 | 8.9 | 29.3 | 6.8 | 52.8 | 5.1 | 20.1 | 8.8 | 18.3 | 6.1 |
| P | 0.533 | | 0.854 | | 0.786 | | 0.478 | | 0.926 | | 0.798 | | 0.288 | |

*Mean* mean value of three measurements, *SD* standard deviation of three measurements
*Statistically significant difference (P < .05)

measurement carried out in time zero and 1 week later. In case of the remaining three parameters (TK, LL, HP), we could not find such a trend (Table 3).

**Variability of photographic coronal parameters over time** There was no statistically significant difference between measurements ($p > 0.05$) for ATSI in zero time, after 1 h, and after 1 week. There was no statistically significant difference between measurements ($p > 0.05$) for POTSI parameters in zero time, after 1 h, and after 1 week (Table 4). A slight tendency regarding the difference between the 1-week measurement and the zero and 1-h measurement was not statistically significant. This observation needs further study in a bigger sample ($p$ values in post hoc tests were between 0.15 and 0.30).

**Normative values of sagittal photographic parameters for children 7–10** Five sagittal photographic parameters (SS, LL, TK, CI, HP) were measured for each child. The data was analyzed separately for boys and girls and for each year of age, ranging from 7 to 10. Numerical values based on the tables (Additional file 2: Appendix 2A) and percentile charts for sex and age (Additional file 2: Appendix 2B) are presented in Additional file 2: Appendix 2. Table 4 contains the exemplary numerical values of the five photographic parameters (all values presented in degrees).

**Table 4** Exemplary table based on numerical values for 7-year-old girls (N = 1083)

| Percentile | SS | LL | TK | CI | HP |
|---|---|---|---|---|---|
| 97 | 44 | 52 | 62 | 41 | 71 |
| 90 | 39 | 45 | 55 | 36 | 66 |
| 75 | 33 | 37 | 48 | 32 | 63 |
| 50 | 27 | 29 | 42 | 27 | 58 |
| 25 | 22 | 23 | 35 | 22 | 54 |
| 10 | 17 | 18 | 28 | 18 | 49 |
| 3 | 12 | 13 | 23 | 14 | 45 |

**Pitfalls and sources of errors in photogrammetry used for posture evaluation** Errors may occur during photographic examination and photography evaluation. Attention should be paid to prepare and position the child according to the protocol. The incorrect preparation or positioning is illustrated below with the examples identified within our study group of 7782 children participating in the local school screening program. In total, 46,595 digital photos were analyzed.

The following problems were noted and are reported below in the following way: (1) type of error and (2) consequence for posture assessment. Figures are illustrating the following:

- Protraction of the shoulders—the upper limbs cover the body contours and anatomical points (Fig. 15)
- Incorrect head position and gaze direction—impact on cervical spine parameters (Fig. 16)
- Inability to adopt spontaneous relaxed posture—impact on lumbar lordosis and thoracic kyphosis angles (Fig. 17)
- Hair covering the body contours—impossibility of measuring photographic parameters (Fig. 18)
- Gluteal cleft covered with underpants—impossible calculation of POTSI index (Fig. 19)
- Bra or swimsuit with limited body contact and obscuring the trunk—sagittal angles design and calculation not possible (Fig. 20)
- One-leg standing—impact on coronal plane symmetry (Fig. 21)
- Incorrect rotational foot positioning—introduction of rotation to the whole body (Fig. 22)
- Digital camera not level—possible photographic parameters modification (Fig. 23)
- Limited communication with the child can be treated as a contraindication for photographical measurements—standardized position not possible (Fig. 24)
- Insufficient image sharpness—difficulties with photographic angle measurement (Fig. 25)

These errors can influence the photographic evaluation and should be avoided.

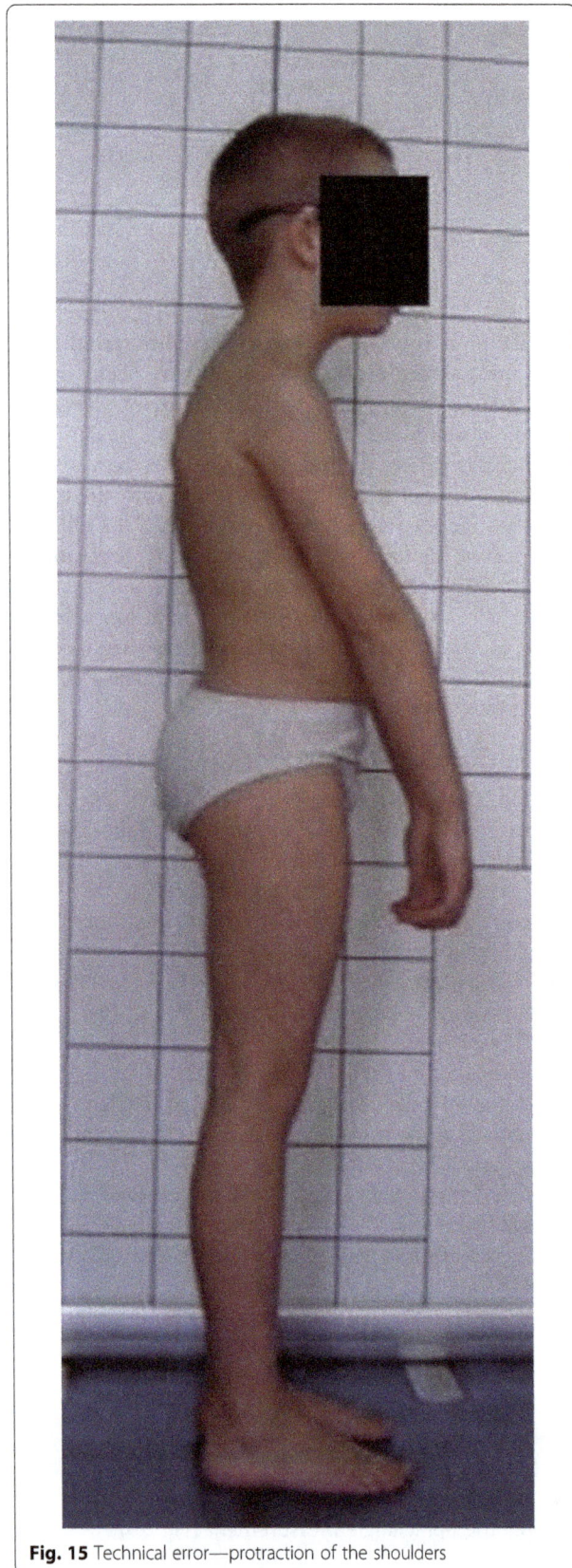

**Fig. 15** Technical error—protraction of the shoulders

## Discussion

### Radiological assessment as the current gold standard for scoliosis evaluation but not for child body posture evaluation

The radiological imaging remains the gold standard for idiopathic scoliosis (IS) diagnosis and evaluation [34–37]. It enables the primary and secondary curves identification, Cobb angle measurement, axial vertebral rotation assessment, and Risser sign grading. It differentiates the idiopathic scoliosis from the congenital one. However, for the large cohort studies or for the school screening purpose, the children are not exposed to radiography because of the radiation risk [38, 39]. In the screening conditions, the suspicion of idiopathic scoliosis is detected with manual anthropometric devices, such as the scoliometer [40–43] or smartphone with a specific device [44–46]. The basic method of school screening for idiopathic scoliosis is a clinical examination in the forward bending position (Adam's test) with the use of scoliometer [47, 48]. Surface topography methods based on computerized image capturing and digitally calculated parameters are also proposed for the evaluation of patients suffering from idiopathic scoliosis. These techniques utilize raster stereography based on distortion of a grid projected onto the back [49–51] or body scanning using light beam and its distortion analysis [49, 52, 53].

Evaluation of physical deformity developing in idiopathic scoliosis presents some common areas together with the body shape evaluation in postural disorders. Similar diagnostic tools are often used. In children, it is especially important to apply the techniques which do not involve exposure to x-ray radiation. Several methods have been proposed for body posture assessment: simple photographic techniques and plumbline measures [54–57], goniometers, inclinometers and linear devices [58–60], computer-assisted methods including electrogoniometers [61], electromagnetic movement systems [62, 63], computer-assisted digitization systems [64–66], or 3D ultrasound-based motion analysis device [67]. Finally, digital photography is gaining grounds in the assessment of trunk alignment [68].

### Overview of photographic parameters proposed for posture evaluation

Photographic parameters for posture evaluation were presented by several authors. The parameters proposed in this study were selected based on the authors' personal experience and the careful analysis of previous publications.

Canales et al. [69] reported the following posterior and sagittal parameters: head position, thoracic kyphosis, lumbar lordosis, pelvic inclination, and knee position

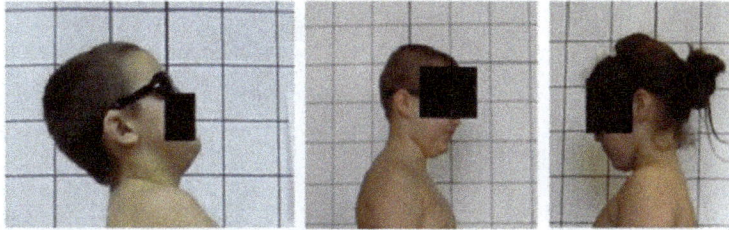

**Fig. 16** Technical error—incorrect head position and/or gaze direction

together with the following anatomical points to be considered: scapulas, shoulders, and ankles (Fig. 26).

Cerrutto et al. [70] reported the following anterior, posterior, and sagittal parameters: P1, P2, L1, L2, L3, AR, and AL angles which were measured based on the lines drawn from the anatomical points: superior and inferior scapular angles, vertical lines related to ear lobe, acromion and scapular prominence, and vertical lines related to manubrium and coracoid process (Fig. 27).

Pausić et al. [71] proposed assessment based on the following anatomical points: head and neck, trunk, pelvis, knee joints, and ankle joints (for the coronal plane) or head and neck, trunk, pelvis, and knee joints for the sagittal plane (Fig. 28).

Penha et al. [8] reported the following posterior and sagittal parameters: lumbar lordosis, thoracic kyphosis, pelvic inclination, head position, and lateral spinal deviations based on anatomical points to be considered (Fig. 29).

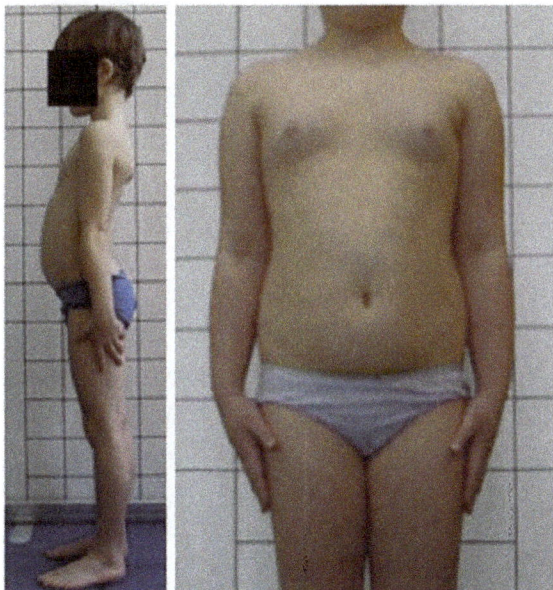

**Fig. 17** Technical error—lack of spontaneous relaxed posture

Ruivo et al. [72] reported the following sagittal parameters: head angle, cervical angle, and shoulder angle (Fig. 30).

Sacco et al. [73] reported the following sagittal parameters: tibiotarsal angle, knee extension/flexion angle, Q angle, and subtalar angle (Fig. 31).

Canhadas et al. [74] proposed the following anatomical points to be considered: external orbicularis, commissura labiorum, acromioclavicular joint, sternoclavicular joint, ear lobe, antero-superior iliac spines, postero-superior and postero-inferior iliac spines, inferior angles of the scapula, olecranon central region, and popliteal line. In addition, the following angles were evaluated: bilateral foot inclination, forward inclination of the fibula, knee angle, cervical lordosis, thoracic kyphosis, lumbar lordosis, knee flexor, tibiotarsal angle, forward head position, and sternal angles (Fig. 32).

Matamalas et al. [75] reported the following posterior parameters: waist height angle, waist angle, and waistline distance ratio (Fig. 33).

Matamalas et al. [76] published the following anterior and posterior parameters: trapezium angle, shoulder height angle, and axilla height angle (Fig. 34).

### Current opinions on digital photography technique

Digital photography completed with analyzing software can be viewed as digital photogrammetry and can be found in several areas of life and technology: architecture, psychology, medicine, rehabilitation, and other fields [77–80]. For the purpose of posture assessment, this technique is easy to access and cost-effective [81, 82]. The technique provides measurement of body angles or distances, which allows for a quantitative posture assessment. Remaining non-invasive, digital photography is becoming an increasingly popular tool for assessing the musculoskeletal system, including the sagittal and coronal curvatures of the spine, in both clinical practice and research [83, 84]. In recent years, the photographic technique has been used to assess the posture of healthy and unhealthy children and adults [69, 74, 85]. Digital photography was applied to assess body posture of children carrying heavy backpacks [86], to evaluate the quality of posture while standing [87, 88] and siting [89], or

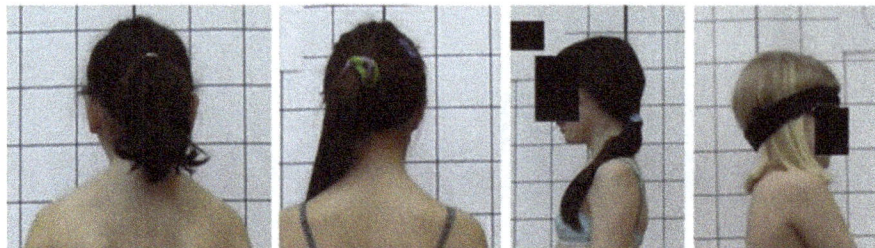

**Fig. 18** Technical error—body contours covered by hair

for quantifying the foot shape [90]. Several studies described usefulness of the photographic technique to assess patients with idiopathic scoliosis [75, 91–94].

### Technical procedures of posture photogrammetry
#### Camera resolution

Different resolutions of digital cameras were used in the previous studies, ranging from 2.0 megapixels (Mpx) [73], 4.1 Mpx [95, 96], through 5.1 Mpx [84], 6.0 Mpx [81], 6.3 Mpx [97] to 7.2 Mpx [98]. For this study, CANON POWER SHOT A590 IS, 1/2.5 CCD matrix, 8.3 megapixels, 35–140-mm lens (Canon Incorporation, Tokyo, Japan) was used. The resolution of $1600 \times 1200$ [2 Mpx] provided sufficient photo quality [99].

#### Camera position—distance and height

In previous photographic studies, the distance between the camera and the object was reported to be 173 cm [97, 100], 300 cm [73, 81, 95, 101], or 400 cm [55]. The camera was positioned at the height of 70, 127, 80 or 90 cm [81], while other authors set the camera by centering the lens at half of the child's height [81, 95, 98]. In our previous experiments, the camera was placed on a stabile tripod at the height of 90 cm and the distance of 300 cm. These settings were previously suggested for children aged 7–10 [81, 98]. Such a combination of distance and height enabled covering the whole silhouette without moving the camera [12].

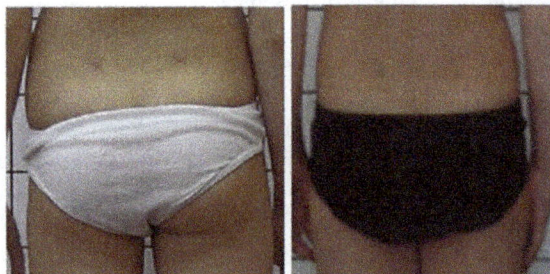

**Fig. 19** Technical error—gluteal cleft upper contour covered by underpants

#### Child positioning

Some authors proposed to practice the photographic examination of the standing child wearing casual clothes, sportswear (shorts and a T-shirt) [87], just shorts [64], or the swimsuit [102]. Unfortunately, the clothes may slightly distort the body contour. Producing and registering images of undressed children seems to be a potential challenge for posture photogrammetry. Nowadays, it involves both the imperative to adopt procedures respecting individual sensitivity and the protection of image processing and storing. Yet, here we are, proposing the evaluation of the child body posture without any T-shirt, thigh or socks, wearing only underwear and bra [103], which is not

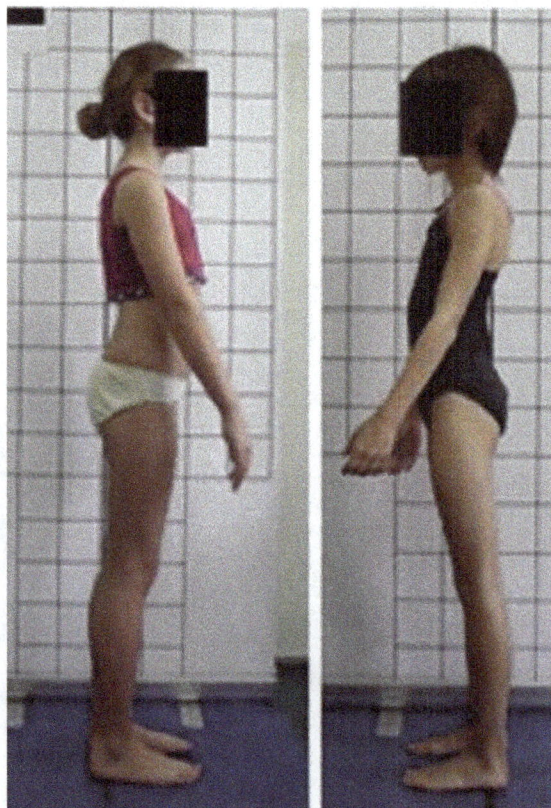

**Fig. 20** Technical error—the trunk obscured by bra or swimsuit

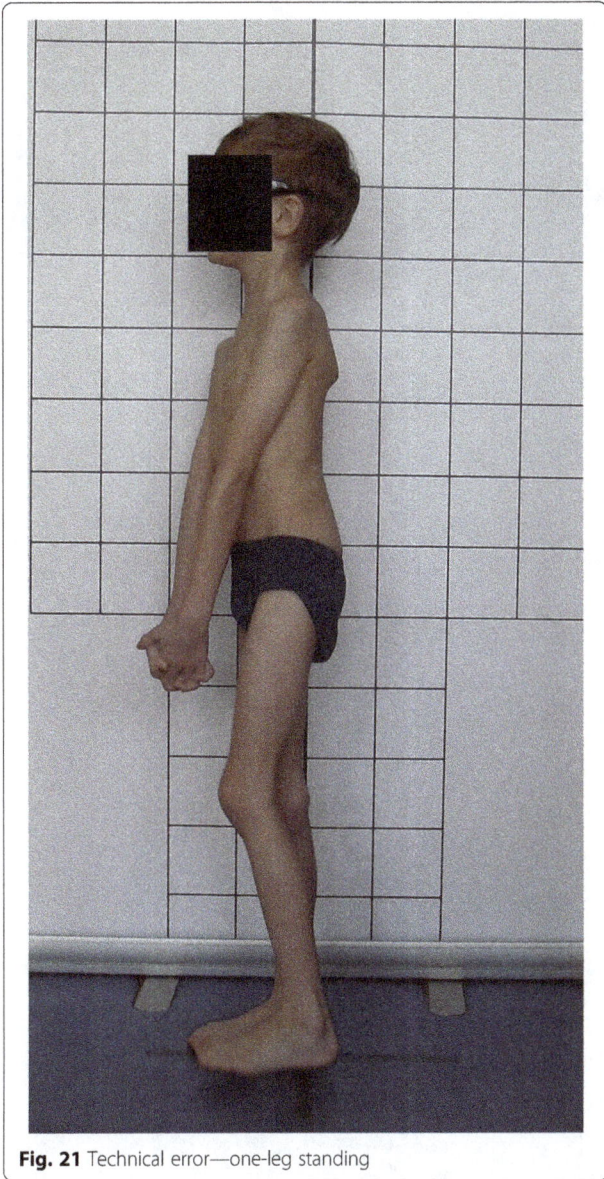

**Fig. 21** Technical error—one-leg standing

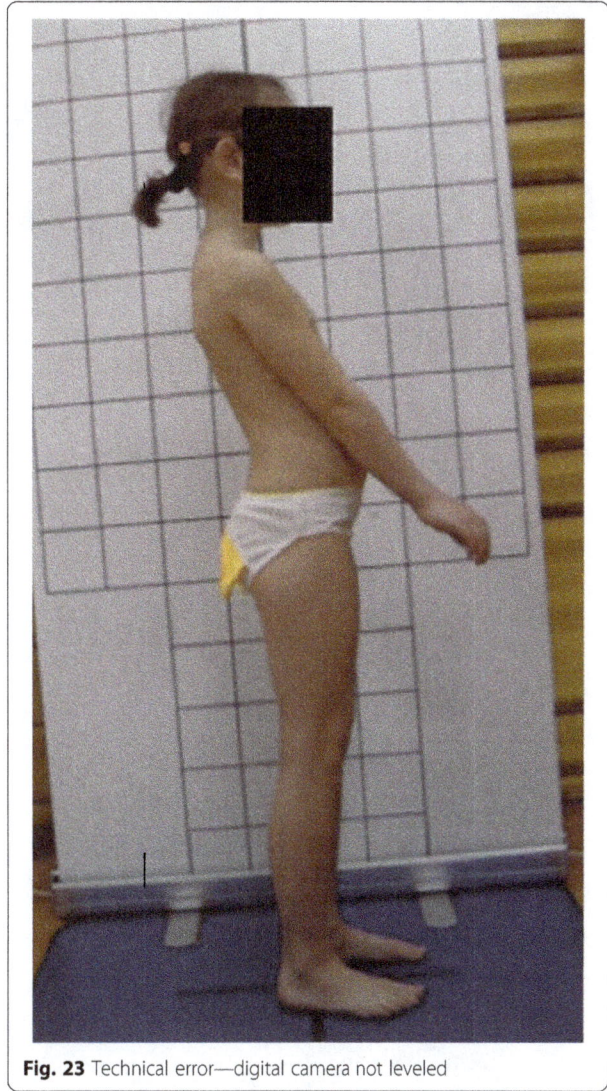

**Fig. 23** Technical error—digital camera not leveled

commonly accepted in our society (with individual cases of parents refusal noted). However, the local cultural background should be considered. Longer hair of the person examined should be tied or curled with a clip so as not to cover the external auditory meatus or neck contour.

### Lower limb positioning—the feet
In previous studies, some authors proposed to set the feet at the 30-degree external rotation in drawn triangles [97] or freely within the defined field lines [84]. In our observation, the 30-degree external rotation of the feet may undesirably impact the position of other parts of the body, especially the ankle joint in relation to the vertical projection of the quadrangle support.

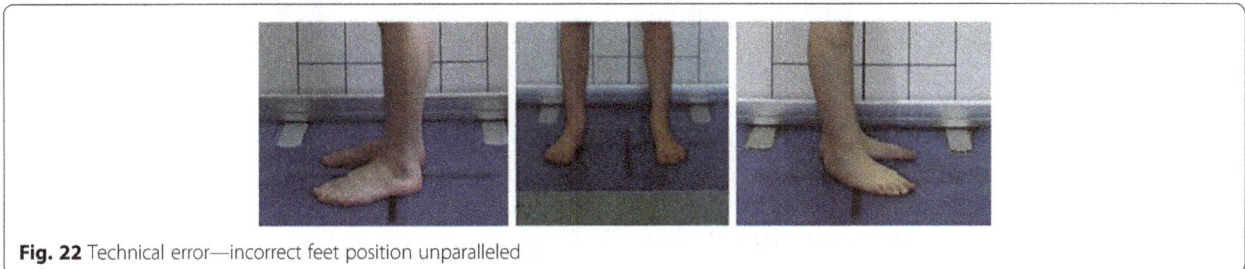

**Fig. 22** Technical error—incorrect feet position unparalleled

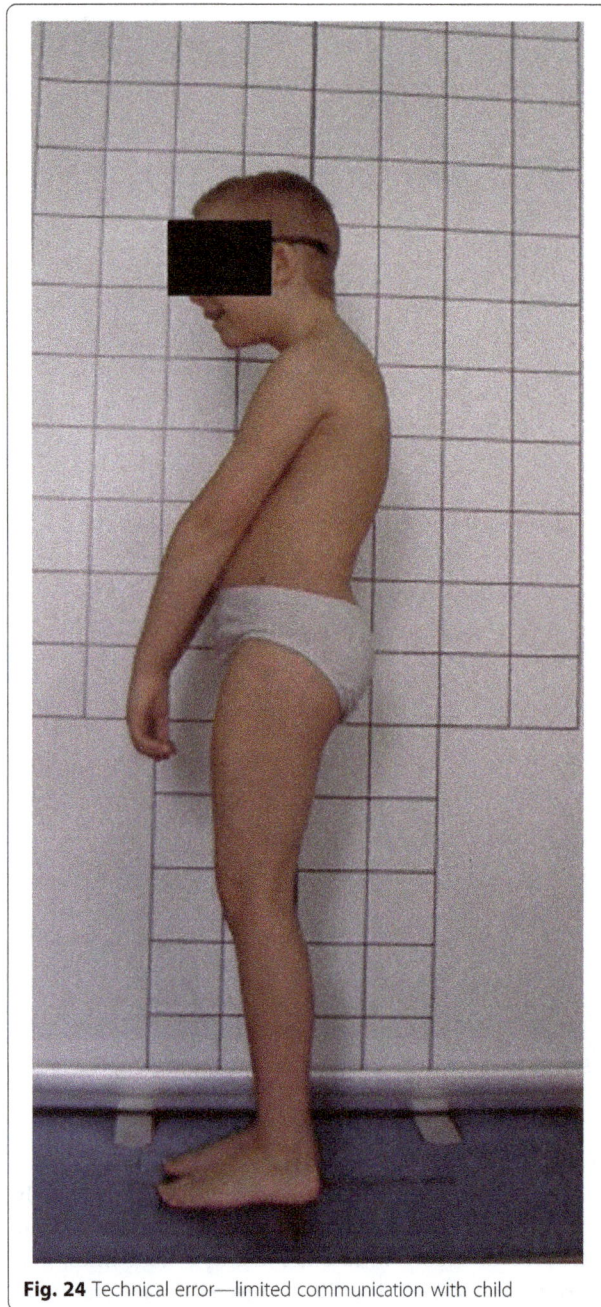

**Fig. 24** Technical error—limited communication with child

We decided to position the feet over the longitudinal and crosswise lines marked on the ground so that the lateral malleoli were situated over the center of crosswise line, and the feet were parallel to the longitudinal line and hip-width apart. We found such setting to be the most neutral feet position which does not interfere with the spontaneous posture [63]. It has also the advantage of being suitable for assessing the tibio-calcaneal angle. In our experiments, most children needed assistance to place the feet correctly.

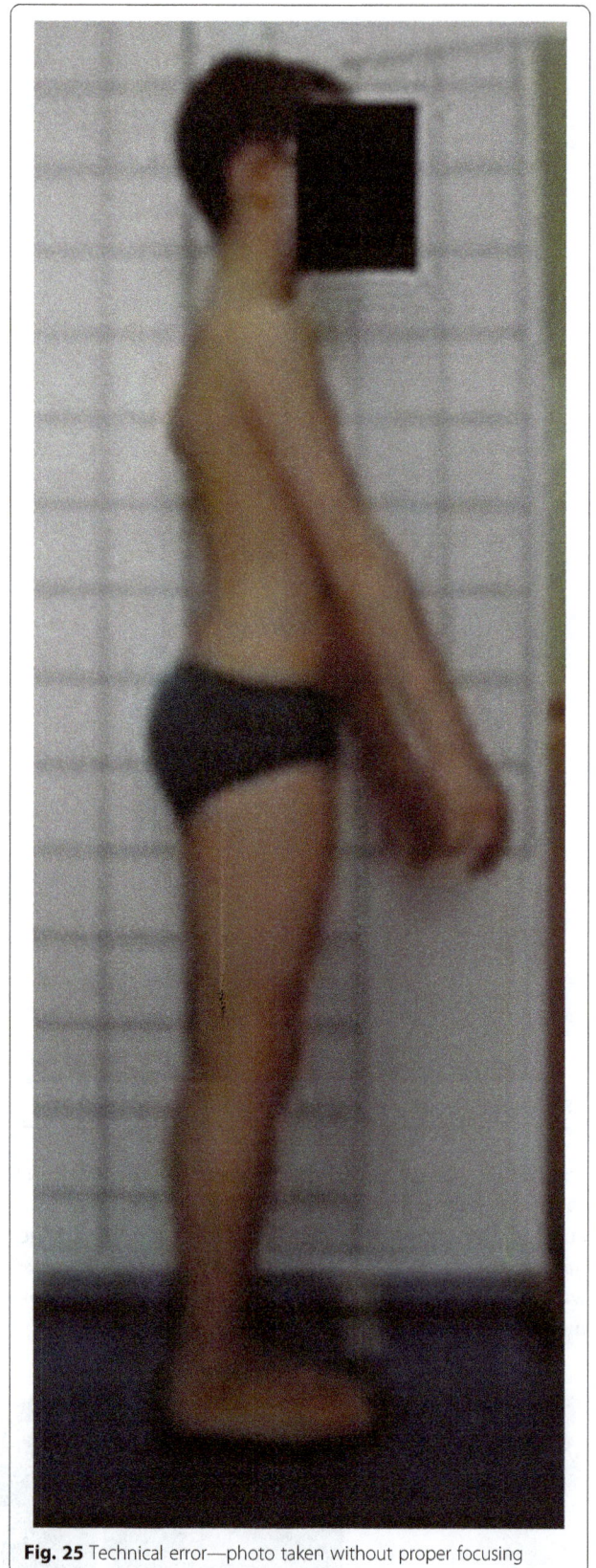

**Fig. 25** Technical error—photo taken without proper focusing

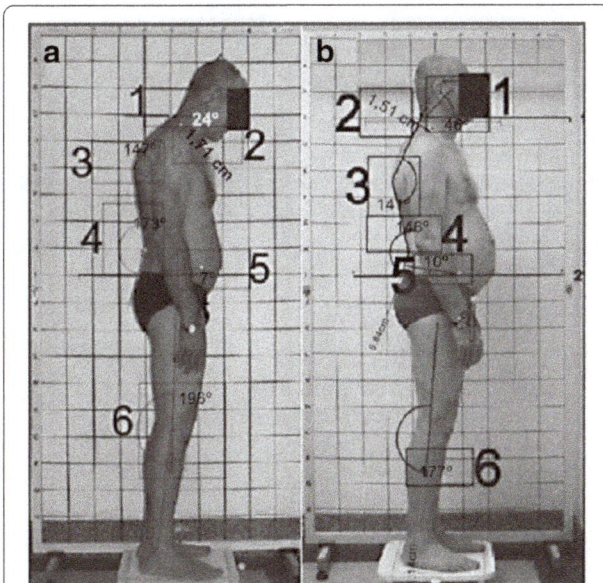

**Fig. 26 a–b** Photographic assessment as proposed by Canales et al. in 2010 ([69], reprinted by permission)

### Lower limbs positioning—the knees

The position of the knee joint and the symmetric lower limbs loading are also objects for standardization as some children tend to stand for the photographic evaluation having one lower limb more loaded or one knee more visibly bended. Such a position would influence the whole body posture, especially the trunk. We recommend positioning the child with equally loaded feet, in neutral setting of the knees, without flexion or hyperextension.

### Upper limb positioning—the elbows

Most authors suggest using the position with upper limbs hanging loosely [87, 96, 98, 102, 104, 105] in order not to influence the trunk [106]. The problem of the upper limb positioning is well-studied in the case of lateral spine radiography and different solutions are proposed to avoid the spine being obscured by the upper limbs [106–108]. Moreover, in the course of the standardization studies, we observed that the relaxed upper limbs sometimes covered the lumbar lordosis contour and greater trochanter. Similar observations have been made by other authors who suggested carrying out photographic sagittal evaluation with the elbow joints bent at 90° [73, 87, 109]. Finally, we recommend setting the upper limbs slightly flexed at about 10°–20° at the gleno-humeral joints and at about 20°–30° at the elbow joints. The movement of the upper limb flexion in the gleno-humeral and the elbow joints is performed slowly to avoid any involuntary trunk movement towards trunk hyperextension [87], which is the way to increasing

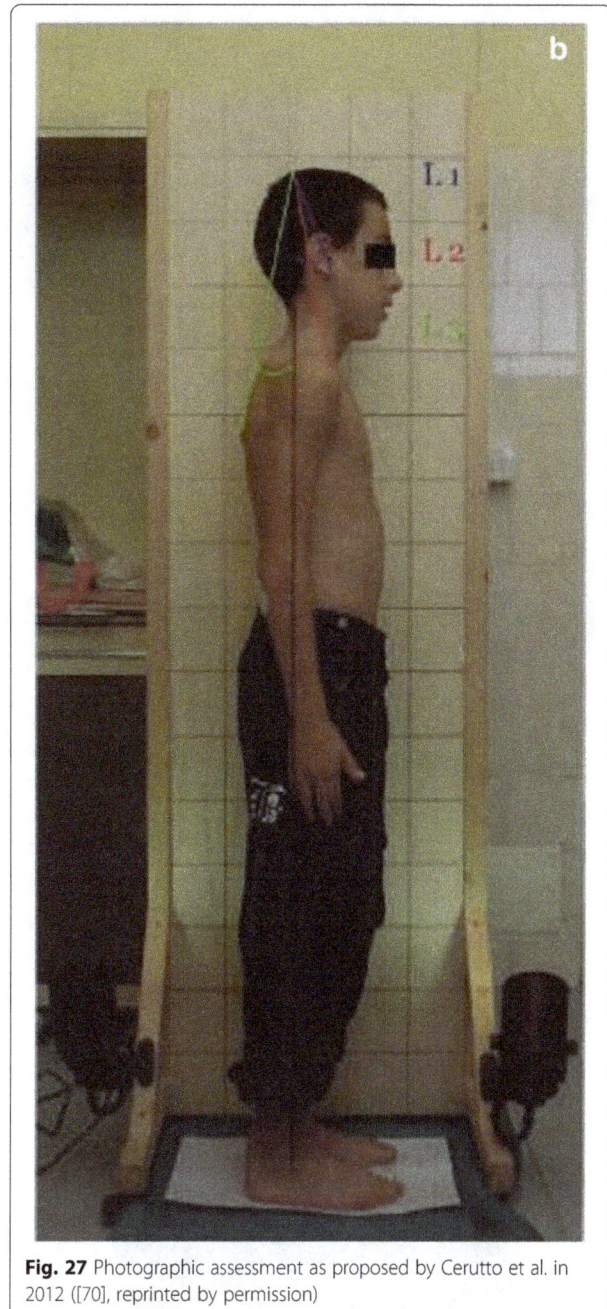

**Fig. 27** Photographic assessment as proposed by Cerutto et al. in 2012 ([70], reprinted by permission)

lower thoracic spine [110] or even creating a pathological lordosis in this region [111]. During this movement, the child is watched, and if any accompanying trunk movement happens, the child is asked to repeat the upper limb movement. In some cases, passive positioning of the upper limbs is needed. In addition, we observed that during the upper limb movement, some children performed elevation or protraction of the shoulders which covered the neck contour and the upper thoracic spine contour. Therefore, during the positioning of the upper limbs, we make sure that the

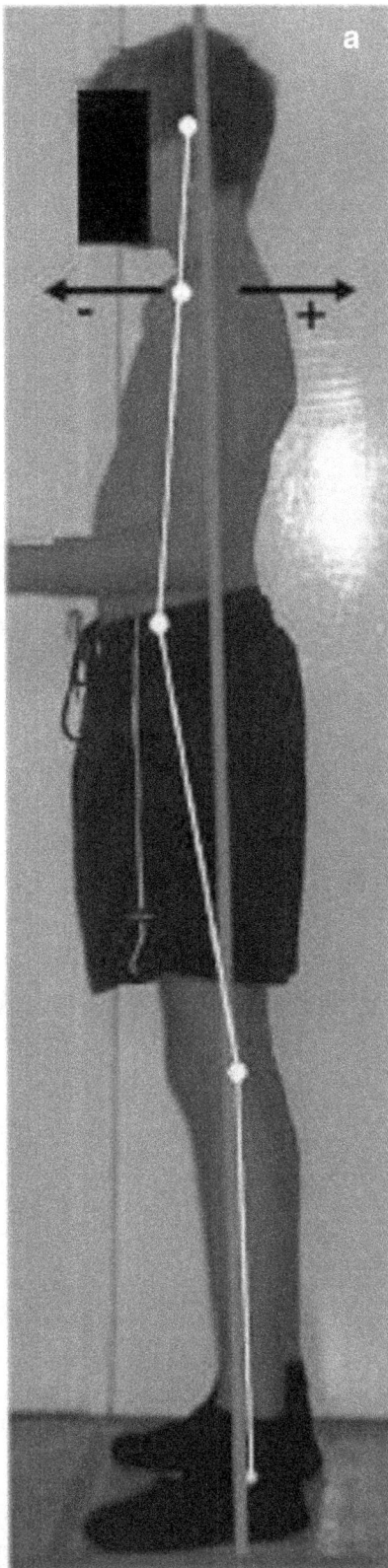

**Fig. 28** Photographic assessment as proposed by Pausić et al. in 2010 ([71], reprinted by permission)

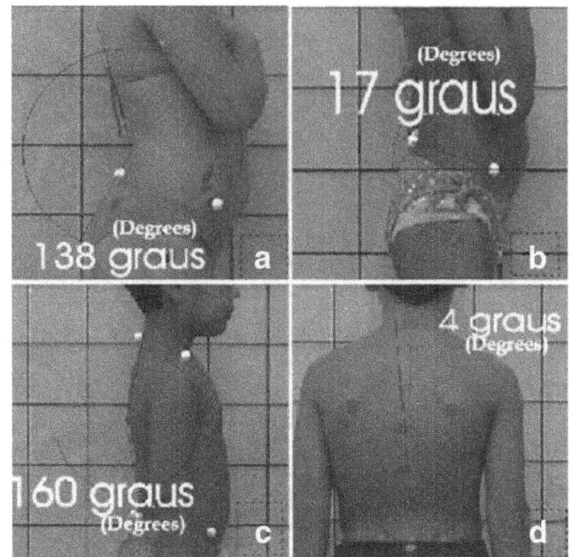

**Fig. 29 a–d** Photographic assessment as proposed by Penha et al. in 2009 ([8], reprinted by permission)

shoulder girdle stays down. It is important to note that the presence of shoulder protraction in loosely hanging upper limbs is common in the population of children aged 7–10 [8].

### Head position and gaze direction

During the standardization of the photographic technique, we checked the effect of the head position and the gaze direction on postural parameters. Our preliminary studies have shown that the head position affects the angular size of thoracic kyphosis and lumbar lordosis. Initially, we were planning to ask the child to look at a specific point marked in front of her/him as proposed in the literature [87]. Then, we noted this created an additional problem because of differences in children's height, which is why we proceeded with the "look ahead" command. Nevertheless, we noticed that some children, even when looking ahead, maintained voluntary lowered head position with the flexion of the cervical spine. Therefore, in order to achieve standardized conditions, each child was instructed to keep the eyes open and to direct the gaze at the eye level the moment it receives the "look ahead" command [71, 109, 112, 113]. Consequently, if an inappropriate voluntary head position was observed, we explained to the child once again how the head should be set. In rare situations, we helped the child by modifying the head position in a gentle way, trying not to trigger any artificially corrected position. In our practice, we also found it useful to ask children not to smile or laugh while taking the photos as it could affect postural parameters [112].

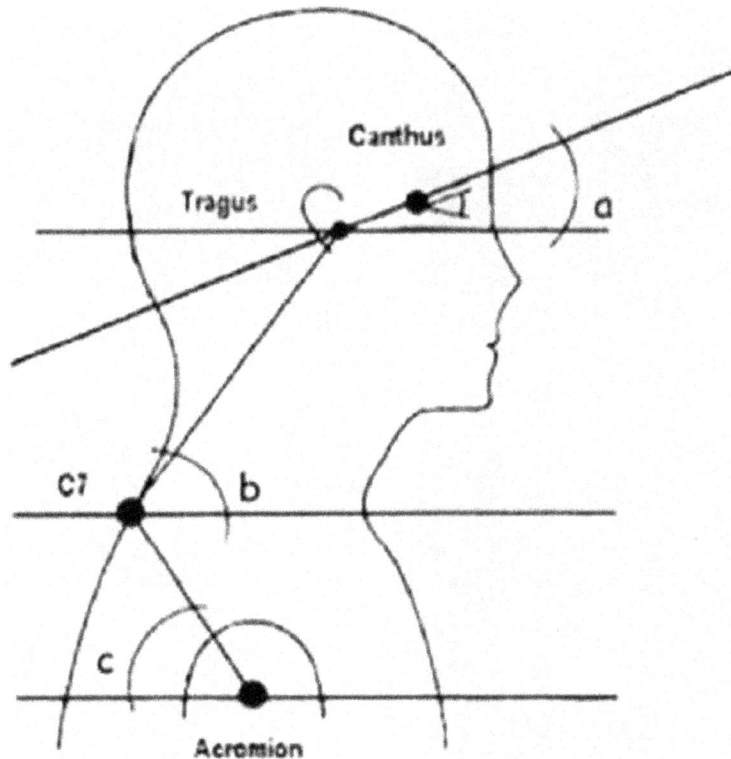

**Fig. 30** Photographic assessment as proposed by Ruivo et al. in 2015 ([72], reprinted by permission)

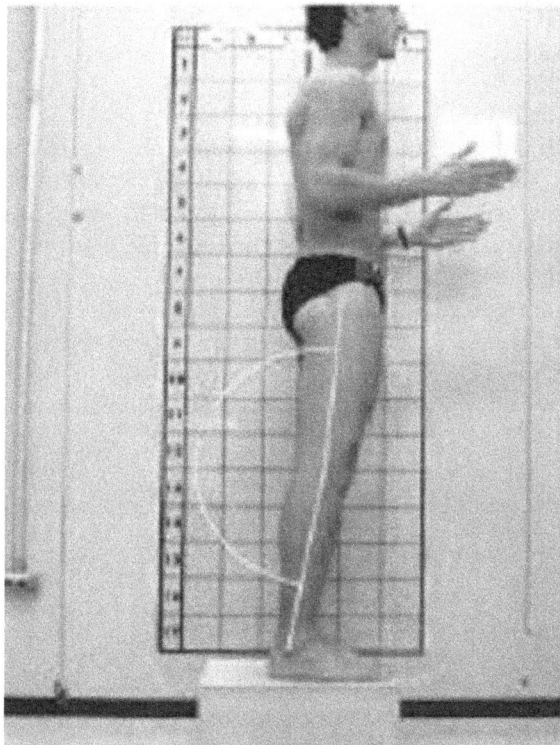

**Fig. 31** Photographic assessment as proposed by Sacco et al. in 2007 ([73], reprinted by permission)

## Digital photography technique for body posture evaluation and documentation

During this study, the postural photogrammetry revealed a simple and quick procedure. One can possibly perform photographic measurements with the use of a simple digital camera or a mobile camera in consideration of the standardized conditions for photographic evaluation. The tripod revealed a helpful device to stabilize the camera and control its position. The time needed for preparing the child for examination together with the time for taking photographic exposures in two sagittal projections was ca. 5 min, whereas the time required for calculation of five standardized sagittal parameters was ca. 3 min. This study confirmed the usefulness of photographic method for body posture documentation and evaluation. Digital photography technique can be used in research on the development and variability of posture in children. The developed procedure allows for the accurate and uniform filling of photographic documentation by physiotherapists and to obtain good quality research which is in line with the EBM rules. Due to its non-invasiveness, the technique can be promoted in scientific and clinical research. Parents' concerns regarding the use of radiography are avoided. The low cost of producing and archiving digital photos has a beneficial effect on technology. There is no need to acquire expensive, specialized equipment or software. Digital photogrammetry

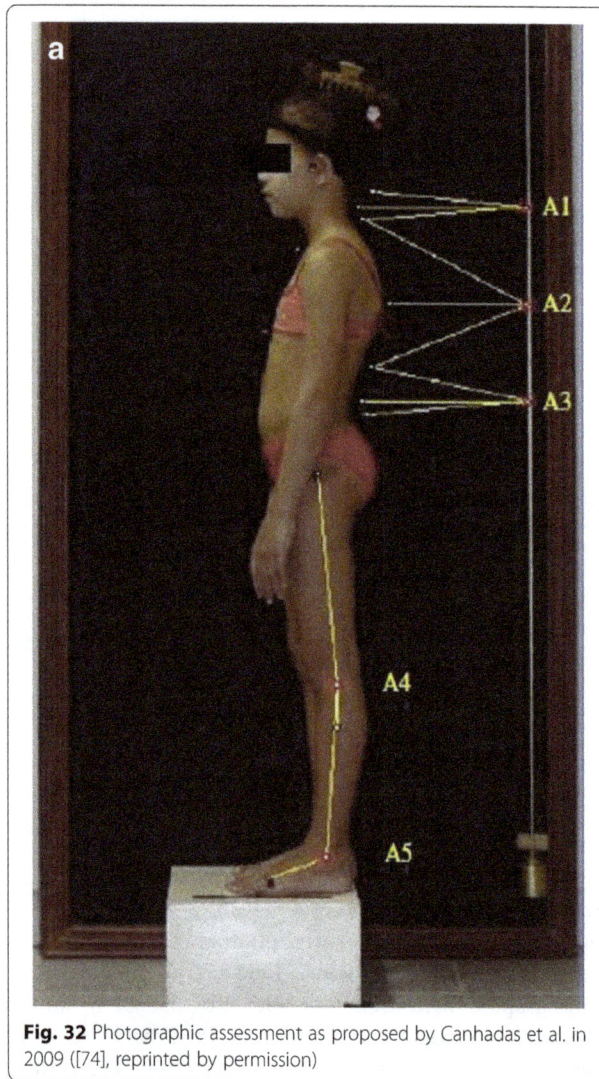

**Fig. 32** Photographic assessment as proposed by Canhadas et al. in 2009 ([74], reprinted by permission)

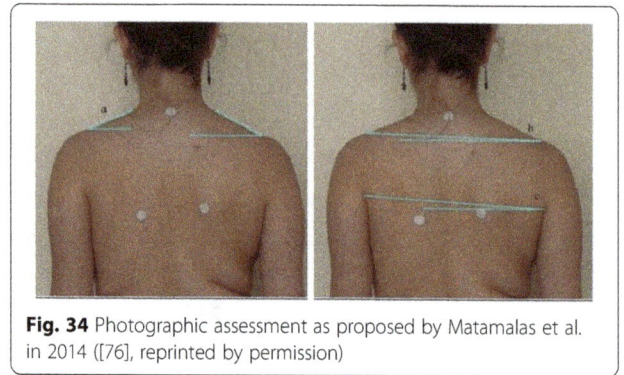

**Fig. 34** Photographic assessment as proposed by Matamalas et al. in 2014 ([76], reprinted by permission)

the simplicity of assessing the posture on the photos is at the core of this technique—it is objective, easy to use, and of low cost [114]. For Cobb et al. [90], the digital photography for a two-dimensional assessment of the body shape is a valuable method for recording the body posture and calculating quantitative parameters in everyday clinical practice. Fortin et al. [109] claim that digital photography technique can be used for scientific assessment provided that the procedures in question are taken into account. Galera et al. mention that the current studies present new diagnostic possibilities of digital photography, which is a common procedure for two-dimensional evaluation of body posture [71]. Digital photography has some limitations. The major limitation of the technique is the two-dimensional body posture assessment, as it is not impossible to measure trunk rotation. The method may not be suitable for children under 7 years of age.

## Conclusions

In summary, although both the surface topography and the radiological evaluation cannot be replaced with digital photography—the former for the 3D imaging, the latter for skeletal imaging—this technique offers a new additive value to human posture imaging. The development of digital photography technique allows for its regular use in the assessment of body posture. The method of child preparation and positioning described above allows us to avoid incidentally modified posture.

screening can be significant for the budget savings of individual units which organize screening (e.g., the local government), which is often crucial in financing various types of research projects. Specific numerical values of the normal range for quantitative and validated parameters are presented in this paper. According to van Maanem et al.,

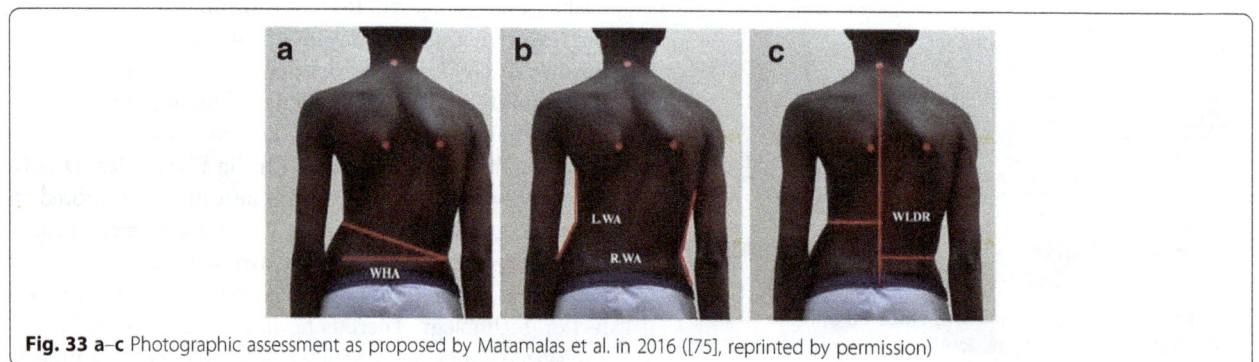

**Fig. 33 a–c** Photographic assessment as proposed by Matamalas et al. in 2016 ([75], reprinted by permission)

The registration of images is simple, quick, harmless and cost-effective. The semi-automatic image analysis has been developed. The choice of postural parameters was based on previous publications and on personal experience and can be modified. The photographic method of body posture assessment developed during this study is characteristic of high reliability of measurements. The five developed and calculated photographic parameters (sacral slope, thoracic kyphosis, lumbar lordosis, chest inclination, and head protraction) describe the child body posture in the sagittal plane and demonstrate good repeatability and reproducibility, which may become a standard for body posture evaluation in children. Performing such a large series of measurements in children resulted in the preparation of normal values and percentile charts for age and sex, making it possible for us to employ the photographic parameters possible in the diagnosis of child posture pathology as well as to monitor the effects of corrective therapy.

## Abbreviations

AA: Acromion-ankle angle; ASIS: Anterior superior iliac spine; ATSI: Anterior Trunk Symmetry Index; C7: Seventh cervical vertebra; CI: Chest inclination angle; EA: Ear-ankle angle; EBM: Evidence-based medicine; FAI-A: Frontal Asymmetry Index at axilla level; FAI-C7: Frontal Asymmetry Index at C7 level; FAI-SN: Frontal Asymmetry Index at sternal notch level; FAI-T: Frontal Asymmetry Index at trunk level; HDI-A: Height Difference Index for axillas; HDI-S: Height Difference Index for shoulders; HDI-T: Height Difference Index for trunk waistline; HP: Head protraction angle; ICC: Intraclass correlation coefficient; IS: Idiopathic scoliosis; L1: First lumbar vertebra; L5: Fifth lumbar vertebra; LL: Lumbar lordosis angle; POTSI: Posterior Trunk Symmetry Index; PSIS: Posterior superior iliac spine; S1: First sacral vertebra; SEM: Standard error for single measurement; SPT: Sagittal pelvic tilt; SS: Sacral slope angle; T12: Twelfth thoracic vertebra; TA: Trochanter-ankle angle; TCA: Tibiocalcaneal angle; TFA: Tibio-femoral angle; TK: Thoracic kyphosis angle

## Acknowledgements

The authors would like to thank Prof. Pawel Ulman for his contribution to statistical analysis, Mr. Krzysztof Korbel, PT, and Ms. Katarzyna Politarczyk, PT, for assistance in the measurements.
The study was performed as part of the local prevention project "Skierniewice Chooses Health – Bad Posture and Postural Defects Prophylaxis in Class I-III Primary School Children" and "Poznan Chooses Health – Bad Posture Prophylaxis in Class I-IV Primary School Children".

## Funding

No sources of funding were utilized for the study.

## Authors' contributions

LS performed the study design, developed the study protocol, data collection, and compilation, described the result analysis and manuscript, drafting and revision, critical revision of the manuscript. MK described result analysis, participated in the acquisition of the data, critical revision of the manuscript. DC performed the study design, developed the study protocol, data collection and compilation, described result analysis and manuscript, drafting and revision, critical revision of the manuscript. MT participated in the acquisition of the data and the critical revision of the manuscript. PC prepared the computer software for the study. NS developed the study protocol, critical revision of the manuscript, TK performed the study design, developed the study protocol, data collection and compilation, described result analysis and manuscript, drafting and revision, as well as the critical revision of the manuscript. All authors read and approved the final manuscript.

## Competing interests

The authors declare that they have no competing interests.

## Author details

[1]Department of Spine Disorders and Pediatric Orthopedics, University of Medical Sciences, 28 Czerwca 1956r. no. 135/147, 61-545 Poznan, Poland. [2]Rehasport Clinic, Poznan, Poland. [3]Rehasport Clinic Licensed Rehabilitation Center, Skierniewice, Poland. [4]Department of Physiotherapy, Józef Rusiecki University College, Olsztyn, Poland. [5]Center of Body Posture, Olsztyn, Poland. [6]Department of Orthopaedics, Pediatric Orthopaedics and Traumatology, The Centre of Postgraduate Medical Education in Warsaw, Otwock, Poland. [7]Faculty of Health Studies, University of West Bohemia, Pilsen, Czech Republic. [8]Faculty of Physical Education and Sport, Charles University, Prague, Czech Republic. [9]ORTOTIKA, s. r. o, Faculty at Motol University Hospital, Prague, Czech Republic. [10]Scoliosis Center, Medical Scanning Tokyo, Tokyo, Japan.

## References

1. Kendall FP, McCreary EK, Provance PG. Muscles testing and function with posture and pain. 4th ed. USA: Lippincott Williams and Wilkins; 2005.
2. Kiebzak W, Szmigiel C, Kowalski I, Sliwinski Z. Importance of risk factors in detecting psychomotor development disorders in children during their first year of life. Advances in Rehabilitation. 2008;22:29–33.
3. Blaszczyk JW, Cieslinska-Swider J, Plewa M, Zahorska-Markiewicz B, Markiewicz A. Effects of excessive body weight on postural control. J Biomech. 2009;42:1295–300. https://doi.org/10.1016/j.jbiomech.2009.03.006.
4. Kowalski IM, Protasiewicz-Falowska H. Trunk measurements in the standing and sitting posture according to evidence based medicine (EBM). J Spine Surg. 2013;1:66–79.
5. Kowalski IM, Protasiewicz-Faldowska H, Siwik P, Zaborowska-Sapeta K, Dabrowska A, Kluszczynski M, Raistenskis J. Analysis of the sagittal plane in standing and sitting position in girls with left lumbar idiopathic scoliosis. Pol Ann Med. 2013;20:30–4. https://doi.org/10.1016/j.poamed.2013.07.001.
6. Komro KA, Tobler AL, Delisle AL, O'Mara RJ, Wagenaar AC. Beyond the clinic: improving child health through evidence-based community development. BMC Pediatr. 2013;13:172. https://doi.org/10.1186/1471-2431-13-172.
7. Sitarz K, Senderek T, Kirenko J, Olszewski J, Taczala J. Sensomotoric development assessment in 10 years old children with posture defects. Polish. J Phys. 2007;3:232–40.
8. Penha P, Joao S, Casarotto R, Amino C, Penteado D. Postural assessment of girls between 7 and 10 years of age. Clinics. 2005;60:9–16.
9. Vrtovec T, Pernus F, Likar B. A review of methods for quantitative evaluation of spinal curvature. Eur Spine J. 2009;18:593–607. https://doi.org/10.1007/s00586-009-0913-0.
10. Vrtovec T, Janssen MMA, Likar B, Castelein RM, Viergever MA, Pernus F. A review of methods for evaluating the quantitative parameters of sagittal pelvic alignment. Spine J. 2012;12:433–46. https://doi.org/10.1016/j.spinee.2012.02.013.

11. Gangnet N, Pomero V, Dumas R, Skalli W, Vital JM. Variability of the spine and pelvis location with respect to the gravity line: a three-dimensional stereoradiographic study using a force platform. Surg Radiol Anat. 2003;25:424–33. https://doi.org/10.1007/s00276-003-0154-6.

12. Lamartina C, Berjano P. Classification of sagittal imbalance based on spinal alignment and compensatory mechanisms. Eur Spine J. 2014;23:1177–89. https://doi.org/10.1007/s00586-014-3227-9.

13. Araujo F, Lucas R, Alegrete N, Azevedo A, Barros H. Individual and contextual characteristics as determinants of sagittal standing posture: a population-based study of adults. The Spine J. 2014;14:2373–83. https://doi.org/10.1016/j.spinee.2014.01.040.

14. Gorecki A, Kiwerski J, Kowalski IM, Marczynski W, Nowotny J, Rybicka M, Jarosz U, Suwalska M, Szelachowska-Kluza W. Prophylactics of postural deformities in children and youth carried out within the teaching environment—experts recommendations. Pol Ann Med. 2009;16:168–77.

15. Czaprowski D, Pawlowska P, Gebicka A, Sitarski D, Kotwicki T. Intra- and interobserver repeatability of the assessment of anteroposterior curvatures of the spine. using Saunders digital inclinometer Ortop Traumatol Rehabil. 2012;14:145–53. https://doi.org/10.5604/15093492.992283.

16. Stolinski L, Kotwicki T, Czaprowski D, Chowanska J, Suzuki N. Analysis of the anterior trunk symmetry index (ATSI). Preliminary report. Stud Health Technol Inform. 2012;176:242–6.

17. Suzuki N, Inami K, Ono T, Kohno K, Asher MA. Analysis of posterior trunk symmetry index (POTSI) in scoliosis. Part 1. Stud Health Technol Inform. 1999;59:81–4. https://doi.org/10.3233/978-1-60750-903-5-81.

18. Inami K, Suzuki N, Ono T, Yamashita Y, Kohno K, Morisue H. Analysis of posterior trunk symmetry index (POTSI) in scoliosis. Part 2. Stud Health Technol Inform. 1999;59:85–8.

19. Culik J, Marik I. Nomograms for determining the tibia-femoral angle. Locomotor System J. 2002;9:81–90.

20. Cheng J, Chan P, Chiang S, Hui P. Angular and rotational profile of the lower limb in 2,630 Chinese children. J Pediatr Orthop. 1991;11:154–61.

21. Fortin C, Feldman DE, Cheriet F, Denis E, Gravel D, Gauthier F, Labelle H. Reliability of a quantitative clinical posture assessment tool among persons with idiopathic scoliosis. Physiotherapy. 2012;98:64–75. https://doi.org/10.1016/j.physio.2010.12.006.

22. Wiltse LL, Winter RB. Terminology and measurement of spondylolisthesis. J Bone Joint Surg. 1983;65:768–72.

23. Stagnara P, DeMauroy JC, Dran G, Gooon GP, Costanzo G, Dimnet J, Pasquet A. Reciprocal angulation of vertebral bodies in a sagittal plane: approach to references for the evaluation of kyphosis and lordosis. Spine. 1982;7:335–42.

24. Boulay C, Tardieu C, Hecquet J, Benaim C, Mouilleseaux B,Marty C, Prat-Pradal D, Legaye J, Duval-Beaupe're G, Pe´lissier J Sagittal alignment of spine and pelvis regulated by pelvic incidence: standard values and prediction of lordosis Eur Spine J 2006;15:415–422. doi: https://doi.org/10.1007/s00586-005-0984-5.

25. Kuo YL, Tully EA, Galea MP. Video analysis of sagittal spinal posture in healthy young and older adults. J Manip Physiol Ther. 2009;32:210–5. https://doi.org/10.1016/j.jmpt.2009.02.002.

26. Bolzan GP, Souza JA, Boton LM, da Silva AMT, Corrêa ECR. Facial type and head posture of nasal and mouth-breathing children. J Soc Bras Fonoaudiol. 2011;23:315–20.

27. Preece SJ, Willan P, Nester CJ, Graham-Smith P, Herrington L, Bowker P. Variation in pelvic morphology may prevent the identification of anterior pelvic tilt. J Man Manip Ther. 2008;16:113–7. https://doi.org/10.1179/106698108790818459.

28. Cerny P, Stolinski L, Drnkova J, Czaprowski D, Kosteas A, Marik I. Skeletal deformities measurements of x-ray images and photos on the computer. Locomotor System J. 2016;23(Suppl 2):32–6. ISSN 2336-4777.

29. Cerny P, Marik I. Anglespine–program for metrology of spinal and knee deformities in growth period. Locomotor System J. 2014;21:276–84.

30. Weir JP. Quantifying test-retest reliability using the intraclass correlation coefficient and the SEM. J Strength Cond Res. 2005;19:231–40.

31. Bland JM, Altman DG. Statistics notes: Cronbach's alpha. BMJ. 1997;314:572.

32. Keszei AP, Novak M, Streiner DL. Introduction to health measurement scales. J Psychosom Res. 2010;68:319–23. https://doi.org/10.1016/j.jpsychores.2010.01.006.

33. Shrout PE, Fleiss JL. Intraclass correlations: uses in assessing rater reliability. Psychol Bull. 1979;86:420–8.

34. Knott P, Pappo E, Cameron M, deMauroy JD, Rivard C, Kotwicki T, Zaina F, Wynne J, Stikeleather L, Bettany-Saltikov GTB, Durmala J, Maruyama T, Negrini S, O'Brien JP, Rigo M. SOSORT 2012 consensus paper: reducing x-ray exposure in pediatric patients with scoliosis. Scoliosis. 2014;9:4. https://doi.org/10.1186/1748-7161-9-4.

35. Kotwicki T, Durmała J, Czaprowski D, Głowacki M, Kolban M, Snela S, Sliwinski Z, Kowalski IM. Conservative management of idiopathic scoliosis—guidelines based on SOSORT 2006 Consensus. Ortop Traumatol Rehabil. 2009;5:379–95.

36. Czaprowski D, Kotwicki T, Durmała J, Stolinski L. Physiotherapy in the treatment of idiopathic scoliosis—current recommendations based on the recommendations of SOSORT 2011 (society on scoliosis orthopaedic and rehabilitation treatment). Advances in Rehabilitation. 2014;1:23–9. https://doi.org/10.2478/rehab-2014-0030.

37. Kotwicki T, Chowanska J, Kinel E, Czaprowski D, Tomaszewski M, Janusz P. Optimal management of idiopathic scoliosis in adolescence. Adolesc Health Med Ther. 2013;4:59–73. https://doi.org/10.2147/AHMT.S32088.

38. Richards SB, Vitale MG. Screening for idiopathic scoliosis in adolescents. An Information tatement J Bone Joint Surg. 2008;90:195–8. https://doi.org/10.2106/JBJS.G.01276.

39. Dutkowsky JP, Shearer D, Schepps B, Orton C, Scola F. Radiation exposure to patients receiving routine scoliosis radiography measured at depth in an anthropomorphic phantom. J Pediatr Orthop. 1990;10:532–4.

40. Fong DY, Lee CF, Cheung KM, Cheng JC, Ng BK, Lam TP, Mak KH, Yip PS, Luk KD. A meta-analysis of the clinical effectiveness of school scoliosis screening. Spine (Phila Pa 1976). 2010;35:1061–71. https://doi.org/10.1097/BRS.0b013e3181bcc835.

41. Sabirin J, Bakri R, Buang SN, Abdullah AT, Shapie A. School scoliosis screening programme—a systematic review. Med J Malaysia. 2010;65:261–7.

42. Sox HC Jr, Berwick DM, Berg AO, Frame PS, Fryback DG, Grimes DA, Lawrence RS, Wallace RB, Washington AE, Wilson MEH, Woolf SH. Screening for adolescent idiopathic scoliosis: review article. JAMA. 1993;269:2667–72. https://doi.org/10.1001/jama.1993.03500200081038.

43. Bunnell WP. An objective criterion for scoliosis screening. J Bone Joint Surg. 1984;66:1381–7.

44. Balg F, Juteau M, Theoret C, Svotelis A, Grenier G. Validity and reliability of the iPhone to measure rib hump in scoliosis. J Pediatr Orthop. 2014;34:774–9. https://doi.org/10.1097/BPO.0000000000000195.

45. Izatt MT, Bateman GR, Adam CJ. Evaluation of the iPhone with an acrylic sleeve versus the scoliometer for rib hump measurement in scoliosis. Scoliosis. 2012;7:14. https://doi.org/10.1186/1748-7161-7-14.

46. Driscoll M, Fortier-Tougas F, Labelle H, Parent S, Mac-Thong J. Evaluation of an apparatus to be combined with a smartphone for the early detection of spinal deformities. Scoliosis. 2014;25:10. https://doi.org/10.1186/1748-7161-9-10.

47. Grivas TB, Vasiliadis ES, Mihas C, Triantafyllopoulos G, Kaspiris A. Trunk asymmetry in juveniles. Scoliosis. 2008;3:13. https://doi.org/10.1186/1748-7161-3-13.

48. Kotwicki T, Chowanska J, Kinel E, Lorkowska M, Stryla W, Szulc A. Sitting forward bending position versus standing position for studying the back shape in scoliotic children. Scoliosis. 2007;2(Suppl 1):S34. https://doi.org/10.1186/1748-7161-2-S1-S34.

49. McCarthy RE. Evaluation of the patient with deformity. In: Weinstein SL, editor. The pediatric spine. New York: Raven Press; 1994. p. 185–224.

50. Drerup B, Hierholzer E, Ellger B. Shape analysis of the lateral and frontal projection of spine curves assessed from rasterstereographs. In: Sevastik JA, Diab KM, editors. Research into spinal deformities. Amsterdam: IOS Press; 1997. p. 271–5.

51. Zubairi J. Applications of computer-aided rasterstereography in spinal deformity detection. Image Vis Comput. 2002;20:319–24.

52. Upadhyay SS, Burwell RG, Webb JK. Hump changes on forward flexion of the lumbar spine in patients with idiopathic scoliosis. Spine (Phila Pa 1976). 1988;13:146–51.

53. Turner-Smith AR, Harris JD, Houghton GR, Jefferson RJA. Method for analysis of back shape in scoliosis. J Biomech. 1988;21:497–509.

54. Zonnenberg AJJ, Maanen V, Elvers JWH, Oostendorp RAB. Intra/interrater reliability of measurements on body posture photographs. J Craniomandibular Pract. 1996;14:326–31. https://doi.org/10.1080/08869634.1996.11745985.

55. Raine S, Twomey LT. Head and shoulder posture variations in 160 asymptomatic women and men. Arch Phys Med Rehabil. 1997;78:1215–21. https://doi.org/10.1016/S0003-9993(97)90335-X.

56. Vernon H. An assessment of the intra- and inter-reliability of the posturometer. J Manipulative and Physiol Ther. 1983;6:57–60.

57. Bullock-Saxton J. Postural alignment in standing: a repeatable study. Austr J Physiother. 1993;39:25–9. https://doi.org/10.1016/S0004-9514(14)60466-9.

58. Braun BL, Amundson LR. Quantitative assessment of head and shoulder posture. Arch Phys Med Rehabil. 1989;70:322–9.

59. Grimmer K. An investigation of poor cervical resting posture. Aust J Physiother. 1997;43:7–16. https://doi.org/10.1016/S0004-9514(14)60398-6.

60. Nilsson BM, Soderlund A. Head posture in patients with whiplash-associated disorders and the measurement method's reliability—a comparison to healthy subjects. Adv Physiother. 2005;7:13–9. https://doi.org/10.1080/14038190510010278.

61. Christensen HW, Nilsson N. The ability to reproduce the neutral zero position of the head. J Manip Physiol Ther. 1999;22:26–8. https://doi.org/10.1016/S0161-4754(99)70102-8.

62. Swinkels A, Dolan P. Regional assessment of joint position sense in the spine. Spine. 1998;23:590–7.

63. Swinkels A, Dolan P. Spinal position sense is independent of the magnitude of movement. Spine. 2000;25:98–105.

64. Dunk NM, Chung YY, Compton DS, Callaghan JP. The reliability of quantifying upright standing postures as a baseline diagnostic clinical tool. J Manip Physiol Ther. 2004;27:91–6. https://doi.org/10.1016/j.jmpt.2003.12.003.

65. Dunk NM, Lalonde J, Callaghan JP. Implications for the use of postural analysis as a clinical diagnostic tool: reliability of quantifying upright standing spinal postures from photographic images. J Manip Physiol Ther. 2005;28:386–92. https://doi.org/10.1016/j.jmpt.2005.06.006.

66. Beaudoin L, Zabjek KF, Leroux MA, Coillard C, Rivard CH. Acute systematic and variable postural adaptations induced by an orthopaedic shoe lift in control subjects. Eur Spine J. 1999;8:40–5. https://doi.org/10.1007/s005860050125.

67. Strimpakos N, Sakellari V, Gioftsos G, Papathanasiou M, Brountzos E, Kelekis D, Kapreli E, Oldham J. Cervical spine ROM measurements: optimizing the testing protocol by using a 3D ultrasound-based motion analysis system. Cephalgia. 2005;25:1133–45. https://doi.org/10.1111/j.1468-2982.2005.00970.x.

68. Zaina F, Atanasio A, Negrini S. Clinical evaluation of scoliosis during growth: description and reliability. In: Grivas TB, editor. The conservative scoliosis treatment. Studies in health technology and informatics, vol. 135. Amsterdam: IOS Press; 2008. p. 123–54.

69. Canales JZ, Cordas TA, Fiquer JT, Cavalcante AF, Moreno RA. Posture and body image in individuals with major depressive disorder: a controlled study. Rev Bras Psiquiatr. 2010;32:375–80. https://doi.org/10.1590/S1516-44462010000400010.

70. Cerruto C, Di Vece L, Doldo T, Giovannetti A, Polimeni A, Goracci C. Computerized photographic method to evaluate changes in head posture and scapular position following rapid palatal expansion: a pilot study. J Clin Pediatr Dent. 2012;37:213–8. https://doi.org/10.17796/jcpd.37.2.11q670.

71. Pausic J, Pedisic Z, Dizdar D. Reliability of a photographic method for assessing standing posture of elementary school students. J Manip Physiol Ther. 2010;33:425–31. https://doi.org/10.1016/j.jmpt.2010.06.002.34vlw000wx.

72. Ruivo RM, Pezarat-Correia P, Carita AI. Intrarater and interrater reliability of photographic measurement of upper-body standing posture of adolescents. J Manip Physiol Ther. 2015;38:74–80. https://doi.org/10.1016/j.jmpt.2014.10.009.

73. Sacco ICN, Alibert S, Queiroz BWC, Pripas D, Kieling I, Kimura AA, Sellmer AE, Malvestio RA, Sera MT. Reliability of photogrammetry in relation to goniometry for postural lower limb assessment. Rev Bras Fisioter. 2007;11:411–7. https://doi.org/10.1590/S1413-35552007000500013.

74. Canhadas Belli JF, Chaves TC, Siriani de Oliveira A, Grossi DB. Analysis of body posture in children with mild to moderate asthma. Eur J Pediatr. 2009;168:1207–16. https://doi.org/10.1007/s00431-008-0911-y.

75. Matamalas A, Bago J, D'Agata E, Pellise F. Validity and reliability of photographic measures to evaluate waistline asymmetry in idiopathic scoliosis. Eur. Spine J. 2016;25:3170–9. https://doi.org/10.1007/s00586-016-4509-1.

76. Matamalas A, Bago J, D'Agata E, Pellise F. Reliability and validity study of measurements on digital photography to evaluate shoulder balance in idiopathic scoliosis. Scoliosis. 2014;9:23. https://doi.org/10.1186/s13013-014-0023-6.

77. Yoder J. Review: photographic architecture in the twentieth century, by Claire Zimmerman. J Soc Archit Hist. 2016;75:110–2. https://doi.org/10.1525/jsah.2016.75.1.110.

78. Beilin H. Understanding the photographic image. J Appl Dev Psychol. 1999;20:1–30. https://doi.org/10.1016/S0193-3973(99)80001-X.

79. Ellenbogen R, Jankauskas S, Collini FJ. Achieving standardized photographs in aesthetic surgery. Plast Reconstr Surg. 1990;86:955–61.

80. do R'r JLP, Nakashima IY, Rizopoulos K, Kostopoulos D, Marques AP. Improving posture: comparing segmental stretch and muscular chains therapy. Clin Chiropr. 2012;15:121–8. https://doi.org/10.1016/j.clch.2012.10.039.

81. Santos MM, Silva MPC, Sanada LS, Alves CRJ. Photogrammetric postural analysis on healthy seven to ten-year-old children: interrater reliability. Rev Bras Fisioter. 2009;13:350–5. https://doi.org/10.1590/S1413-35552009005000047.

82. Giglio CA, Volpon JB. Development and evaluation of thoracic kyphosis and lumbar lordosis during growth. J Child Orthop. 2007;1:187–93. https://doi.org/10.1007/s11832-007-0033-5.

83. do Rosário JLP. Photographic analysis of human posture: a literature review. J Bodyw Mov Ther. 2014;18:56–61. https://doi.org/10.1016/j.jbmt.2013.05.008.

84. Ferreira EAG, Duarte M, Maldonado EP, Burke TN, Marques AP. Postural assessment software (PAS/SAPO): validation and reliability. Clinics. 2010;65:675–81. https://doi.org/10.1590/S1807-59322010000700005.

85. Neiva PD, Kirkwood RN, Godinho R. Orientation and position of head posture, scapula and thoracic spine in mouth-breathing children. Int J Pediatr Otorhinolaryngol. 2009;73:227–36. https://doi.org/10.1016/j.ijporl.2008.10.006.

86. Grimmer-Somers K, Milanese S, Louw Q. Measurement of cervical posture in the sagittal plane. J Manip Physiol Ther. 2008;31:509–17. https://doi.org/10.1016/j.jmpt.2008.08.005.

87. McEvoy MP, Grimmer K. Reliability of upright posture measurements in primary school children. BMC Musculoskelet Disord. 2005;6:35. https://doi.org/10.1186/1471-2474-6-35.

88. Gadotti IC, Magee DJ. Validity of surface measurements to access craniocervical posture in the sagittal plane: a critical review. Phys Ther Rev. 2008;13:258–68. https://doi.org/10.1179/174328808X309250.

89. Perry M, Smith A, Straker L, Coleman J, O'Sullivan P. Reliability of sagittal photographic spinal posture assessment in adolescents. Adv Physiother. 2008;10:66–75. https://doi.org/10.1080/14038190701728251.

90. Cobb SC, James R, Hjertstedt M, Kruk J. A digital photographic measurement method for quantifying foot posture: validity, reliability, and descriptive data. J Athl Train. 2011;46:20–30. https://doi.org/10.4085/1062-6050-46.1.20.

91. Guan X, Fan G, Wu X, Zeng Y, Su H, Gu G, Zhou Q, Gu X, Zhang H. Photographic measurement of head and cervical posture when viewing mobile phone: a pilot study. Eur Spine J. 2015;24:2892–8. https://doi.org/10.1007/s00586-015-4143-3.

92. Matamalas A, Bago J, D' Agata E, Pellise F. Does patient perception of shoulder balance correlate with clinical balance? Eur Spine J. 2016;25:3560–7. https://doi.org/10.1007/s00586-015-3971-5.

93. Sai-hu M, Benlong S, Xu S, Zhen L, Ze-zhang Z, Bang-ping Q, Yong Q. Morphometric analysis of iatrogenic breast asymmetry secondary to operative breast shape changes in thoracic adolescent idiopathic scoliosis. Eur Spine J. 2016;25:3075–81. https://doi.org/10.1007/s00586-016-4554-9.

94. Saad KR, Colombo AS, Ribeiro AP, Joao SMA. Reliability of photogrammetry in the evaluation of the postural aspects of individuals with structural scoliosis. J Bodyw Mov Ther. 2012;16:210–6. https://doi.org/10.1016/j.jbmt.2011.03.005.

95. Souza JA, Pasinato F, Basso D, Castilhos Rodrigues Correa E, Toniolo da Silva AM. Biophotogrammetry: reliability of measurementsobtained with a posture assessment software (SAPO). Rev Bras Cineantropom Desempenho Hum. 2011;13:299–305. https://doi.org/10.5007/1980-0037.2011v13n4p299.

96. Penha PJ, Baldini M, Amado João SM. Spinal postural alignment variance according to sex and age in 7- and 8-year-old children. J Manip Physiol Ther. 2009;32:154–9. https://doi.org/10.1016/j.jmpt.2008.12.009.

97. Fortin C, Feldman DE, Cheriet F, Labelle H. Validity of a quantitative clinical measurement tool of trunk posture in idiopathic scoliosis. Spine. 2010;35:E988–94. https://doi.org/10.1097/BRS.0b013e3181cd2cd2.

98. Milanesi JM, Borin G, Corrêa ECR, da Silva AMT, Bortoluzzi DC, Souza JA.

Impact of the mouth breathing occurred during childhood in the adult age: biophotogrammetric postural analysis. Int J Pediatr Otorhinolaryngol. 2011; 75:999–1004. https://doi.org/10.1016/j.ijporl.2011.04.018.

99. Young S. Research for medical photographers: photographic measurement. J Audiov Media Med. 2002;25:94–8. https://doi.org/10.1080/014051102320376799.

100. Fortin C, Feldman DE, Cheriet F, Labelle H. Differences in standing and sitting postures of youth with idiopathic scoliosis from quantitative analysis of digital photographs. Phys Occup Ther Pediatr. 2013;33:1–14. https://doi.org/10.3109/01942638.2012.747582.

101. Galera S, Nascimento L, Teodoro E, Tomazini J. Comparative study on the posture of individuals with and without cervical pain. IFMBE Proc. 2009;25: 131–4. https://doi.org/10.1007/978-3-642-03889-1_36.

102. Lafond D, Descarreaux M, Normand MC, Harrison DE. Postural development in school children: a cross-sectional study. Chiropr Osteopat. 2007;15:1–7. https://doi.org/10.1186/1746-1340-15-1.

103. O'Sullivan PB, Grahamslaw KM, Kendell M, Lapenskie SC. Mo"ller NE, Richards KV. The effect of different standing and sitting postures on trunk muscle activity in a pain-free population. Spine. 2002;27:1238–44.

104. Normand MC, Descarreaux M, Harrison DD, Harrison DE, Perron DL, Ferrantelli JR. Three dimensional evaluation of posture in standing with the posture print: an intra- and inter-examiner reliability study. Chiropr Osteopat. 2007;15:1–11. https://doi.org/10.1007/s00586-005-0984-5.

105. Smith A, O'Sullivan P, Straker L. Classification of sagittal thoraco-lumbo-pelvic alignment of the adolescent spine in standing and its relationship to low back pain. Spine. 2008;33:2101–7. https://doi.org/10.1097/BRS.0b013e31817ec3b0.

106. Vedantam R, Lenke LG, Bridwell KH, Linville DL, Blanke K. The effect of variation in arm position on sagittal spinal alignment. Spine. 2000;25:2204–9.

107. Tyrakowski M, Janusz P, Mardjetko S, Kotwicki T, Siemionow K. Comparison of radiographic sagittal spinopelvic alignment between skeletally immature and skeletally mature individuals with Scheuermann's disease. Eur Spine J. 2015;24:1237–43. https://doi.org/10.1007/s00586-014-3595-1.

108. Tyrakowski M, Mardjetko S, Siemionow K. Radiographic spinopelvic parameters in skeletally mature patients with Scheuermann disease. Spine (Phila Pa 1976). 2014;39:E1080–5. https://doi.org/10.1007/s00586-014-3595-1.

109. Fortin C, Feldman DE, Cheriet F, Labelle H. Clinical methods for quantifying body segment posture: a literature review. Disabil Rehabil. 2011;33:367–83. https://doi.org/10.3109/09638288.2010.492066.

110. Czaprowski D, Pawlowska P, Stolinski L, Kotwicki T. Active self-correction of back posture in children instructed with 'straighten your back' command. Man Ther. 2014;19:392–8. https://doi.org/10.1016/j.math.2013.10.005.

111. Stolinski L, Kotwicki T, Czaprowski D. Active self correction of child's posture assessed with plurimeter and documented with digital photography. Progress in Medicine. 2012;25:484–90.

112. Grimmer KA, Williams MT, Gill TK. The associations between adolescent head-on-eck posture, backpack weight and anthropometric features. Spine. 1999;24:2262–7.

113. Solow B, Sandham A. Cranio-cervical posture: a factor in the development and function of the dentofacial structures. Eur J Orthod. 2002;5:447–56. https://doi.org/10.1093/ejo/24.5.447.

114. Van Maanen CJ, Zonnenberg AJ, Elvers JW, Oostendorp RA. Intra/interrater reliability of measurements on body posture photographs. Cranio. 1996;14: 326–31.

# Permissions

All chapters in this book were first published in SSD, by BioMed Central; hereby published with permission under the Creative Commons Attribution License or equivalent. Every chapter published in this book has been scrutinized by our experts. Their significance has been extensively debated. The topics covered herein carry significant findings which will fuel the growth of the discipline. They may even be implemented as practical applications or may be referred to as a beginning point for another development.

The contributors of this book come from diverse backgrounds, making this book a truly international effort. This book will bring forth new frontiers with its revolutionizing research information and detailed analysis of the nascent developments around the world.

We would like to thank all the contributing authors for lending their expertise to make the book truly unique. They have played a crucial role in the development of this book. Without their invaluable contributions this book wouldn't have been possible. They have made vital efforts to compile up to date information on the varied aspects of this subject to make this book a valuable addition to the collection of many professionals and students.

This book was conceptualized with the vision of imparting up-to-date information and advanced data in this field. To ensure the same, a matchless editorial board was set up. Every individual on the board went through rigorous rounds of assessment to prove their worth. After which they invested a large part of their time researching and compiling the most relevant data for our readers.

The editorial board has been involved in producing this book since its inception. They have spent rigorous hours researching and exploring the diverse topics which have resulted in the successful publishing of this book. They have passed on their knowledge of decades through this book. To expedite this challenging task, the publisher supported the team at every step. A small team of assistant editors was also appointed to further simplify the editing procedure and attain best results for the readers.

Apart from the editorial board, the designing team has also invested a significant amount of their time in understanding the subject and creating the most relevant covers. They scrutinized every image to scout for the most suitable representation of the subject and create an appropriate cover for the book.

The publishing team has been an ardent support to the editorial, designing and production team. Their endless efforts to recruit the best for this project, has resulted in the accomplishment of this book. They are a veteran in the field of academics and their pool of knowledge is as vast as their experience in printing. Their expertise and guidance has proved useful at every step. Their uncompromising quality standards have made this book an exceptional effort. Their encouragement from time to time has been an inspiration for everyone.

The publisher and the editorial board hope that this book will prove to be a valuable piece of knowledge for researchers, students, practitioners and scholars across the globe.

# List of Contributors

Rebecca J. Crawford
Institute for Health Sciences, School of Health Professions, Zürich University of Applied Sciences, Technikumstrasse 81, Winterthur CH-8401, Switzerland
Faculty of Health and Exercise Sciences, Curtin University, Perth, Australia

Quentin J. Malone
Centre for Neurological Surgery, Perth, Australia

Roger I. Price
Department of Medical Technology and Physics, Sir Charles Gairdner Hospital, Perth, Australia
School of Physics, University of Western Australia, Perth, Australia

Jean Théroux, Ariane Ballard, Christelle Khadra, Hubert Labelle and Sylvie Le May
Research Center, Sainte-Justine University Hospital Center, Montreal, QC, Canada

Norman Stomski and Stanley Innes
School of Health Profession, Murdoch University, 90, South Street, Murdoch, WA 6150, Australia

Ariane Ballard, Christelle Khadra and Sylvie Le May
Faculty of Nursing, University of Montreal, Montreal, QC, Canada

Hubert Labelle
Faculty of Medicine, University of Montreal, Montreal, Canada

Satoshi Suzuki, Nobuyuki Fujita, Tomohiro Hikata, Akio Iwanami, Ken Ishii, Masaya Nakamura, Morio Matsumoto and Kota Watanabe
Department of Orthopaedic Surgery, Keio University School of Medicine, 35 Shinanomachi, Shinjyuku, Tokyo 160-8582, Japan

Sabrina Donzelli, Fabio Zaina, Francesca Di Felice and Alberto Negrini
ISICO, Via R Bellarmino 13/1, 20141, Milan, Italy

Gregorio Martinez
ISICO, Barcelona, Spain

Stefano Negrini
University of Brescia, Don Gnocchi Foundation, Milan, Italy

Christos Topalis, Anna Grauers, Elias Diarbakerli and Paul Gerdhem
Department of Clinical Science, Intervention and Technology (CLINTEC), Karolinska Institutet, Stockholm, Sweden

Anna Grauers
Department of Orthopaedics, Sundsvall and Härnösand County Hospital, Sundsvall, Sweden

Elias Diarbakerli and Paul Gerdhem
Department of Orthopaedics, Karolinska University Hospital, Stockholm, Sweden

Aina Danielsson
Department of Orthopaedics, Sahlgrenska University Hospital, Gothenburg, Sweden

Christos Topalis
Department of Clinical Science, Intervention and Technology, Karolinska Institutet, K54, Karolinska University Hospital, SE-141 86 Stockholm, Sweden

Rob C. Brink, Dino Colo, Tom P. C. Schlösser and René M. Castelein
Department of Orthopaedic Surgery, University Medical Center Utrecht, 3508 GA Utrecht, The Netherlands

Koen L. Vincken
Image Sciences Institute, University Medical Center Utrecht, Utrecht, The Netherlands

Marijn van Stralen
Imaging Division, University Medical Center Utrecht, Utrecht, The Netherlands

Steve C. N. Hui and Winnie C. W. Chu
Department of Imaging and Interventional Radiology, Prince of Wales Hospital, The Chinese University of Hong Kong, Shatin, Hong Kong

Lin Shi
Department of Diagnostic Radiology and Organ Imaging, Prince of Wales Hospital, The Chinese University of Hong Kong, Shatin, Hong Kong

Jack C. Y. Cheng
Department of Orthopaedics and Traumatology, Prince of Wales Hospital, The Chinese University of Hong Kong Shatin, Hong Kong

**Edmond H. Lou, Doug L. Hill, Douglas Hedden and Marc Moreau**
Department of Surgery, University of Alberta, 6-110F, Clinical Science Building, 8440-112 Street, Edmonton, Alberta T6G 2B7, Canada

**Edmond H. Lou and Doug L. Hill**
Department of Research and Innovation Development, Glenrose Rehabilitation Hospital, Edmonton, Alberta T5G 0B7, Canada

**Andreas Donauer and Melissa Tilburn**
Department of Prosthetics and Orthotics, Glenrose Rehabilitation Hospital, Edmonton, Alberta T5G 0B7, Canada

**Arnold YL Wong**
Department of Rehabilitation Sciences, Faculty of Health and Social Sciences, The Hong Kong Polytechnic University, Hung Hom, Hong Kong, SAR, China

**Jaro Karppinen**
Medical Research Center Oulu, Department of Physical and Rehabilitation Medicine, University of Oulu and Oulu University Hospital, Oulu, Finland
Finnish Institute of Occupational Health, Oulu, Finland

**Dino Samartzis**
Department of Orthopaedics and Traumatology, The University of Hong Kong, Pokfulam, Hong Kong, SAR, China

**A. Stępień, K. Graff and and A. Wit**
Department of Rehabilitation, Józef Piłsudski University of Physical Education, Warsaw, Poland

**K. Fabian**
Regional Children's Hospital, Jastrzębie Zdrój, Poland

**M. Podgurniak**
Department of Physiological Sciences, University of Life Science, Warsaw, Poland

**Yawara Eguchi, Munetaka Suzuki, Hajime Yamanaka, Hiroshi Tamai and Tatsuya Kobayashi**
Department of Orthopaedic Surgery, Shimoshizu National Hospital, 934-5, Shikawatashi, Yotsukaido, Chiba 284-0003, Japan

**Sumihisa Orita, Kazuyo Yamauchi, Miyako Suzuki, Kazuhide Inage, Kazuki Fujimoto, Hirohito Kanamoto, Koki Abe, Kazuhisa Takahashi and Seiji Ohtori**
Department of Orthopaedic Surgery, Graduate School of Medicine, Chiba University, 1-8-1 Inohana, Chuo-ku, Chiba 260-8670, Japan

**Yasuchika Aoki**
Department of Orthopaedic Surgery, Eastern Chiba Medical Center, 3-6-2, Okayamadai, Togane, Chiba 283-8686, Japan

**Tomoaki Toyone and Tomoyuki Ozawa**
Department of Orthopaedic Surgery, Showa University School of Medicine, 1-5-8 Hatanodai, Shinagawa-ku, Tokyo 142-8555, Japan

**Yawara Eguchi, Munetaka Suzuki, Hajime Yamanaka, Hiroshi Tamai and Tatsuya Kobayashi**
Department of Orthopeadic Surgery, Shimoshizu National Hospital, 934-5, Shikawatashi, Yotsukaido, Chiba 284-0003, Japan

**Toru Toyoguchi**
Department of Orthopaedic Surgery, Chiba Qiball Clinic, 4-5-1, Chuo-ku, Chiba 260-0013, Japan

**Masao Koda, Sumihisa Orita, Kazuyo Yamauchi, Miyako Suzuki, Kazuhide Inage, Kazuki Fujimoto, Hirohito Kanamoto, Koki Abe, Kazuhisa Takahashi and Seiji Ohtori**
Department of Orthopaedic Surgery, Graduate School of Medicine, Chiba University, 1-8-1 Inohana, Chuo-ku, Chiba 260-8670, Japan

**Yasuchika Aoki**
Department of Orthopaedic Surgery, Eastern Chiba Medical Center, 3-6-2, Okayamadai, Togane, Chiba 283-8686, Japan

**Sanja Schreiber**
Faculty of Rehabilitation Medicine, University of Alberta, Edmonton, Alberta, Canada

**Eric C Parent**
Department of Physical Therapy, University of Alberta, Edmonton, Alberta, Canada

**Doug L Hill, Douglas M Hedden, Marc J Moreau and Sarah C Southon**
Department of Surgery, University of Alberta, Edmonton, Alberta, Canada

**Jennifer C. Theis and Allan Abbott**
Faculty of Health Science and Medicine, Bond Institute of Health and Sport, Bond University 2 Promethean Way, Robina, Queensland 4226, Australia

**Jennifer C. Theis, Anna Grauers, Elias Diarbakerli, Panayiotis Savvides and Paul Gerdhem**
Department of Orthopaedics, Department of Clinical Science, Intervention and Technology (CLINTEC), Karolinska Institutet, Karolinska University Hospital, SE-141 86 Stockholm, Sweden

**Anna Grauers**
Department of Orthopaedics, Sundsvall and Härnösand County Hospital, 85186 Sundsvall, Sweden

**Allan Abbott**
Department of Physical Therapy, Karolinska University Hospital, SE-141 86 Stockholm, Sweden
Division of Physiotherapy, Department of Neurobiology, Care Sciences and Society, Karolinska Institutet, SE-141 86 Stockholm, Sweden
Department of Medical and Health Sciences, Division of Physiotherapy, Faculty of Health Sciences, Linköping University, SE-58183 Linköping, Sweden

**Søren Ohrt-Nissen, Dennis Winge Hallager, Martin Gehrchen and Benny Dahl**
Spine Unit, Department of Orthopedic Surgery, Rigshospitalet, University of Copenhagen, Blegdamsvej 9, Copenhagen East 2100, Denmark

**Jason Pui Yin Cheung, Kenny Kwan, Kenneth M. C. Cheung and Dino Samartzis**
Department of Orthopedics and Traumatology, The University of Hong Kong, Professorial Block, 5th Floor 102 Pokfulam Road, Hong Kong, SAR, China

**Niranjan Kavadi, Richard A. Tallarico and William F. Lavelle**
Department of Orthopedic Surgery, SUNY Upstate Medical University, 750 E. Adams Street, Syracuse, NY 13210, USA

**William F. Lavelle**
6620 Fly Road, Suite 200, East Syracuse, NY 13057, USA

**Jason Pui Yin Cheung, Karen Ka Man Ng, Prudence Wing Hang Cheung, Dino Samartzis and Kenneth Man Chee Cheung**
Department of Orthopaedics and Traumatology, Queen Mary Hospital, The University of Hong Kong, Pokfulam Road, Hong Kong, SAR, China

**Adrian Gardner and Fiona Berryman**
The Royal Orthopaedic NHS Foundation Trust, Bristol Road South, Northfield, Birmingham B31 2AP, UK

**Adrian Gardner and Paul Pynsent**
Department of Anatomy, Institute of Clinical Science, University of Birmingham, Edgbaston, Birmingham B15 2TT, UK

**Yew Long Lo**
Department of Neurology, National Neuroscience Institute, Singapore General Hospital, Outram Road, Academia Level 4, Singapore 169608, Singapore
Duke-NUS Medical School, Singapore, Singapore

**Yam Eng Tan, Sitaram Raman, Adeline Teo, Yang Fang Dan and Chang Ming Guo**
Singapore General Hospital, Singapore, Singapore

**Dariusz Czaprowski**
Department of Physiotherapy, Józef Rusiecki University College in Olsztyn, Bydgoska 33, 10-243 Olsztyn, Poland
Center of Body Posture, Bydgoska 33, 10-243 Olsztyn, Poland

**Łukasz Stoliński**
Spine Disorders Center, Rehasport Licensed Rehabilitation Center, Al. Niepodległości 4, 96-100 Skierniewice, Poland

**Łukasz Stoliński, Mateusz Kozinoga and Tomasz Kotwicki**
Spine Disorders and Pediatric Orthopedics Department, University of Medical Sciences, 28 Czerwca 1956 135/147 Street, 61-545 Poznań, Poland

**Łukasz Stoliński and Mateusz Kozinoga**
Rehasport Clinic, Górecka 30, 60-201 Poznań, Poland

**Marcin Tyrakowski**
Department of Orthopaedics, Pediatric Orthopaedics and Traumatology, The Center of Postgraduate Medical Education in Warsaw, Konarskiego 13, 05-400 Otwock, Poland

**Hasan Ghandhari, Ebrahim Ameri, Farshad Nikouei, Milad Haji Agha Bozorgi, Shoeib Majdi and Mostafa Salehpour**
Bone and Joint Reconstruction Research Center, Shafa Orthopedic Hospital, Iran University of Medical Sciences, Tehran, Iran

**John Thometz and XueCheng Liu**
Department of Orthopedic Surgery, Children's Hospital of Wisconsin, Medical College of Wisconsin, Milwaukee, WI, USA

**John Thometz and XueCheng Liu**
Musculoskeletal Functional Assessment Center, Children's Hospital of Wisconsin, Medical College of Wisconsin, Milwaukee, WI, USA

**Robert Rizza and Ian English**
Department of Mechanical Engineering, Milwaukee School of Engineering, Milwaukee, WI, USA

**Sergery Tarima**
Division of Biostatistics, Institution for Health and Society, Medical College of Wisconsin, Milwaukee, WI, USA

**John Thometz**
Pediatric Orthopaedics, 9000 W. Wisconsin Ave., Suite 360, Milwaukee, WI 3201, USA

**L. Stolinski, M. Kozinoga and T. Kotwicki**
Department of Spine Disorders and Pediatric Orthopedics, University of Medical Sciences, 28 Czerwca 1956r. no. 135/147, 61-545 Poznan, Poland

**L. Stolinski and M. Kozinoga**
Rehasport Clinic, Poznan, Poland

**L. Stolinski**
Rehasport Clinic Licensed Rehabilitation Center, Skierniewice, Poland

**D. Czaprowski**
Department of Physiotherapy, Józef Rusiecki University College, Olsztyn, Poland
Center of Body Posture, Olsztyn, Poland

**M. Tyrakowski**
Department of Orthopaedics, Pediatric Orthopaedics and Traumatology, The Centre of Postgraduate Medical Education in Warsaw, Otwock, Poland

**P. Cerny**
Faculty of Health Studies, University of West Bohemia, Pilsen, Czech Republic
Faculty of Physical Education and Sport, Charles University, Prague, Czech Republic
ORTOTIKA, s. r. o, Faculty at Motol University Hospital, Prague, Czech Republic

**N. Suzuki**
Scoliosis Center, Medical Scanning Tokyo, Tokyo, Japan

# Index

www.ingramcontent.com/pod-product-compliance
Lightning Source LLC
Chambersburg PA
CBHW080639200326
41458CB00013B/4679